Grid Technologies for E-Health:

Applications for Telemedicine Services and Delivery

Ekaterina (Eka) Kldiashvili
Georgia Telemedicine Union (Association), Georgia

Medical Information Science
REFERENCE

MEDICAL INFORMATION SCIENCE REFERENCE

Hershey · New York

Director of Editorial Content:	Kristin Klinger
Director of Book Publications:	Julia Mosemann
Acquisitions Editor:	Lindsay Johnston
Development Editor:	Christine Bufton
Publishing Assistant:	Casey Conapitski
Typesetter:	Travis Gundrum
Production Editor:	Jamie Snavely
Cover Design:	Lisa Tosheff

Published in the United States of America by
Medical Information Science Reference (an imprint of IGI Global)
701 E. Chocolate Avenue
Hershey PA 17033
Tel: 717-533-8845
Fax: 717-533-8661
E-mail: cust@igi-global.com
Web site: http://www.igi-global.com

Library of Congress Cataloging-in-Publication Data

Grid technologies for e-Health : applications for telemedicine services and delivery / Ekaterina (Eka) Kldiashvili, editor.
p. cm.
Summary: "This book presents applications of the possibilities of Grid technologies for telemedicine and eHealth as well as presentation of ongoing projects and achievements"--Provided by publisher. Includes bibliographical references and index.
ISBN 978-1-61692-010-4 (hardcover) -- ISBN 978-1-61692-011-1 (ebook) 1. Medical telematics. 2. Telecommunication in medicine. 3. Computational grids (Computer systems) I. Kldiashvili, Ekaterina, 1973- R119.95.G75 2010
610.28--dc22

British Cataloguing in Publication Data
A Cataloguing in Publication record for this book is available from the British Library.

Table of Contents

Preface ... xiv

Chapter 1
The Application of Virtual Organization Technology for eHealth ... 1
Ekaterina Kldiashvili, Georgian Telemedicine Union (Association), Georgia

Chapter 2
Grid Technology: E-Learning in Telemedicine and Organizational Collaboration ... 18
I. H. Monrad Aas, Vestfold Mental Health Care Trust, Norway

Chapter 3
Health and Health Care Grid Services and Delivery Integrating eHealth and Telemedicine ... 36
Thomas Clark, Global Telemed Limited, UK

Chapter 4
The Teams of Leaders (ToL) Concept: The Grid, the Mesh, and the People in the World of Information and Knowledge-Based Global Healthcare ... 65
Dag von Lubitz, MedSMART, Inc., USA & Bieda Poco Dargante Institute, Denmark

Chapter 5
Grid Architecture and Components in Diagnostic Pathology ... 105
Gloria Bueno García, Universidad de Castilla-La Mancha, Spain
Marcial García Rojo, Hospital General de Ciudad Real, Spain
Roberto González Morales, Universidad de Castilla-La Mancha, Spain
Oscar Déniz Suárez, Universidad de Castilla-La Mancha, Spain
Jesús García González, Hospital General de Ciudad Real, Spain

Chapter 6
Grid Technology in Telepatology and Personalised Treatment ... 117
O. Ferrer-Roca, University of La Laguna, Spain
F Marcan, University of La Laguna, Spain
M. E. Vidal, University Simon Bolivar, Venezuela
E. Ruckhaus, University Simon Bolivar, Venezuela
X. Santos, University of La Laguna, Spain
E. Iglesias, University Simon Bolivar, Venezuela

Chapter 7
Gridifying Neuroscientific Pipelines: A SOA Recipe and Experience from the neuGRID Project............ 129
David Manset, maatG, France
The neuGRID Consortium

Chapter 8
Computational Grids: An Introduction to Potential Biomedical Uses and Future Prospects in Oncology: Neuro-Oncology Applications as a Model for Cancer Sub-Specialties............ 152
Ribhi Hazin, Harvard University, USA
Ibrahim Qaddoumi, St. Jude's Children's Research Hospital, USA
Francisco Pedrosa, Instituto Integrado de Medicina Prof Fernando Figueira - IMIP, Brazil

Chapter 9
Grid for Post Operative Care through Wireless Sensor Networks............ 164
N.P Chowdhry, Mehran University of Engineering and Technology, Pakistan
Adnan Ashraf, Mehran University of Engineering and Technology, Pakistan
B.S Chowdhry, Mehran University of Engineering and Technology, Pakistan
A.K Baloch, Mehran University of Engineering and Technology, Pakistan
A.W Ansari, University of Sindh, Pakistan
H. De Meer, University of Passau, Germany

Chapter 10
Data Security in Electronic Health Records............ 182
Stefane M. Kabene, Ecole des Hautes Etudes en Sante Publique (EHESP), France
Raymond W. Leduc, University of Western Ontario, Canada
Candace J. Gibson, University of Western Ontario, Canada

Chapter 11
A Secure Teleradiology Grid............ 195
Robert Rudowski, Medical University of Warsaw, Poland
Michal Dzierzak, Medical University of Warsaw, Poland
Bartosz Kaczynski, Medical University of Warsaw, Poland

Chapter 12
Tele-Audiology in the United States: Past, Present, and Future............ 205
John Ribera, Utah State University, USA

Chapter 13
Global Health Network Supercourse and Cancer Epidemiology: Free Cancer Epidemiology Resources on the Internet 215
Faina Linkov, University of Pittsburgh Cancer Institute, USA
Elizabeth Radke, University of Pittsburgh Graduate School of Public Health, USA
Mita Lovalekar, University of Pittsburgh Graduate School of Public Health, USA
Ronald LaPorte, University of Pittsburgh Graduate School of Public Health, USA

Compilation of References 224

About the Contributors 254

Index 262

Detailed Table of Contents

Preface xvi

Chapter 1
The Application of Virtual Organization Technology for eHealth.. 1
Ekaterina Kldiashvili, Georgian Telemedicine Union (Association), Georgia

Several years ago any talk related to the Internet would have to be proceeded by an explanation of what it is and how it works. At present information and communication technologies became the essential part of our life and practical activity. eHealth can be designated as a special form of information and communication technologies. It is obvious that eHealth has a great potentiality; however today there are unfortunately only a few examples of its large services. Efficient, effective and reliable systems for remote consultations and distance education are the top requirements for eHealth. Grid technologies have emerged as an important new field, distinguished from conventional distributed computing by its focus on large-scale sharing, innovative applications, and, in some cases, high-performance orientation. "Grid technology" we are going to define as flexible, secure, coordinated resource sharing among dynamic collections of individuals, institutions, and resources – what can be described as "virtual organizations". The present chapter will discuss the application of Virtual Organization technology for eHealth purposes. Over the past five years, research and development efforts within the mentioned technology have produced protocols, services, and tools. Virtual Organization technology will offer the opportunity for improving healthcare services and for making healthcare expertise available to underserved locations.

Chapter 2
Grid Technology: E-Learning in Telemedicine and Organizational Collaboration 18
I. H. Monrad Aas, Vestfold Mental Health Care Trust, Norway

The present chapter is about telemedicine, but not about software and hardware. It is about humanware. Telemedicine's greatest problem is not to make the technology work. It is organizations and humans in organizations who will decide the future of telemedicine. Telemedicine is not just a simple success story and the diffusion of telemedicine has been slower than many expected. For the future of telemedicine, a shift in the way we think may be necessary. Few authors have focused on learning in telemedicine (with what is here considered as associated aspects: team organization; learning organizations; network organization). The learning potential connected to telemedicine is significant. Learning may constitute an important argument for telemedicine. In the present chapter, focus is on the role learning and collaboration may have for the future of telemedicine. To take the full advantage of the learning potential a higher volume of telemedicine is necessary, but this requires more organizational collaboration. Improved collaboration is obtainable by implementing collaboration measures. The chapter shows that focus on learning and collaboration may well be important for the future of telemedicine. It is recommended that managers lead change processes in their organizations, where the different aspects of importance for realization of learning benefits of telemedicine are treated. For telemedicine, it is important that future research includes: investigations on how to obtain learning benefits and which collaboration measures are relevant for the different telemedicine applications. Objectives of the present chapter are to propose: (1) more international research on learning in telemedicine (with mentioned associated aspects) and telemedicine collaboration problems and (2) to show the background for this proposal.

Chapter 3
Health and Health Care Grid Services and Delivery Integrating eHealth and Telemedicine 36
Thomas Clark, Global Telemed Limited, UK

Health Grids offer new solutions and alternatives to existing models for the delivery of Healthcare Services to diverse Populations across dissimilar Geographical and Political Regions. Incorporating new medical science, legal systems, systems and networks, financing, technologies, processes, procedures, business and government participation, competitive, cost-effective integration with existing, experimental and competing delivery models is a basic requirement. Integration is likely to be performed locally and may be required to avoid the disruption of existing models, e.g., Patient, Practitioner and Payer choice. This chapter addresses a selection of issues that have been encountered in other high-technology integrations. Less-complex and more limited-in-scope than Health Grids they indicate a need for adaptability and multiple solutions. Choice and options will be important. The ability for Users to personalize, and re-structure as needed or desired, a Health Grid will be paramount.

Chapter 4
The Teams of Leaders (ToL) Concept: The Grid, the Mesh, and the People in the World
of Information and Knowledge-Based Global Healthcare.. 65
Dag von Lubitz, MedSMART, Inc., USA & Bieda Poco Dargante Institute, Denmark

The revolution in computer, information, and telecommunication sciences facilitated revolution in "the way we do business." Despite the wealth of new actionable information and actionable knowledge that this revolution created in healthcare, it was not enough to break the barriers of thought, bureaucracy, and politics. Thus, although the knowledge and professional expertise that are required to avert the threatening collapse of global healthcare are readily available, they remain locked in isolated pools separated by historical barriers, increasing intra- and interdisciplinary specialization, and by stiflingly narrow perception of healthcare complexity. Based on maximum integration of CT, IT, IM, KM, and multidimensional human expertise, the concept of "Teams of Leaders" (ToL) has been employed with rapidly growing success. Implementation of ToL leads to the development of "actionable understanding" that converts highly capable but isolated islands of creative power, into unified mission and task oriented "swarms" endowed with a vastly expanded, collective expertise and operational capabilities. With its roots deep in the advanced technologies of IT/IM/KM, Teams of Leaders transcend bureaucracies and politics, and the collaborative outputs generated through ToL-based operations may constitute one of the pivotal elements of the desperately needed healthcare restructuring.

Chapter 5
Grid Architecture and Components in Diagnostic Pathology 105
Gloria Bueno García, Universidad de Castilla-La Mancha, Spain
Marcial García Rojo, Hospital General de Ciudad Real, Spain
Roberto González Morales, Universidad de Castilla-La Mancha, Spain
Oscar Déniz Suárez, Universidad de Castilla-La Mancha, Spain
Jesús García González, Hospital General de Ciudad Real, Spain

The Grid vision has described as a world in which computational power (resources, services, data) is a readily available as different utilities. They are available to users by means of computational, data, application, information and knowledge services at different levels and areas. These services can interact to perform specified tasks in an efficient and secure way. Their main applications include large-scale computational and data intensive problems in science and engineering. Therefore, Grids are likely to have a deep impact on health related applications. Moreover, they seem to be suitable for tissue-based diagnosis. This chapter analyzes the general structures and functions of a Grid environment implemented for tissue-based diagnosis on digital images. Moreover, it describes the web-based automated image analysis system developed by the authors for diagnostic pathology.

Chapter 6
Grid Technology in Telepatology and Personalised Treatment 117
O. Ferrer-Roca, University of La Laguna, Spain
F Marcan, University of La Laguna, Spain
M. E. Vidal, University Simon Bolivar, Venezuela
E. Ruckhaus, University Simon Bolivar, Venezuela
X. Santos, University of La Laguna, Spain
E. Iglesias, University Simon Bolivar, Venezuela

Histopathology requires automation, quality control and global collaborative tools. Usually the PIMS (Pathology information management system) automates samples, images and reports and progressively incorporates the PI (Pathology informatics), the D-PATH (digital pathology), e-PATH (electronic pathology), the PPH (Patho-pharmacology), virtual autopsy (VA) and all type of translational research in the PMIS. Not being subject to a specific standard, quality control follows ISO-13485:2003 on services and medical devices, ISO 17025:2005 on technical aspects; and ISO-15198:2003 for automate and quantifiable procedures that will be affected by the new European Directive on medical devices. For the non-standardized pathology procedures, consumer's requirements are what define test and calibration procedures. The paper analysed the non-standardized procedures: VS (Virtual Slides), GRID networking and Literature Based Discovery as tools for knowledge discovery of relevant relationships on image-diagnosis and personalized treatments. Standardized procedures available for search and annotation are the ISO/IEC 11179 Information Technology Metadata Registries specification, the ISO/IEC 13250:2003 for topics maps or MPEG-7 & 21 for images and the ISO/IEC 24800-3 for JPEG query search. The forthcoming innovations prepare to quality certify the so called "solo-pathology" robotic labs, supported by telepathology to reduce diagnostic errors and carrying out a relevant task on personalized treatment through GRID technology. In this environment the JPEG query search play a relevant role on images which metadata can be annotated on natural language.

Chapter 7
Gridifying Neuroscientific Pipelines: A SOA Recipe and Experience from the
neuGRID Project 129
David Manset, maatG, France
The neuGRID Consortium

In recent times, innovative new e-Infrastructures have materialized all around the globe to address the compelling and unavoidably increasing demand on computing power and storage capacity. All fields of science have entered an era of digital explosion and thus need to face it with appropriate and scalable instruments. Amongst century's cutting-edge technologies, the grid has become a tangible candidate which several initiatives have harnessed and demonstrated the added value of. Turning the concept into a concrete solution for Neurosciences, the neuGRID project aims to establish a grid-based e-Infrastructure providing neuroscientists with a powerful tool to address the challenge of developing and testing new markers of neurodegenerative diseases. In order to optimize the resulting grid and to deliver a user-friendly environment, neuGRID has engaged the process of migrating existing imaging and data mining toolkits to the grid, the so-called gridification, while developing a surrounding service oriented architecture of agnostic biomedical utilities. This chapter reports on a preliminary analysis of the issues faced in the gridification of neuroimaging pipelines and attempts to sketch an integration model able to cope with the several and heterogeneous applications used by neuroscientists.

Chapter 8
Computational Grids: An Introduction to Potential Biomedical Uses and Future Prospects
in Oncology: Neuro-Oncology Applications as a Model for Cancer Sub-Specialties 152
Ribhi Hazin, Harvard University, USA
Ibrahim Qaddoumi, St. Jude's Children's Research Hospital, USA
Francisco Pedrosa, Instituto Integrado de Medicina Prof Fernando Figueira - IMIP, Brazil

A network of interconnected computers, or "computational grids," can facilitate the ability of users to complete complex computational tasks that would be virtually impossible with a single computer. By leveraging the computational strength of grids, individual users can efficiently disseminate, exchange, and retrieve information as easily as if it were stored locally. As we found in this study, the possibilities computational grids present for highly specialized medical fields such as neuro-oncology are limitless. By harnessing the power of grids, neuro-oncologists can link to sophisticated interactive medical images around the world, perform complicated statistical analyses, create larger collaborative research projects, and improve delivery of care to patients around the globe. Thus, utilization of grid computing modules will inevitably lead to marked improvements in clinicians' ability to detect, manage, and prevent complications associated with brain tumors.

Chapter 9
Grid for Post Operative Care through Wireless Sensor Networks.. 164
N.P Chowdhry, Mehran University of Engineering and Technology, Pakistan
Adnan Ashraf, Mehran University of Engineering and Technology, Pakistan
B.S Chowdhry, Mehran University of Engineering and Technology, Pakistan
A.K Baloch, Mehran University of Engineering and Technology, Pakistan
A.W Ansari, University of Sindh, Pakistan
H. De Meer, University of Passau, Germany

To address the solution for problems of e-health systems, the various new algorithms are developed. Today, the parallel and distributed programming concepts have motivated the doctors and technology experts for the development of e-health grid systems. This e-health grid system is expected to provide more efficient patient care system, better security and more dedicated links among patients, pharmaceutical companies and their experts. The chapter discusses the project significance of grid computing with its past, present and future in the perspective of e-health. The interdisciplinary research and development in the field of biochemistry, health care, information technology and biomedical engineering has enabled technologists to develop equipments and systems for patient monitoring at distances. The pharmaceutical companies, doctors and technology experts have been working for platforms with continuous connectivity for the treatment and post operative care for patients in homes and in hospitals. The practical significance of such developments shall be discussed in the Chapter including the exponential growth and exploration of new areas in post operative care systems where Wireless Sensor Network (WSN) is playing a vital role. Moreover, the chapter explains that 'how video conferencing or face to face examination of patient can be performed in the preview of e-learning'. Since, this e-health grid system contains varied parametric input and output and there is a need of data fusion system. The last, but not least, we discuss here the challenges and process of acquisition and retrieval of the abstract data types (medical images and different sonic beats) using web-portal and MIS e-health care systems.

Chapter 10
Data Security in Electronic Health Records 182
Stefane M. Kabene, Ecole des Hautes Etudes en Sante Publique (EHESP), France
Raymond W. Leduc, University of Western Ontario, Canada
Candace J. Gibson, University of Western Ontario, Canada

Traditionally, patient information has been recorded on paper and stored in file folders at healthcare facilities and within physicians' offices. The implementation of electronic health records (EHRs), the lifetime record of an individual's health and health services delivered, allows for information to be stored on computers and offers the opportunity to store considerably more data, in much less space, with new efficiencies and value added as information is easier to access, legible, timely, non-redundant and readily available. However, there are many issues to consider with the implementation of a fully shared EHR. The protection of the information contained in the record is of the utmost importance as individuals stand to become quite vulnerable if that personal health information is compromised or accessed by unauthorized users. Therefore, one of the goals of this chapter is to uncover ways in which personal health information is being protected in EHR systems. The second objective, a broader one, examines what regulations, legislation and policies are in place that remove some of the uncertainty and risk and make the use of shared information safe and secure. Many of the techniques and technologies used so far are adopted from the corporate world, where data security has been an issue for some time. Current legislation in the United States and Canada at both the federal and state/provincial levels has addressed the general principles of data security and privacy but are still lacking in specifics with regard to cross-jurisdictional sharing of health information and the implementation and use of EHRs. Many of the researchers and studies on the subject find this to be one of the most important areas of concern moving forward. The opportunities for EHR implementation and use are exciting as they have the strong potential to improve both individual health care and population health, but without proper regulation and policies in place it is possible that the risks may outweigh the benefits.

Chapter 11
A Secure Teleradiology Grid 195
Robert Rudowski, Medical University of Warsaw, Poland
Michal Dzierzak, Medical University of Warsaw, Poland
Bartosz Kaczynski, Medical University of Warsaw, Poland

A modern secure teleradiology grid consists of several important parts. The first part is to ensure the highest security of storing the medical data. At present time the old fashioned storage solutions are replaced by Grid Storage and Content Addressable Storage (CAS) infrastructure of archiving medical records in a flexible and secure way. The second part of secure teleradiology grid is related to applying appropriate data transmission security protocols and digital signatures in the various nodes of grid. Also human and law aspects of security need to be taken into account because of international nature of teleradiology development. The law should be consistent in different nodes of teleradiology grid.

Chapter 12
Tele-Audiology in the United States: Past, Present, and Future 205
John Ribera, Utah State University, USA

The incorporation of telehealth into the daily clinical practice of audiologists in the United States is in its early stages of development. Some initial research has been conducted in order to validate the use of telehealth technologies in providing hearing and balance evaluation and management services (Krumm, Huffman, Dick, & Klich, 2008; Krumm, Ribera, & Klich, 2007;Krumm, Ribera, & Schmiedge, 2005; Lancaster, Krumm, & Ribera, 2008). More research is needed. This chapter suggests possible applications using existing technology and explores the possibility of virtual audiology clinics nation-wide and internationally.

Chapter 13
Global Health Network Supercourse and Cancer Epidemiology: Free Cancer
Epidemiology Resources on the Internet 215
Faina Linkov, University of Pittsburgh Cancer Institute, USA
Elizabeth Radke, University of Pittsburgh Graduate School of Public Health, USA
Mita Lovalekar, University of Pittsburgh Graduate School of Public Health, USA
Ronald LaPorte, University of Pittsburgh Graduate School of Public Health, USA

There have been even fewer scientific studies examining the translation of prevention research into the classroom. In order to improve global cancer education, global cancer educators need access to good educational lectures and existing data in the area of cancer morbidity and mortality. This chapter will concentrate on describing several resources of cancer information available on the Internet: the Supercourse, SEER, CANCERMondiale, and Cancer Atlas.

Compilation of References 224

About the Contributors 254

Index 262

Preface

The manuscript represents the most current development in application of Grid technologies for telemedicine and eHealth purposes. The popularity of the Internet as well as the availability of powerful computers and high-speed network technologies as low-cost commodity components has led to the development of Grid computing. The term Grid is chosen as an analogy to a power Grid that provides consistent, pervasive, dependable, transparent access to electricity irrespective of its source. A detailed analysis of this analogy can be found. Grids enable the sharing, selection, and aggregation of a wide variety of resources including supercomputers, storage systems, data sources, and specialized devices that are geographically distributed and owned by different organizations. The Grid infrastructure can benefit different applications. It can be viewed as a seamless, integrated computational and collaborative environment. Grid applications often couple resources that cannot be replicated at a single site, or which may be globally located for other practical reasons. These are some of the driving forces behind the foundation of global Grids. In this light, the Grid allows users to solve larger or new problems by pooling together resources that could not be easily coupled before. Hence, the Grid is not only a computing infrastructure, for large applications, it is a technology that can bind and unify remote and diverse distributed resources.

Research using population-based data repositories gains increasing importance of Grid technologies in academia, industry and governmental bodies. In life sciences, e.g., there is a compelling demand for the integration and exploitation of heterogeneous biomedical information for improved clinical practice, medical research, and personalized healthcare. In this context Grid technologies are becoming a common infrastructure in order to federate different data sources to enable researchers as well as medical professionals to query and access distributed information in a unified and integrated way and to seamlessly provide computing resources. Various Grid-related research projects focus on the development, enhancement and implementation of Grid infrastructures in healthcare.

The present publication presents application of possibilities of Grid technologies for telemedicine and eHealth as well as presentation of ongoing projects and achievements. Having in mind the vision for the manuscript, I have asked some of the best and the experienced in Grid technologies and telemedicine and eHealth to help me put together this manuscript, which should be understandable, informative, and comprehensive. I am grateful to everyone who has contributed to the manuscript. I hope this publication will reflect the current status of application of Grid technologies for telemedicine and eHealth purposes.

Ekaterina Kldiashvili, Ph.D.
Executive Director
Georgian Telemedicine Union (Association)

Chapter 1
The Application of Virtual Organization Technology for eHealth

Ekaterina Kldiashvili
Georgian Telemedicine Union (Association), USA

ABSTRACT

Several years ago any talk related to the Internet would have to be proceeded by an explanation of what it is and how it works. At present information and communication technologies became the essential part of our life and practical activity. eHealth can be designated as a special form of information and communication technologies. It is obvious that eHealth has a great potentiality; however today there are unfortunately only a few examples of its large services. Efficient, effective and reliable systems for remote consultations and distance education are the top requirements for eHealth. Grid technologies have emerged as an important new field, distinguished from conventional distributed computing by its focus on large-scale sharing, innovative applications, and, in some cases, high-performance orientation. "Grid technology" we are going to define as flexible, secure, coordinated resource sharing among dynamic collections of individuals, institutions, and resources – what can be described as "virtual organizations". The present chapter will discuss the application of Virtual Organization technology for eHealth purposes. Over the past five years, research and development efforts within the mentioned technology have produced protocols, services, and tools. Virtual Organization technology will offer the opportunity for improving healthcare services and for making healthcare expertise available to underserved locations.

INTRODUCTION

The term globalization involves a complex series of economic, social, technological and political changes seen as increasing interdependence and interaction between people and companies in disparate locations. The phenomenon of globalization has already reached the medical field, most importantly in the areas of knowledge, diagnosis and therapy. The access of as many people as possible to these areas should be guaranteed by a technically efficient man-machine interacting

DOI: 10.4018/978-1-61692-010-4.ch001

system and by an effective organization of specialists around the world. An efficiently operational and organized exchange of medical information increases the quality of diagnosis and therapy, and assures the training and continuous education of the medical personnel. The main task of a medical informatics system is to enable medical non-experts to gather, exchange and discuss relevant data at any time with experts at any place of the world. A wise conception of such a structured dialogue for consultations and continuing medical education is based on a user-friendly, fast, simple, efficient and sustainable system for the exchange of medical information.

Several years ago any talk related to the Internet would have to be proceeded by an explanation of what it is and how it works, but at present information and communication technologies (ICT) became the essential part of our life and practical activity. eHealth can be designated as a special form of ICT; as a method of delivering medical services by electronic means of communication, with the provider and the recipient of these services being at different places.

The introduction of eHealth applications often result in substantial changes in healthcare practices. Investments in eHealth are usually accompanied by improvement in the quality of care and services, shorter turnaround times and more availability of information. As a consequence there are significant changes in health outcomes and patient satisfaction. A continuous assessment is required to appreciate and respond to changes after the introduction of eHealth in a healthcare system. A proper evaluation should include: assessment of advantages, disadvantages, costs (transaction and incremental costs), investment schedules, fluency and quality of communication, needs of and access to different services, changes in work process, and the division of work evoked by the new "instrument". Since telemedicine can also influence the conventional decision making of clinicians, the legal and ethical consequences of telemedicine and eHealth should also be assessed.

Efficient, effective and reliable systems for remote consultations and distance education are the top requirements for eHealth. However, solutions have so far proved elusive and the deployment of ICT in many health sectors has required major transformational changes. One of the major problems for a full potential delivery of telemedicine is to provide the tools for the world-wide access. Thus, it is necessary to make radical improvements in service productivity, access to medical services, and improved quality of diagnostic with acceptable levels of patient safety. A well developed ICT could serve to breakdown many of the existing barriers to the access of eHealth in the world.

The term "Grid" was coined in the middle 1990s to denote a proposed distributed computing infrastructure for advanced science and engineering. Considerable progress has since been made on the construction of such an infrastructure, but the term "Grid" has also been conflated, at least in popular perception, to embrace everything from advanced networking to artificial intelligence. One might wonder whether the term has any real substance and meaning. Is there really a distinct "Grid problem" and hence a need for new "Grid technologies"? If so, what is the nature of these technologies, and what is their domain of applicability? While numerous groups have interest in Grid concepts and share, to a significant extent, a common vision of Grid architecture, there is no consensus on the answers to these questions. One of the main strategies of grid computing is using software to divide and apportion pieces of a program among several computers, sometimes up to many thousands.

The purpose of the present chapter is to argue that the Grid concept is indeed motivated by a real and specific problem and that there is an emerging, well-defined Grid technology base that addresses significant aspects of this problem. In the process, it develops a detailed architecture and roadmap for current and future Grid technologies. Furthermore, the chapter asserts that while Grid technologies are currently distinct from other major technology trends, such as Internet, enterprise, distributed, and peer-to-peer computing, these other trends can benefit significantly from growing into the problem space addressed by Grid technologies.

The real and specific problem that underlies the Grid concept is coordinated resource sharing and problem solving in dynamic, multi-institutional virtual organizations. The sharing that the chapter is concerned with is but primarily file exchange but rather direct access to computers, software, data, and other resources, as is required by a range of collaborative problem-solving and resource-brokering strategies emerging in industry, science, and engineering. This sharing is, necessarily, highly controlled, with resource providers and consumers defining clearly and carefully just what is shared, who is allowed to share, and the conditions under which sharing occurs. A set of individuals and/or institutions defined by such sharing rules from what is called a virtual organization (VO).

The present chapter will discuss the application of Virtual Organization (VO) technology for eHealth purposes. It is well known, that Virtual Organizations are a set of individuals and/or institutions that have direct access to computers, software, data, and other resources, and to share resources in a highly controlled manner, with resource providers and consumers defining clearly and carefully just what is shared, who is allowed to share, and the conditions under which sharing occurs. VOs vary tremendously in their purpose, scope, size, duration, structure, community, and sociology yet they all involve a broad set of common concerns and requirements, namely: the need for highly flexible sharing relationships, ranging from client-server to peer-to-peer; for sophisticated and precise levels of control over how shared resources are used, including fine-grained and multi-stakeholder access control, delegation, and application of local and global policies; for sharing of varied resources, ranging from programs, files, and data to computers, sensors, and networks; and for diverse usage modes, ranging from single user to multi-user and from performance sensitive to cost-sensitive and hence embracing issues of quality of service, scheduling, co-allocation, and accounting.

Current distributed computing technologies do not address the above concerns and requirements, and it is here precisely where VOs' approach comes on the scene. Over the past five years, research and development efforts within the VOs community have produced protocols, services, and tools that address the challenges that arise when we seek to build scalable networks. Basic technologies supporting VOs include the Internet and the World Wide Web telecommunications, electronic mail, groupware, and video conferencing.

It is obvious that eHealth has a great potentiality; however today there are unfortunately only a few examples of its large services. The benefits of expanding eHealth and telemedicine use are threefold: it can improve the quality of healthcare services; it will allow a better exploitation of limited hospital resources and of expensive medical equipment; it will help to address the problem of unequal access to healthcare. VO technology will offer the opportunity for improving healthcare services and for making healthcare expertise available to underserved locations.

BACKGROUND

It is well known, that eHealth is a rapidly developing application of clinical medicine where medical information is transferred via application of ICT for the purpose of consulting, remote medical procedures or examinations. It can be as simple as discussing of a case by two healthcare professionals by using of web technologies or as complex as using satellite technology and videoconferencing equipment to conduct a real-time consultation between medical specialists. eHealth encompass all applications of ICT in healthcare (telemedicine, electronic patient records, health information on the Internet, distance education, etc.).

eHealth has a longer history. The National Aeronautics and Space Administration (NASA) played an important role in the early development of this field. NASA's efforts in eHealth began in the early 1960s when humans began flying in space. Physiological parameters were telemetered from both the spacecraft and the space suits during missions. These early efforts and the enhancement in communication satellites fostered the development of telemedicine and many of the medical devices in the delivery of healthcare today. At 90s of last century it became clear that ICT in general had developed much. The speed of transmission of larger amounts of information had increased and the usability of ICT for healthcare became larger. A new era for telemedicine started. The number of possible applications of the new technology developed much and continues to develop. Telemedicine is now an enabler to transcend both distance and time barriers for collaboration. As a result requests to possibilities and resources of ICT increase. Grid computing and Virtual Organization technologies have been developed.

Virtual Organizations (VO) are a set of individuals and/or institutions that have direct access to computers, software, data and other resources, and to share resources in a highly controlled manner, with resource providers and consumers defining clearly and carefully just what is shared, who is allowed to share, and the conditions under which sharing occurs. VOs vary tremendously in their purpose, scope, size, duration, structure, community, and sociology yet they all involve a broad set of common concerns and requirements, namely: the need for highly flexible sharing relationships, ranging from client-server to peer-to-peer, for sophisticated and precise levels of control over how shared resources are used, including fine-grained and multi-stakeholder access control, delegation, and application of local and global policies; for sharing of varied resources, ranging from programs, files and data to computers, sensors, and networks; and for diverse usage modes, ranging from single user to multi-user and from performance sensitive to cost-sensitive and hence embracing issues of quality of service, scheduling, co-allocation, and accounting. Current distributed computing technologies do not address the above concerns and requirements, and it is here precisely where VO technology comes on the scene.

Healthcare is more and more complex and the fast turnover of accurate knowledge is a constant challenge. eHealth as well as application of VO for healthcare purposes can address this. Most specialists have the resources to attend national and international scientific meetings, however most primary care team members do not have this opportunity. Developing of telemedicine networks, virtual conferences and streaming of scientific events provides an opportunity to reach front-line healthcare professionals. Virtual Organization technology can be used as a tool to facilitate the sharing of healthcare knowledge and expose the world community to outstanding achievements, resources and knowledge.

Virtual Organization Technology for eHealth

From the review and analysis of first attempts of application of VO technology for eHealth it has become obvious that there is a variety of problems and challenges. The healthcare systems, and the education of healthcare personnel, have to be re-organized to systems that function in a cross-border fashion. Prerequisites for this development shall be a specific emphasis on equity of access, interoperability and standardization of systems and protocols, security and legal aspects. There are technical, legal, organizational and financial problems to be solved.

Technical problems. Although the VO technology needed mostly does exist already today, there are still area-specific technical barriers that have to be overcome. The most prominent barriers are easy-to-use, intuitive, robust and smooth user interfaces and devices. The services must be offered to all users through such interfaces, and all of them have to be implemented in a uniform way. The access to the technology and systems must be smooth and transparent to the users. Otherwise they won't achieve a good acceptance.

Legal problems. The legal barriers that have to be overcome are essentially the general ones applying to eHealth field. Responsibility, confidentiality, liability and access only to certified professionals are some of the key issues.

Organizational problems. There are serious organizational barriers, however such as eHealth at home require smooth collaboration of different organizations. This requires a significant redesign of processes, which means a change from the enterprise-centric view to a system-wide perspective with patient at the center. Today the paradigm of service chains in healthcare built on VO-based collaboration of service providers linked in a service provision network is still in its infancy. However, the increasing interest in recent approaches like managed care, disease management, and case management, which are strongly related to this paradigm shift, shows that the necessity of changing the way in which healthcare systems are organized is more and more recognized and continually becomes transparent. Country-specific factors, such as roles of different providers of health and social care services, insurance companies, housing providers, local authorities, and eHealth providers, need to be taken into account when introducing healthcare at home.

Financial problems. The financial barriers largely depend on the different countries' policies. In countries with national healthcare systems these services will be a part of the overall healthcare system. In insurance based countries, where services are reimbursed on a fee-for service basis, new codes will have to be established. In countries with market-driven healthcare systems the prices need to be adapted to market prices driven by the healthcare consumers. At this time there is a little evidence on how the broad implementation of VO based eHealth services will affect the financial situation of healthcare system in total, and its participants in particular. The challenge is to create comprehensive systems (networks of services offering the basis for patient-individual service chains) which are financially beneficial for all players.

Other problems. The application of VO technology for eHealth purposes can help to solve the huge problem of an 'elderly society'. Stakeholders, including health professionals, researchers, public officials, and the lay public must collaborate on a range of activities. These activities include initiatives to build robust health information system that provides equitable access, development of high-quality, audience-appropriate information and support services for specific health problems, and health-related decisions for all segments of the population, especially for underserved persons, training of health professionals in the science of communication and the use of communication technologies, evaluation of interventions, promotion of a critical understanding and practice of effective health communication both for end-users and for health professionals, and initiatives to gain knowledge about eHealth consumers' use of and their needs and attitudes with regards to VO technology in eHealth.

In spite of the potential which application of VO technology for eHealth has as mechanism too support health systems, a number of barriers, at various levels, would need to be overcome for health systems to take full advantage of these opportunities. These barriers are not unidimensional, focusing on technical knowledge as previously assumed, but rather a multidimensional construct, encompassing technical knowledge, economic viability, organizational support and behavior modification. Three most important barriers to VO technology application for eHealth adoption were identified as the problem of interoperability, acceptance of a 'new' health system, and regulatory constraints.

Interoperability is a key challenge. This is the fragmentation problem – many pieces of information, in many formats, on many platforms, in many stakeholder environments both physically (stored in different locations) and logically (not organized in the same fashion) accentuating issues of interoperability that are raised by lack of compatibility of systems and equipment. The problem of interoperability is not limited to technical standardization as typically assumed, but encompasses the complex issues of integrating cultural, financial and workflow systems. Ensuring that the 'ways of working' of health systems are interoperable is a major challenge.

Acceptance of VO technology in eHealth presents a particular challenge. It is important to promote the use of automated tailoring of information access and summaries to accommodate variations in culture, language, literacy, and health-related goals, as well as integrated decision-support systems that can proactively foster best practices. Unfortunately, collection and delivery of the necessary epidemiological and patient data on which such systems must be built are problematic. However, once collected, VO technology can be used for timely transfer of data to central services for planning and management purposes. At the organizational level, revolutionary advances in medicine and technology as a whole during the past few decades have resulted in shifts in the boundaries between hospitals, primary healthcare, and community care. In the future, VO in eHealth is likely to add to this by changing the way in which health services are provided, from clinical messaging (advice, results and referrals), to distributed electronic health records, increased connectivity between health services, patient appliances to assist self-management, and the use of technology to improve communication. These changes need to be sensitive to acceptance concerns related to changing established medical traditions, professional autonomy and loss of control.

Liability in connection with standards of care and medical malpractice, responsibility for security and confidentiality of patient-specific information are major legal challenges. Owing to be computerized communications involved in eHealth, determining where transactions occurred, which laws apply and which courts have jurisdiction will be problematic. At the policy level, challenges include professional standards of providing care and licensing of care givers, and regulation of medical devices and VO and eHealth application software. Application of VO technology in eHealth as well as eHealth is currently unregulated, unlike all other aspects of the health system.

VO technology in eHealth raises or accentuates ethical, legal and policy issues. Confidentiality of information, protecting the privacy of patients and safeguarding the integrity of information will present significant challenges with increasing use of eHealth. There will also be gender issues to be addressed and model guidelines will be needed to resolve problems brought on by cultural differences among countries engaged in eHealth activities.

Interconnectivity comprises a lot more than merely devising and installing the technological infrastructure so as to be able to communicate and spread medical data through defined secured channels from one point on the earth to another. Interconnectivity is responsible for several aspects of VO technology application for eHealth purposes when installing and running it:

- Technical aspects;
- Organizational aspects;
- Psychological aspects;
- Social and socio-cultural aspects;
- Financial aspects;
- Legal aspects;
- Political aspects;
- Security aspects.

All these aspects are intertwined with all the sections and contributions are briefly described below. It is important to mention major features since they may serve as important criteria to be observed and integrated for the development of 'running eHealth systems".

Technical aspects. With the availability of electronic patient record systems which try to integrate not merely both the stationary and the ambulatory medical workflow of diagnostics and therapy, but deliver real-time medical patient data in a ubiquitous fashion to hold these data available at any time and any location, the basis for a global data exchange in the field of medicine is given. The main stakes today comprise HL7 (HL7 2004) and information servers, CDA (CDA 2004), SCIPHOX (SCIPHOX 2004), and many other existing and to become documentation standards. More and more, the availability and performance of terrestrial communication lines becomes continually better: back from analogue telephone line to digital ISDN and nowadays xDSL lines. Whereas these communication line types are financially affordable usually for private and small business applications and services, such lines of even better quality (e.g. optical fiber) are today too expensive to compete adequately for a substantial market share in medicine.

Organizational aspects. The necessary forms of organization within hospitals and the medical practices are only partially compatible with each other. As of yet, there are no general recommendations as how to organize services which have to deal with a more thought digitalization of medicine. This however, is independent of the underlying communication technology used.

Psychological aspects. Many staff members in a medical setting – irrelevant of their hierarchical position – are still reluctant to use computer-based help in their daily routine work. It has clearly been shown that for physicians, the 'option to possess a gadget' to handle medical instructions is interesting, but the interest soon enough looses intensity after a very short period of time. For the paramedics, however, such gadgets often become integrated for good into their medical routine, and they are thought to use them much longer, much more intensely, and with a greater understanding of the gadget's practical value.

Social and socio-cultural aspects. Many studies have shown that socio-cultural changes of a society towards the incorporation of electronic gadgets into daily life have great influence on the way people think and even expect how medicine should work. Technocracy has become one of the outstanding features of medicine in the opinion of most people. Irrelevant of whether this view is correct or adequate, medicine now is no longer in a condition to reluctantly defy all technological advances made. The standard of ubiquitous communicability for man has to become a feature of medicine as well. Furthermore, hierarchical structures no longer being accepted the way they used to be, a tendency can be noted which strengthens the individual's 'home right'. More and more applications and services are directly integrated into the consumers' homes, and they are expected to be both safe and trustworthy.

Financial aspects. The ongoing everyday usage of ICT has given rise to VO technology solutions associated with continually decreasing and thus affordable prices which make this technology usable for the large majority of users.

Legal aspects. The heterogeneity of legal preconditions for carrying out eHealth applications and services, invariant of the used technology still in many countries forms a broad barrier with a national and an international component.

Political aspects. Adjourning to the legal problems, the general attitude towards an ongoing digitalization in many countries is apparent, the way and direction, however, in which these developments are brought to flourish, are potentially different. In this situation, some coordination actions on an international level are mandatory.

Security aspects. Security threats – not merely in the sense of a technological impact (virus attacks, worms, malicious scripts, etc.), but also concerning human behavior in carrying out national or international conflicts – are most imminent in people's minds when it comes to data security. This issue, however, has nothing to do with the underlying method of communication, but refers to the application and service layers to be applied.

The most important aspects which enable 'new' technologies to be widely accepted are:

- User-friendliness;
- Reliability;
- Error tolerance;
- Security and privacy;
- Service availability;
- Quality of service;
- Quality of workflow realization.

Existing solutions must be integrated into more modern software concepts. Concerning the availability of VO technology, ad-hoc networks must be installable within short periods of time. Adequate Quality of Service shall be provided. Different technological gadgets and equipments must be interoperable so as to work together and be compatible to each other on a large scale.

Access to medical data must be authorized by the informed patient. The physician is not the proprietor of these data, whereby he may edit and manipulate them according to their 'load of truth'. Medical data must be ubiquitous for mobility's and flexibility's sake.

Clear structures of medical workflows must be elaborated and installed into both software and hardware concepts which allow for a digitalization of medical data in every respect. The acceptance that by ongoing digitalization routine aspects of work can be simplified and made more efficacious is crucial for the onset of technology apart from the postulation of user-friendliness and cognitive transparency.

The use of VO technology for eHealth must go out of the hospitals and go into the homes of the health consumers. Healthcare is already being deliverable at home and the electronic documentation needs to follow. Thus, the concept of continuous socialization (with the family, with friends etc.) can be upheld better than before, and cases of hospitalization with all their aspects of microbiological contamination and psychological deprivation and depersonalization can be reduced significantly.

Establishing real world applications and services will, in the near future, definitively have the potential to help to save money, reduce redundancies, avoid a waste of resources, reduce the system-specific administrative overload and keep up and foster international bonds and treaties. Models will have to be developed which offer the same range of applications and services at the same or even better conditions (upstream and downstream velocity, data scrambling etc.) for both the health consumer and the healthcare professional based on the most suitable access technology.

A unification of legal preconditions has to be proposed by each country. In the world a general legal framework will have to be imposed for developing the legal background for eHealth applications and services dealing with the transport of medical data both nationally and internationally.

Regardless of each country's healthcare policy, the general direction shall be an 'opening of data transfer through closed channels' to transmit data safely from one point to another. Therefore, on the side of the policy makers, medically expert advisors and consultants who not only know the individual healthcare situation perfectly well, but also have idea deep knowledge of the technology to be used together with a vision of where the whole development is heading to, shall be introduced to offset up the new basic laws to foster the understanding eHealth on the one hand and help the development of the needed applications and services on the other.

Data transfer has to be made safe and trustworthy. On the one side for the health consumer who wants to be assured that his medical data are not disclosed to anybody else but himself or herself. On the other side for the healthcare professional who does not want his medical workflow data exposed to unauthorized or forbidden benchmarking or other manipulation. Technologies must be developed which guarantee adequate amounts of privacy for all users of eHealth applications and services. Communication networks, thus, must exclude the possibility that their data stream is being logged and 'reverse engineered' to something human readable and something which can be associated to a real human being. Furthermore, patients can have access to the log files of their medical data viewed by 'authorized' persons thus implying a control mechanism for the accuracy and integrity of his/her own data.

The technological basis to support the communication and integration of VO technology for management of medical patient data exists and can be used. However, the heterogeneity of middleware in the healthcare sector reflects the real problems for the introduction, installation, and maintenance of such technology. And this situation seems to be mostly independent of the technological nature. But apart from technological questions, the main stakes are to seamlessly integrate all of the mentioned aspects into one singular, possibly globally usable concept which enables the empowered citizen to take part in the best medical quality everywhere on the planet. Therefore, some challenges and opportunities are addressed:

- The basic technology deals with management of medical data. Thus a standardized document format is needed.
- The applications and services presently used and to be developed are independent of underlying communication carrier.
- Utilities to integrate existing middleware and to convert 'older' data sets are needed. The software used has to be transparent and user-friendly to the maximum for all users.
- Technology has to go hand in hand with the health consumers' and the healthcare professionals' needs and demands and must not be used 'role of technology push versus demand pull'.
- Socio-cultural changes need to be implicitly taken into account when it comes to developing systems which shall not only be used in a clinical context, but also be able to be integrating able into the health consumers' home.
- Legal and political aspects have to be harmonized on both a national and an international level. This is the more important on behalf of the growing mobility and flexibility of today's populations.
- The basic demand for the individual's right to be proprietor of his or her own data is that adequate data security is a mandatory step which no longer needs any arguments. The medical data are owned by the patients. External interceptions cannot be tolerated.

Therefore, interconnectivity for healthcare services has many aspects (technical, organization, psychological, social and socio-cultural, financial, legal, political, security-associated) which play a substantial intertwined role in application of VO technology for eHealth. Only this application enables an efficient and efficacious performance of exchanging medical data through existing structures. With adequate definitions of both existing demand and available technology software applications and established services can be used to minimize efforts and redundancy and to maximize output and efficiency in medical data handling.

FUTURE

The possibilities of Grid technologies and VOs presented in the present chapter are of course not the only view that can be taken. Below are summarized and reviewed some alternative perspectives.

The Grid is a next-generation Internet – "The Grid" is not an alternative to "the Internet". It is rather a set of additional protocols and services that build on Internet protocols and services to support the creation and use of computation- and data-enriched environments. Any resource that is "on the Grid" is also, by definition, "on the Net".

The Grid is a source of free cycles – Grid computing does not imply unrestricted access to resources. Grid computing is about controlled sharing. Resource owners will typically want to enforce policies that constrain access according to group membership, ability to pay, and so forth. Hence, accounting is important, and a Grid architecture must incorporate resource and collective protocols for exchanging usage and cost information, as well as for exploiting this information when deciding whether to enable sharing.

The Grid requires a distributed operating system – Grid software should define the operating system services to be installed on every participating system, with these services providing for the Grid what an operating system provides for a single computer: namely, transparency with respect to location, naming security, and so forth. Put another way, this perspective views the role of Grid software as defining a virtual machine. However, we feel that this perspective is inconsistent with primary goals of broad deployment and interoperability. There are arguments those prove that the appropriate model is rather the Internet Protocol suite, which provides largely orthogonal services that address the unique concerns that arise in networked environments. The tremendous physical and administrative heterogeneities encountered in Grid environments means that the traditional transparencies are unobtainable; on the other hand, it does appear feasible to obtain agreement on standard protocols. The architecture proposed in the chapter is deliberately open rather than prescriptive: it defines a compact and minimal set of protocols that a resource must speak to be "on the Grid"; beyond this, it seeks only to provide a framework within which many behaviors can be specified.

The Grid requires new programming models – Programming in Grid environments introduces challenges that are not encountered in sequential (or parallel) computers, such as multiple administrative domains, new failure modes, and large variations in performance. However, the chapter argues that these are incidental, not central, issues and that the basic programming problem is not fundamentally different. As in other contexts, abstraction and encapsulation can reduce complexity and improve reliability. But, as in other contexts, it is desirable to allow a wide variety of higher-level abstractions to be constructed, rather than enforcing a particular approach. So, for example, a developer who believes that a universal distributed shared memory model can simplify Grid application development should implement this model in terms of Grid protocols, extending or replacing those protocols only if they prove inadequate for this purpose. Similarly, a developer who believes that all Grid resources should be presented to users as objects needs simply to implement an object-oriented "Application Program Interface" in terms of Grid protocols.

The Grid makes high-performance computers superfluous – The hundreds, thousands, or even millions of processors that may be accessible within a VO represent a significant source of computational power, if they can be harnessed is a useful fashion. This does not imply, however, that traditional high-performance computers are obsolete. Many problems require tightly coupled computers, with low latencies and high communication bandwidths; Grid computing may well increase, rather than reduce, demand for such systems by making access easier.

The most important and perspective application of VO technology for eHealth is education of healthcare professionals at a distance, so called distance education (eLearning). It may be defined as the application of ICT to acquire new knowledge or skills across the whole range of areas which will affect healthcare professionals, and enrich their experience in rendering the best possible care to patients throughout the process of medical care. eHealth education has the abilities to apply new concepts, and ideas in which the learner becomes an owner of that knowledge, without any respect to distance. As such, eHealth overall, and in particular eHealth education, is significant part of healthcare development, since the event of modern medicine. eHealth education process as a culture, uses for the most part, distance learning as the medium of dissemination of advanced information, and while it is an important aspect of today's education process, this medium should not be distracting, and the principles of learning and education should be unchanged. The addition of technology should not substitute for failed pedagogical process, but technology should allow that educational process, and the message to be disseminated, and tailored to individual groups and professionals, by retaining along some of the educational principles of traditional education. eHealth education centers on the following issues:

- Distance learning;
- Continuous Medical Education (CME) for medical professionals;
- Advanced eHealth professionals education in the changing environment;
- Patient's education in health related issues in the information age.

While distance learning benefits are not challenged by most, it is difficult to estimate the impact on education overall. Nonetheless, it is becoming more and more prevalent around the world. In a survey of Internet found more than 3,000 programs and 1,100 accredited institutions using distance learning in 1,400 fields of studies, represented by over 50,000 courses. The impact of distance learning should be measured by the content of the curriculum which should be based on the process, perception, product and the mode of delivery. As such distance learning and distance education process should be scrutinized just as traditional curriculum has been in the past and continue to be so. The only 'change' should really be the medium of dissemination. Not the content per se, not the overall approach, and certainly not the end product, which is the education of the students, health professional and, the patients themselves. The differences between classical teaching and learning, and new and modern form of teaching as well as learning is substantial in this new era. Instead of confined classroom teaching and learning, the entire universe has become a workplace, a learning environment, anywhere, anytime, 24 hours in a day. This creates a sense of shared knowledge and virtual networking alliances.

The demand for distance learning stems from the common sense of its applicability, but it requires the same standards of production, and evaluation of such programs. The main reasons to implement distance learning in health education are:

- Healthcare professional, in the information age, will acquire new skills and new knowledge without major disruption of their work.
- The need to reduce the cost of obtaining such education on new information (travel expenses, lodging, registration fees on venues like clinical conferences, congresses, and other forms of meetings).
- Need for better convergence of information age healthcare professional in ICT and VO technology.

CME is an important aspect of healthcare professionals in order for them to maintain the acquired knowledge, and to gain new information, which will make possible:

- To offer the best possible care to their patients implementing current standards of care.
- To satisfy governmental, institutional and scientific and clinical societies requirements for licensing, membership, and good standing in societies, associations

and other organized forms of healthcare professionals.
- To ensure that, they are up to speed with current medical practices.

Distance learning and advances in VO technology allows healthcare professionals to participate in CME programs without disrupting their daily routine work to participate in the traditional meetings. Furthermore, it allows and ensures consistency throughout the educational process among peers, institutions and countries.

The question how technology will change our world is not any more relevant. The answer to this question is obvious. The advances in eHealth education have brought significant changes in health education overall. Advanced technologies such as computers, diagnostic imaging, robotics, voice-activating machines, and remote controls have changed hospitals and operating theatres in hospitals around the western world. In parallel with these developments, the patient has become an educated and informed consumer who:

- Questions the decisions of the practitioner and demand explanations and an evidence based medicine approach.
- Validates his or her expertise through web sites and other forms.
- Requires that the doctor offers care, current with world standards.

Furthermore, today's patient can consult any expert in the field, in any country of the world, at any time without respect to geography and distance. At the same time, the world equilibrium has not followed the punctuation of the industrial world directed by the broad bandwidth rush, and there is a huge discrepancy between countries and continents. Subsequently, there is a great need for eHealth education to become a catalyst of equilibration among countries and nations as we move toward a perfect future and electronic globalization. The wide application of eHealth education programs, will most likely narrow significantly if not eliminate entirely, the gap between the countries delivery health systems, and between the imagination, dreams, and achievements of those who do not have the capability to apply new healthcare standards, and those who have such capabilities. For these radical changes to become a reality it will take time and investment, as well serious international collaboration, but the concept of eHealth education has the potential to offer such radical changes, and for the most part, has been accepted, adopted around the world, and has raised hopes that it will create equality and equilibrium in the education of patients and healthcare professionals.

eHealth education has potential to change the delivery of existing medical care and will create more efficient and economically sound healthcare systems, where advanced medical knowledge will prevent unnecessary transfers of patients to countries who can care for those patients, and/or prevent death and morbidity because country's medical professional will be well prepared. eHealth education will bring together a coalition of new partners with innovative boundaries and clear vision. This last element is most important, especially in countries with middle and low incomes, devastated by wars, suffering, political neglect and poverty.

The concept of eLearning, particularly in the health area, requires leadership. This leadership consists of a new generation of healthcare professional who are:

- Multi-dimensional and multi-tasked;
- Have the passion to change the world;
- Are not afraid to disturb the status quo, and are willing to share the knowledge among institutions and nations of the world;
- View technology as the enabler of change, but not the sole answer itself.

At the same time, this concept is a direct result of demands from the public and the consumers themselves. These demands call for:

- Fundamental reshaping of healthcare education system which needs to become a priority in a global sense, and not of focused, self-limited, institutional or driven by national interests;
- Execution process of electronic learning and teaching in the health area which is no different from other e-leadership challenges that include speed, leverage, adaptation, management and organization of the entire process;
- Creativity and adaptation of new education processes in ever changing environment.

eHealth education is about breaking the old rules, changing the models of education, asking the toughest questions and facing the facts that break the silence, and challenges the assumptions of the status quo.

Education of health providers is a major issue in the current environment, as there is a great need for advancing the education process of all health care professionals. The report of the Institute of Medicine in 2001 states that clinical education simply has not kept pace with or has been responsive enough to shifting patient demographics and desires, changing health system expectations, evolving practice requirements and staffing arrangements, new information, focus on improving quality and new technologies. As such, healthcare providers have not been prepared adequately in either academic or continuing education venues to address these major changes in patient population. Healthcare providers are more and more asked to work on inter-disciplinary teams, often supporting patients with chronic conditions, although they may lack the training and education that is based on a team-based approach. Based on multiple reports and analysis, the twenty first century healthcare provider, and system, should ensure that all healthcare professionals be educated to deliver patient-centered care as members of an inter-disciplinary team, emphasizing evidence-based practice, quality proven approaches and informatics.

The proper techniques and methods of disseminating the existing knowledge and evidence-based medicine education programs and processes from renowned institutions and universities to countries around the world are a matter of some debate. What is not a matter of debate at all anymore is the fact that, this dissemination of knowledge and expertise should be a priority of those who possess the knowledge and skills to disseminate it. Such initiatives should come as an international concerted action and collaboration of eHealth in order to facilitate the implementation of VO networks around the world.

The implementation of eHealth education as an expression of needs and demands from the public and healthcare providers is based on a growing concern for medical errors, advances of patient-centered healthcare systems; need to improve cost-benefit ratios and rationalizations of healthcare.

The entire aspect of needs and demands as pertained to eHealth education process needs to be centered in described issues of distance learning, advanced eHealth professionals education in the changing environment, CME for medical professionals, and patient's education in pathology related issues in the information age, and change. Furthermore, it should be taken in mind, the core competencies needed for healthcare professionals that have been created and required common vision across the topics. These competencies are:

- Patient centered care,
- Work on inter-disciplinary teams,
- Employ evidenced-based practices,
- Apply quality improvement techniques, and
- Utilize informatics.

While all five these competencies are extremely important, the utilization of informatics as an important element of VO can effectively:

- Reduce the medical errors;
- Helps manage the knowledge and information, and support the decisions making process based on evidence based practice guidelines;
- Ensures better communication between healthcare providers and patient;
- Advance the goals of redesigning the healthcare systems.

As a result, the core competencies help implement new evidence-based healthcare protocols and support the notion that, every citizen of the world need to receive the best possible existing care.

The implementation of eHealth education process remains one of the most important issues among current health challenges, that are staggering and numerous, as illustrated by numerous studies:

- Only in the USA each year 98,000 people die from medical errors, more than those who die from motor vehicle crashes, breast cancer, or AIDS.
- Other challenges include the lack of the 'best system', poor accommodation of patients' needs, inability to assimilate the increasingly complex scientific advances, failure to address the growing consumerism among the patients.
- Healthcare provider's workforce shortage and discontent.

These are important issues that have led to medical errors, poor quality of care, and dissatisfaction among patients and healthcare providers. In this environment of technological advances, information technology and evidence based medicine has the potential for transformation of healthcare. The integration of more recent advances and visions with goals of the institutions, nations and more broadly of the world is the main challenge, however.

The use of well defined education programs for healthcare providers will be the cornerstone of the new revolution of the "e-era". Current specific challenges in implementing eHealth education and other revolutionary advances for healthcare professions educations are:

- Lack of funding, lack of faculty and faculty development programs.
- Lack of coordination and integration of accreditation, licensing, and certification process at the governmental and institutional level.
- Lack of application existing evidence based medicine.
- Shortage of visionary leaders and champions.
- Crowded curricula of healthcare education for healthcare professional, often with irrelevant courses.
- Insufficient channels to share the information on the best practices, among medical professionals, governments and institutions.

eHealth in medical training could supplement greatly education of healthcare professionals in countries with middle and low incomes for example, without the expenses of moving those specialists from one country to the other for supplemental education. Eventually, eHealth education could be advanced to healthcare telementoring which could assist in the provision of medical care to underserved areas and potentially facilitate the teaching of advanced medical skills worldwide. Although there are still multiple logistical, technical and legal barriers to the widespread application of healthcare mentoring and telepresence medicine great progress has been achieved in this complex field.

eHealth education is a very important element of overall progress in the application of VO technology. In order to be able to advance this, as an accepted culture and part of the daily practice of healthcare professionals, there are many initiatives that need to be taken, or existing one to be supported. Few issues that need resolved in order for eHealth education to prosper and be accepted are:

- 'Product' acceptance by traditional medical educators, scholars, and legislators.
- Changing the old style of education to the new one and thus breaking the 'traditional' classroom healthcare teaching and learning methods.
- Lack of capability and availability of technology in most of the world for disseminating the knowledge, or in other words lack of communications.
- Language and cultural diversity.
- Socio-economic and political status of the countries in need for eHealth education.
- Legislative policies and championships for new information age.

While technological means for broadcasting and transmission of the eHealth education programs and clinical data is becoming abundant around the world, there is a great part of the planet that is not covered by Internet and will not have the ability to overcome the digital divide for decades to come. This should be our chance to advance the cause, and the issue, of infrastructure and perhaps a vision in some cases.

CONCLUSION

Perspectives and strategies for VO technology for eHealth are currently evolving, as emerging operative requirements would allow self-sustainable large scale exploitation while recent technological developments are available to support integrated and cost-effective solutions to such requirements. However, as far as we know few eHealth services have proceeded to large scale exploitation, even after successful technological demonstration phases. Main exploitation drawbacks, problems and deficiencies have been:

1. Partial solutions approach instead of integrated total approach to healthcare assistance needs.
2. Lack of economical drive and consequently no self-sustainability for large scale exploitation.
3. Insufficient H24 (24 hours/day 365 days/year) medical and social operators support.
4. Insufficient networking approach for medical operators and scientific/clinical structures.

eHealth is the most important for the ensuring the safe medical care. It is well known, that the first contact with patients needing medical help is the contact with the local primary care health center. Second opinions from specialists are often required in primary care health centers. An efficient and appropriate strategy of medical care can be worked out at the initial steps of patient's contact with healthcare. Such an approach can avoid unnecessary hospitalization, and will be a substantial contribution to the reduction of health costs.

eHealth has the potential for offering the worldwide medical community the following qualitative and quantitative improvements:

1. Distance consultations, diagnosis and advice for treatment.
2. Opening up new ways for education and training. Improvement in qualification of national specialists and health technicians, by opening up international medical databases.
3. Overall improvement of service by regional centralization of resources (specialists, hardware and software packages).
4. Effectiveness and efficiency in a management of actions related to reduction of wait-

ing times for consultations, and introduction of medical information systems.

eHealth is able to reduce healthcare costs in the following ways:

1. Reduction of operating costs through centralization and optimization of resources (expertise, laboratories, equipment and etc.).
2. Reduction in travel cost and time for specialists visiting other hospitals and centers for consulting.
3. Reduction in costs for training and updating, improvement of specialists' qualifications through distance learning and access to medical databases.

eHealth by comparison with the usual healthcare service introduces added value and a positive impact at social, economic and cultural levels. As a result, eHealth is initiating to have an important influence on many aspects of healthcare service in countries with low and middle income. By application of Virtual Organization technology this process becomes easier and smoother.

REFERENCES

Banta, D. (2003). The development of health technology assessment. *Health Policy (Amsterdam)*, *63*, 121–132. doi:10.1016/S0168-8510(02)00059-3

Beitiger, J., Johnson, W., Bivens, H., Humphreys, S., & Rhea, R. (2000). Constructing the ASCI Grid. *Proc. 9th IEEE Symposium on High Performance Distributed Computing.*

Detmer, D. (2000). Information technology for quality health care: a summary of United Kingdom and United States experiences. *Quality in Health Care*, *9*, 181–189. doi:10.1136/qhc.9.3.181

Detmer, D. (2001). Transforming health care in the internet era. *World Hospitals and Health Services*, *37*, 2.

Dixon, R., & Stahl, J. (2008). Virtual visits in a general medicine practice: A pilot study. *Telemedicine and e-Health, 14*(6), 525-530.

Gabbay, J., & Walley, T. (2006). Introducing new health interventions. *British Medical Journal*, *332*, 64–65. doi:10.1136/bmj.332.7533.64

Gonzalez, M., Quesada, G., Urrutia, I., & Gavidia, J. (2006). Conceptual design of an e-health strategy for the Spanish health care system. *International Journal of Health Care Quality Assurance*, *19*(2), 146–157. doi:10.1108/09526860610651681

Hjelm, M. (2001). Telemedicine and in-patient. *Hospitals International*, *37*, 2.

Jannett, P., & Jackson, A., & Ho, K., & Healy, T., & Kazanjian, A., & Wollard, R., & Haydt, S., & Bates, J. (2005). The essence of telehealth readiness in rural communities: an organizational perspective. *Journal of Telemedicine and eHealth, 11*, 137-145.

Jannett, P., Yeo, M., Pauls, M., & Graham, J. (2003). Organizational readiness for telemedicine: implications for success and failure. *Journal of Telemedicine and Telecare*, *9*(2), 27–30. doi:10.1258/135763303322596183

Kobb, R., & Lane, R., & Stallings, D. (2008). E-learning and telehealth: Measuring your success. *Telemedicine and e-Health, 14*(6), 576-579.

Lam, D., & MacKenzie, C. (2005). Human and organizational factors affecting telemedicine utilization within U.S. military forces in Europe. *Telemedicine Journal and e-Health*, *11*, 70–78. doi:10.1089/tmj.2005.11.70

Lane, K. (2006). Telemedicine news. *Telemedicine and e-Health, 12*(5), 507-511.

Lareng, L. (2002). Telemedicine in Europe. *European Journal of Internal Medicine*, *13*, 1–13. doi:10.1016/S0953-6205(01)00188-1

Latifi, R., & Muja, S., & Bekhteshi, F., & Merrell, R. (2006). The role of telemedicine and information technology in the redevelopment of medical systems: The case of Kosova. *Telemedicine and e-Health, 12*(3), 332-340.

Merell, R., & Doarn, C. (2008). Is it time for a telemedicine breakthrough? *Telemedicine and e-Health, 14*(6), 505-506.

Moore, D., Green, J., Jay, S., Leist, J., & Maitland, F. (1994). Creating a new paradigm for CME: Seizing opportunities within the health care revolution. *The Journal of Continuing Education in the Health Professions*, *14*, 4–31. doi:10.1002/chp.4750140102

Moura, A., & Del Giglio, A. (2000). Education via internet. *Revista da Associação Médica Brasileira*, *46*(1), 47–51.

Nannings, B., & Abu-Hanna, A. (2006). Decision support telemedicine systems: A conceptual model and reusable templates. *Telemedicine and e-Health, 12*(6), 644-654.

Pak, H. (2007). Telethinking. *Telemedicine and e-Health, 13*(5), 483-486.

Riva, G. (2000). From telehealth to e-health: Internet and distributed virtual reality in health care. *Journal of CyberPsychology & Behavior*, *3*(6), 989–998. doi:10.1089/109493100452255

Riva, G. (2002). The emergence of e-health: using virtual reality and the internet for providing advanced healthcare services. *International Journal of Healthcare Technology and Management*, *4*(1/2), 15–40. doi:10.1504/IJHTM.2002.001127

Sloot, P., Tirado-Ramos, A., Altintas, I., Bubak, M., & Boucher, C. (2006). From molecule to man: Decision support in individualized E-Health. *Computer*, *39*(11), 40–46. doi:10.1109/MC.2006.380

KEY TERMS AND DEFINITIONS

eHealth: is an emerging field in the intersection of medical informatics, public health and business, referring to health services and information delivered or enhanced through the Internet and related technologies.

Telemedicine: can be defined as rapid access to shared and remote medical expertise by means of telecommunications and information technologies, no matter where the patient or relevant information is located.

Virtual Organizations: are a set of individuals and/or institutions that have direct access to computers, software, data, and other resources, and to share resources in a highly controlled manner, with resource providers and consumers defining clearly and carefully just what is shared, who is allowed to share, and the conditions under which sharing occurs.

Internet: is a global system of interconnected computer networks that interchange data by packet switching using the standardized Internet Protocol Suite (TCP/IP).

World Wide Web: (commonly shortened to the Web) is a system of interlinked hypertext documents accessed via the Internet.

Computing Technology: can be defined as the activity of using and developing computer technology, computer hardware and software.

eLearning: is defined as an approach to facilitate or enhance education by electronic means such as email, computers, or the Internet.

Continuing Medical Education (CME): is the process within the scope of medicine which provides information and activities designed to maintain and improve the ability of the medical professional to provide high quality patient care.

Information and Communication Technologies (ICT): is an umbrella term that includes all technologies for the manipulation and communication of information.

Chapter 2
Grid Technology:
E-Learning in Telemedicine and Organizational Collaboration

I. H. Monrad Aas
Vestfold Mental Health Care Trust, Norway

ABSTRACT

The present chapter is about telemedicine, but not about software and hardware. It is about humanware. Telemedicine's greatest problem is not to make the technology work. It is organizations and humans in organizations who will decide the future of telemedicine. Telemedicine is not just a simple success story and the diffusion of telemedicine has been slower than many expected. For the future of telemedicine, a shift in the way we think may be necessary. Few authors have focused on learning in telemedicine (with what is here considered as associated aspects: team organization; learning organizations; network organization). The learning potential connected to telemedicine is significant. Learning may constitute an important argument for telemedicine. In the present chapter, focus is on the role learning and collaboration may have for the future of telemedicine. To take the full advantage of the learning potential a higher volume of telemedicine is necessary, but this requires more organizational collaboration. Improved collaboration is obtainable by implementing collaboration measures. The chapter shows that focus on learning and collaboration may well be important for the future of telemedicine. It is recommended that managers lead change processes in their organizations, where the different aspects of importance for realization of learning benefits of telemedicine are treated. For telemedicine, it is important that future research includes: investigations on how to obtain learning benefits and which collaboration measures are relevant for the different telemedicine applications. Objectives of the present chapter are to propose: 1) more international research on learning in telemedicine (with mentioned associated aspects) and telemedicine collaboration problems and 2) to show the background for this proposal.

DOI: 10.4018/978-1-61692-010-4.ch002

INTRODUCTION

In a historical perspective, technology has played a fundamental role for society and organizations. For many years, it has been clear that also IT and telecommunications will bring great changes. In many countries, the information society is gradually replacing the industrial society (Castell 2000). The health sector, however, is at an early stage of potential future changes. A number of technological solutions for health care are classifiable as ICT (information and communication technology). When it comes to consequences for the health sector, telemedicine is important. Telemedicine is an enabler to transcend distance barriers for collaboration. The term telemedicine has been given a number of definitions (Aas 2007), such as 'medicine at a distance' and 'the use of telecommunication technology to assist in the delivery of health care'. Early in our century it became clear that many found the term telemedicine difficult and the collective term 'e-Health' was made. E-Health encompasses all applications of ICT in health care.

The physical infrastructure of modern telecommunications consists of computers connected together. We are dealing with an electronic network. In the later years, the term grid technology has become important. Internationally, we find several definitions of grid technology. A grid system can be defined to consist of: 1) resources that are not subject to centralized control, 2) use standard, open, general-purpose protocols and interfaces, and 3) non-trivial quality of services is delivered (Foster, 2002; Plaszczak & Wellner, 2006). Obviously, telemedicine may well mean application of grid technology.

During the 1990ies a considerable enthusiasm for telemedicine was seen. The belief developed that telehealthcare might revolutionize the practice of medicine (Finch et al., 2003), but the diffusion of telemedicine has been slower than many expected. Telemedicine is not just a simple success story (Finch et al., 2003; May et al., 2003) and a telemedicine system implementation that only considers the technology will fail (Buxton, 1999). Since telemedicine has not been spreading like wildfire, the question comes up: why so?

Today we know that organizational issues are important for diffusion and daily use of telemedicine. This knowledge comes from empirical research. The question of telemedicine having organizational consequences, or not, is completely outdated (Aas 2007).

A new way of thinking could be advantageous for the future of telemedicine. Few authors have focused on learning (with what is here considered as associated aspects: team organization; learning organizations; network organization) and collaboration in telemedicine. In the present chapter, focus is limited to the role learning and collaboration may have for the future of telemedicine. To take the full advantage of learning in telemedicine, a higher volume of telemedicine is necessary, but this requires more organizational collaboration. A look at organizational collaboration is necessary to obtain benefits from telemedicine, learning included. Learning and collaboration are connected and they may be connected to the future of telemedicine.

Objectives: The objectives of the present chapter are to propose: 1) more international research on learning in telemedicine (with mentioned associated aspects) and telemedicine collaboration problems and 2) to show the background for this proposal.

LEARNING IN TELEMEDICINE

Telemedicine can be an important source of learning (Aas, 2002; 2007; Abrahamian et al., 2002; Nilsen & Moen, 2008) and learning in telemedicine is classifiable as eLearning. E-Learning is essentially the network-enabled transfer of skills and knowledge and includes digital collaboration (http://www.webopedia.com/TERM/E/e_learning.html). Few health care organizations have taken measures to exploit the learning potential of telemedicine and focus on the learning benefit of telemedicine has been limited in international research. In the following, several examples of learning in telemedicine are given under three headings, i.e. teleradiology, teleconsultations and continuing education. After a summing up of general aspects of learning in telemedicine, the important role of three distinct organizational forms is outlined, i.e. team organization; learning organizations and network organization. Section two is finished with 'General organizational aspects of telemedicine'.

Teleradiology

Radiology has been through a process of complete digitalisation. The digitalisation of radiology technology undoubtedly has a role to play for learning. The new technology can result in more communication. Not at least so between hospitals. People from different radiology departments can learn of each other. A senior radiologist and a younger doctor (located at two different hospitals) can simultaneously look at the same images and by telephone speak together. The senior radiologist is a mentor for the younger. Distance is no longer a barrier for mentoring. Likewise, radiologists from smaller hospitals can access interpretations performed at university hospitals (Aas, 2007). Easy access to specialised radiology competence can result in learning. In radiology, second opinion is important in some cases. When images are transmitted in electronic networks, second opinion is easily obtained (Aas, 2007). At a hospital, radiologists and clinicians can simultaneously look at images and by communicating learn of each other. The radiologists can understand how clinicians solve problems. In general, teleradiology collaboration can be an effective tool for continuous education (Gortiz et al. 2006).

With the digitalisation of radiology, larger and better archives of radiology images can be built up. The archives can be common for all connected hospitals. Such archives can be the basis for development of large teaching archives. The teaching archives can include, for example, specialized archives with interesting cases. At radiology departments, quality assurance can be done by supervision. With new technology, supervision of daily work becomes easier. Managers of departments can easily take a look at images and interpretations, give feedback to the radiologists and learning results. University hospitals can organize remote teaching and transmit this as videoconferences to all interested. Also, smaller hospitals can invite resource persons and transmit lectures. Totally more people have access to resource persons. With new technology, radiologists can access relevant information in electronic patient records (for example diagnosis, interpretations of pathology sections, and treatment result). When own work is viewed in light of such information, learning can occur (Aas 2007).

Teleconsultations

Joint consultations between specialists and GPs (general practitioners), outside of telemedicine, are known to lead to educational gains, improved patient welfare and more efficient use of the health service (Harrison et al 1996). In the joint consultations, specialists and GPs have a master-apprentice relationship. The master-apprentice relationship is a good situation for learning. In remote consultations, we often have a master-apprentice relationship and we know learning occurs (Aas 2002). Teleconsultations can be used by GPs for support from medical specialists. In the collaboration, diagnosis and treatment options are presented and discussed (Nilsen & Moen 2008). A study showed that four of five involved told they learn something new by working with remote consultations (Aas 2002). First of all, they improve their knowledge of the specialty in which they are involved, for example personnel involved in telepsychiatry learn psychiatry. All GPs can tell they learn something new, but (when involved in remote consultations) nurses, psychologists, other categories of personnel, and even medical specialists tell they learn (Aas 2002). When in doubt, second opinion is important. Technologically, second opinion is obtainable with teleconsultations. It is obvious that teleconsultations can be exploited not just for treating patients, but also for mentoring and learning. In the following, examples of telemedicine and learning are given.

Telepsychiatry

International research shows little reason to believe negative treatment consequences of telepsychiatry, but some psychiatrists may believe so (Bee at al. 2008; Cuevas et al. 2006; Modal et al. 2006; Myers et al. 2007; O'Reilly et al. 2007; Voss 2009; Werner 2005). Telepsychiatry can promote learning across locations and different competencies, decrease isolation, and strengthen relationships between colleagues (Cuevas et al. 2006; Voss 2009). A study showed that all involved in telepsychiatry learn something new (Aas, 2002). The technology can result in improved contact between mental hospital and local health care concerning discharge, admission and better follow up after discharge. After discharge to local community, psychiatric patients can receive follow up by telemedicine. The need for patient travel for specialist treatment is reduced. Local ancillary personnel, including nurses, can obtain professional instructions by telematics from a psychiatrist, and this can result in learning (Aas, 2002). The future learning potential of telepsychiatry is promising.

Other Forms of Teleconsultations

In general, we have clear indications that learning results from very different forms of telemedicine. 3D (three-dimensional) technology may be advantageous for trauma medicine as needed expertise can reach the site before transport to hospital. Learning seems to be an indirect benefit (Welch et al. 2009). In frozen-section telepathology, pathologists are consulted by telecommunications to perform evaluation of the microscopic sections. Those who consult the pathologists can learn (Aas 2002). Remote consulations in dermatology and otolaryngology are known to result in learning (Aas 2002; Blum et al 2004; Mars & Dlova 2008). Telehomecare could become an important future application of the technology and result in increased local competence (Gerrard et al. 1999). Midwives can find videoconferences with parents at home useful after early discharge (Lindberg et al. 2007).

When remote consultations are performed, with doctors on both sides of the electronic network, costs are high. Substitution of the GPs by nurses can be considered, but few substitution experiments have been performed. Work boundaries between doctors and nurses may change, with the nurses performing tasks previously done by doctors (Gerrard et al. 1999). There is reason to perform more systematic evaluation of substitution in telemedicine. Nurses can have enthusiastic attitudes to telemedicine (Hebert et al. 2004). In connection with wound care they can consult specialists and find store-and-forward teledermatology acceptable (Binder et al. 2007).

Continuing Education

Telehealth is especially well accepted in continuing education (Vuonovirta et al. 2009). The ideas from the Virtual Health Care Knowledge Center in Georgia show that eLearning has potential to become an important tool in medical education (Burduli et al. 2008; Schrader et al. 2008). Problem based learning with integration of medical education systems, such as virtual classrooms; virtual groups and virtual clinical case libraries (valuable teaching cases with information on patient history of disease, laboratory results, medical imaging, physical examination, differential diagnosis etc) extends the learning possibilities (Burduli et al. 2008; Schrader et al. 2008). In many countries,

Table 1. Applications of telemedicine

Telemedicine has a number of applications, such as telepsychiatry, telehomecare (virtual visits to the home and monitoring in the home), rehabilitation, teleradiology, remote consultations, teledermatology, telcotolaryngology, telepathology, teledialysis, store-and-forward telemedicine, diabetes, wound care, cardiology, stroke, postoperative care, ophthalmology, geriatrics, endoscopic gastroenterology, acute medicine, electronic messages (for example discharge abstracts to primary care), military applications, telemedicine to ships and oil rigs at sea.

data are collected for a MBDS (Minimum Basic Data Set) or EPR (Electronic Patient Record). The databases can be large, but systematic exploitation of stored data for learning is modest. Conversion of the information into usable knowledge and continuous learning from the knowledge could have been more in focus (Goodfellow et al. 2008). Likewise, little has been done concerning quality standards for education through telemedicine (Shershneva & Olson 2005).

General Aspects of Learning in Telemedicine

Table 1 shows a number of applications of telemedicine. What is known today makes it likely that learning is not limited to applications where learning has been studied. With the new technology, the learning potential for different applications, education and continuing education seems to be significant. It should have been more explored. Research on learning effects of the new technology is at an early stage. Telemedicine can mean cooperation between levels of care, inter-professional, and inter-specialty work. The involved may get new knowledge and add knowledge to their group's collective knowledge. They may learn professional knowledge, about different work processes, values and behavior within other disciplines, develop new contacts and networks, modify own practice and generate new ideas. A broader understanding consisting of several perspectives is built up (Haythornthwaite 2005). For example, primary cares combination of knowledge about local health care and broader knowledge of the patients' social situation, with specialist competence, can make a difference in clinical work. Obviously the technology can be systematically exploited for mentoring. When health care organizations connect for telemedicine, they also connect for learning. The learning effect, in itself, can constitute an important argument for telemedicine.

Team Organization

In the 1990ies, teamwork was increasingly emphasised in health care. Team organization can play a positive role for learning, innovativeness and creativity (Greenhalgh et al., 2004; Ovretveit et al., 1997; Mohrman et al., 1995; Sjøvold, 2006; Stead, 1998). A team consists of several people (a group) organized around a set of objectives (Hertog & Tolner, 1997). Telemedicine work is definable as teamwork (Shulman, 1996; Hertog & Tolner, 1997; Ovretveit, 1996). When personnel from different organizations communicate telemedically, they form virtual teams or virtual organizations (Cascio, 1999). In part, learning in telemedicine is a result of people working together in teams. More telemedicine can mean more learning. The increased emphasis on teamwork with telemedicine is an important development. The combination of skills in multidisciplinary teams has potential to add value in diagnosis and treatment (English, 1997; Ovretveit, 1993; 1996; 1997; Wagner, 2000). Virtual teams offer flexibility, responsiveness, and diversity of perspectives, even more so than co-located groups (Walther et al., 2005). Both production of health services by teams and the electronic communication may have positive effect on service quality (Wagner, 2000; Rice et al., 1990). It should be noticed that many of the common problems in multidisciplinary teams are preventable (Ovretveit, 1997).

Learning Organizations

Often learning is an unplanned side product of telemedicine, but we have already shown that health care could take advantage of the learning potential to a greater degree. By taking into consideration the concept of 'learning organizations' we go one step further. In learning organizations, the learning becomes part of a more general organizational thinking. Focus is more on how the total organization learns. Learning organizations have a role to play in promoting new knowledge (Greenhalgh et al., 2004). For learning organizations, management must involve itself. Learning promotes the intellectual capital of organizations. Management to promote the intellectual capital can include management of relationships between employees to promote knowledge sharing and to develop a learning culture and organizational infrastructure (Senge et al., 1994; Snow et al., 1999). Such thinking can be applied to the telemedicine work situation itself, but it should not be forgotten that telemedicine workers have a relationship to own organization. What the involved learn from work with telemedicine can see diffusion in own organization (Aas 2002), but a too hierarchic organization may represent a hurdle for the flow of knowledge in organizations (Nikula, 1999; Nordhaug, 1993; Stead, 1998). Organizations can change structure to a less centralized form, decentralize functions, and use delegation (Aas, 1997).

It is highly wanted that health care organizations follow new developments. An innovation can be considered as: 'a novel set of behaviours, routines, and ways of working that are directed at improving health outcomes--' (Greenhalgh et al., 2004; Rogers, 2003). Telemedicine is, itself, an innovation in service delivery, but this innovation may play a role for change in how work is done. Telemedicine communication can result in diffusion of new knowledge, new treatments and diagnostics and new work procedures. Innovativeness and creativity of health care organizations are improved (Aas, 2002; 2007; Grimshaw et al., 2005; Mohrman et al, 1995; Sjøvold, 2006).

Network Organization

From learning organizations, we can go one step further in our organizational thinking. Telemedicine means involving larger areas and we need to think for larger areas. In telemedicine, electronic networks form an infrastructure for network organization. Telemedicine networks are networks of professional influence and networks for learning. In organization theory, network organization is a well-known and distinct organization form. Thinking from network organization can play a role for organization of telemedicine in areas. Network organization means a formation of alliances between organizations. A network has potential to improve organizational learning and an organizations capability to exploit new forms of knowledge (Grimshaw et al., 2005; Sandkuhl & Fuchs-Kittowski, 1999). Highly interesting for telemedicine and health care organizations. Health care organizations are clearly wanted to follow new developments. Totally we find many different motives for network organization, such as enhanced human and social capital, development of new services, more standardized patient treatment for similar patients, joint projects for new developments, research cooperation and economies of scale. All motives are relevant in connection with telemedicine. A network can be especially useful for the exchange of know-how or a particular approach to production (Powell, 1990). Networks are also suited to deal with complex problems that are sometimes ill defined (Chisholm, 1998). Not an unknown problem in health care. For the importance of inter-company networks on company performance, of the two perspectives efficiency strategy and learning through networks strategy, the learning strategy has a greater impact (Hagedoorn & Duysters, 2002), i.e. an additional argument for forming telemedicine networks with great learning benefits.

Single health care organizations do not need to develop all kinds of competence. The alliances in network organization can be used to increase organizations' flexibility in what they can do, i.e. capability complementation. Here, capability complementation means pooling of capabilities and resources of organizations collaborating by telecommunications (Schilling, 2005). New skills and human resources can be developed in-house, but with collaboration they can be developed faster and cheaper (Schilling 2005). This means that formation of telemedicine networks should not be based on narrow telemedicine thinking, i.e. that the clinical job is done. Formation of networks can take into consideration the question of which organizational network has the best learning effects. Competence in each organization should be seen in relation to competence in potential collaborating organizations. Communication external to own organization can play a significant role for organizational innovativeness (Greenhalgh et al., 2004; Hagedorn & Duysters, 2002). When formation of telemedicine networks takes this into consideration, we can add one more argument for telemedicine.

To make network organizations work, shared visions and a sense of common purpose are important (Chisholm, 1998; Weinstein et al., 1997). Obviously relations between organizations and people have a role to play. Social capital is about relations and relations matter for development of network organizations. Work in telemedicine networks may enhance social capital of organizations. It should be noticed that communities and societies with high levels of social capital have been proposed to work more productively and cooperatively than those with low levels (Anderson & Boubullian, 1997; Hjelm et al., 2003; Welsh & Pringle, 2001). Once again, we have an argument for telemedicine.

General Organizational Aspects of Telemedicine

That telemedicine can be an important source of learning (Aas 2007) should not be overlooked or just considered an accidental side product. In future, work with telemedicine should include organizational thinking. The three distinct organizational aspects mentioned here (team organization, learning organizations and network organization) all have a role to play for learning. Other, important aspects for formation of telemedicine networks are found under the headings organizational centralization and decentralization (Aas 2006a;b). If skilled organizational thinking is involved, organizational thinking could become decisive for telemedicine's future.

ORGANIZATIONAL COLLABORATION

Collaboration

Health care is fundamentally a collaborative process. Persons working alone do not have all the skills and all the knowledge necessary to solve the diagnostic and treatment problems. In international literature, we find several definitions of collaboration (Cohen & Mankin, 1999; Biggs, 1997; Paul, 2005; Dhar & Olson, 1989). One definition is: making joint cognitive effort toward achieving an agreed upon goal (Chen et al., 2002). The value of collaboration can be said to be a function of the quality, relevance, and complementarity of the employees' knowledge (Paul, 2005).

Collaboration and Telemedicine

Telemedicine requires collaboration between participating parties. We all know that collaboration, in general, does not necessarily work well (Buunk et al., 1998; Chanlat, 1997). Collaboration across organizational borders is a source of significant problems (Wagner, 2000). Telemedical work often occurs across organizational borders. It is then not surprising that availability of technology does not automatically result in telemedicine (Ekeland, 1999; Ogasawara et al., 2001; Voss 2009). It should be noticed that empirical research has shown that telemedicine collaboration can be made to work well. This applies to rather different applications, like telemedicine remote consultations (including telepsychiatry), teleradiology and maritime telemedicine (Aas, 2001; 2005; Axelsson & Axelsson, 2006; Monnier et al., 2003; Puskeppeleit 2008).

Collaboration Measures

Obtaining benefits of telemedicine is dependent on implementing the right collaboration measures (Aas, 2001; 2005). A measure can be defined as: 'any maneuver made as part of progress toward a goal' (http://wordnet.princeton.edu). Collaboration measures are tools to obtain good collaboration. Examples of collaboration measures are given in Tables 2 and 3. What is definable as telemedicine can be discussed (Aas, 2007). We do not know if all applications of technology, which may be definable as telemedicine, are equally requiring when it comes to collaboration measures (examples: Internet sites offering on-line psychotherapy compared to chat groups where patients with mental health problems can communicate with each other compared to telepsychiatry with GP and patient communicating with psychiatrist). It should be noticed that problems related to collaboration are not the only problems of importance for the future of telemedicine (Aas, 2007; Finch et al., 2003; May et al., 2003).

Collaboration and Teleradiology

The production process in radiology has two fundamental elements: capturing images and interpretation of images. Traditionally both are done in the same radiology department. With the new technology, it is relevant to consider reorganizing the production process. Images can be captured in one organization and interpreted in another. This requires more than a well functioning technology. Teleradiology requires implementation of measures of collaboration. Not at least when the volume is large (Aas, 2005). In Table two, 17 measures for collaboration in teleradiology are presented.

Collaboration and Teleconsultations

When the right competence is not present at the site of consultation, the problem can be solved with referral to specialist care. For the patient, travel to specialist care can take time and costs. Remote consultations are an alternative, but remote consultations can also have other applications. For example: a psychiatric nurse, working with a patient who has been transferred to own local community, can have regular follow-up consultations with the psychiatrist who treated the patient at the mental hospital. Psychiatric patients can feel more open and comfortable communicating via telemedicine (Whitten & Kuwahara, 2004) and even prefer telepsychiatry to face-to-face consultations (Detmer, 2000). In Table three, the 10 measures for collaboration in remote consultations (Aas, 2001) are presented merged for four applications, i.e. telepsychiatry, teledermatology, telepathology frozen-section service, and teleotolaryngology. A totally separate presentation for the four specialties was evaluated, but little could be gained by this. Characteristics of collaboration in remote consultations are not necessarily that dependent on specialty (Aas, 2001).

Similarity in Collaboration Measures

Teleradiology and remote consultations are pretty different forms of telemedicine, but we find obvious similarities (and differences) in collaboration measures (see: Table two and three). Three measures for improved collaboration are the same both in teleradiology and remote consultations: make someone responsible and distribute tasks, orga-

Table 2. Overview of 17 measures for improved teleradiology collaboration

1) Make someone responsible and distribute tasks	To make someone responsible for teleradiology is important. Not at least when teleradiology of a greater volume is planned.
2) Knowing each other	Teleradiology means co-operation between individuals from different organizations. Knowing one another plays a positive role for the co-operation. Face-to-face meetings should be organized.
3) Problems of attitude	Co-operation problems are not just software and hardware problems, but also 'humanware' problems. Personality plays a role. Better co-operation when the involved are motivated and interested. Use persons with positive attitudes or motivate personnel for teleradiology.
4) Support from management	Support and involvement from management necessary for teleradiology. Departments with an active and interested leader are more positively evaluated by co-operating departments. Higher management levels should develop departmental managers into champions for teleradiology.
5) Organizational merger	Teleradiology in-between organizationally merged departments works better. Evaluate merger as a tool for problem reduction.
6) Organize time for teleradiology at the radiology departments	Teleradiology can compete with ordinary work tasks for the personnel's time. Pressure to participate in ordinary work can be great. Managers must inform all personnel that teleradiology is an equally legitimate work task. Organize the departments resources both for ordinary work and teleradiology.
7) Distribution of production capacity in-between radiology departments	Teleradiology of a larger volume may lead to significant change in the distribution of workload between co-operating departments. Regional health authorities may have to reconsider distribution of production capacity in-between radiology departments.
8) Experience with teleradiology	Experience plays a positive role. Better co-operation with larger volumes teleradiology. Health authorities can promote larger volumes by deciding criteria for teleradiology, which results in and maintains larger volumes.
9) Good referrals (requests) and good interpretations	Good referrals especially important for teleradiology. They make it easier for the radiologist to get a good idea about patient problem. Competence in referrals can be developed and electronic referrals with standardized contents can be used. Good quality interpretations play a positive role for the co-operation. Interpretations can be written on an electronic form with standardised contents.
10) Quick replies to clinicians	Easier to co-operate when requesting clinician receives the interpretation quickly. Routines should be established securing that clinicians receive interpretations quickly.
11) Improved schooling of radiographers	Competence is necessary when problems with the technology, for assistance with daily use, and teaching of new personnel. Radiographers can be educated into «superusers» taking care of such tasks.
12) Thorough learning of procedures	The involved should be familiar with procedures used. Personnel can be «drilled» in procedures for sending and receiving images.
13) Standardisation of procedures and nomenclature	When radiologists perform interpretations it is important to know how the images were obtained. Radiology departments can communicate and agree to use the same radiology procedures. One and the same procedure must have the same name at co-operating departments. Departments can use standardised nomenclature developed at national level, or communicate to obtain standardised nomenclature.
14) Economic and ethical motivations for teleradiology	Economic incentives can be used to promote teleradiology. Costs should be covered for participating organizations. Teleradiology can improve quality, and it becomes ethically indefensible not to use it. When departments discuss teleradiology co-operation the ethical motivation should be a part of the discussion.
15) Connect all the departments' workstations	It should be possible to transmit images to and from all workstations. All radiology work stations should be integrated in the departments', the hospitals' and the health region's network
16) Knowledge of technology and IT-personnel	Teleradiology co-operation works better when partners have access to good technology knowledge. Hospital IT-personnel should learn about the new technology, have an introduction to how a radiology department works, its needs, relationship to the rest of the hospital, and other parts of the health service. Larger radiology departments can consider employment of IT-personnel at own department.
17) Technology and co operation	Technical problems with communication make teleradiology co-operation difficult. Co-operating departments can have the same technology (hardware and software), require from vendors that technology they buy can communicate, and a region can have a common computer store.

Table 3. Overview of 10 measures for improved collaboration in telemedicine remote consultations

1) Experience with remote consultations	Better co-operation with participants who are experienced. Management can promote larger volumes of remote consultations, use the same set of persons for telemedicine, and use participants with several years of working experience from their discipline. It is also easier to co-operate with persons who are relaxed in front of a camera
2) Meeting at the same time	Telemedicine remote consultations is synchronous work. Employees of different organizations may have highly different schedules and find it difficult to involve on short notice in a simultaneous co-operation. The solution can be long term planning by making half-year schedules for when sessions with remote consultations should take place.
3) Knowing each other	Knowing one another can play a positive role for the co-operation. Face-to-face meetings between participants can be organized. Having met each other personally is not decisive, but the co-operation can become easier.
4) Different personalities	Personality plays a role for the co-operation. Important that participants are reliable, effective, and interested. Use persons with positive attitudes or motivate personnel for remote consultations.
5) Chairman for sessions with several participants	When several speak at the same time what is heard on the other side of the network becomes quite messy. A chairman should be appointed for such sessions. Those who want to speak can be added to a list of speakers, when it is a person's turn the microphone can be passed over, and the camera can be focused on the one speaking.
6) Good preparations	Preparations play a positive role. Easier to co-operate with those who are well prepared and well structured. When necessary participants should prepare for sessions.
7) Make participants responsible and distribute tasks	Easier to co-operate with those who are responsible formally and in reality. With many involved in a session important to decide who should do what. Tasks should be distributed with a following responsibility.
8) Education and level of education	Participants should be educated for the telemedicine work, for example laboratory technicians should be educated for their work with telepathology frozen sections. Level of general education plays a role, for example psychiatrists can prefer patients to be followed to the studio by a general practitioner rather than a nurse.
9) Better co-operation with those who need help	Easier to co-operate with persons who need help. Need for help can be a criteria for connecting personnel to a network.
10) Interest for technology becomes a distraction	Occupation with technology during a session can disturb. Participants should be advised to focus on the patient/ subject during sessions, and not with the technology.

nize face-to- face meetings (knowing each other plays a positive role), and telemedicine should be organized so participants get more experience with telemedicine (the collaboration works better when the volume is larger). Four collaboration measures in teleradiology have some similarity to two collaboration measures in telemedicine remote consultation (the measure called problems of attitude in teleradiology has some similarity to the measure called different personalities in remote consultations, the teleradiology measures improved schooling of radiographers, thorough learning of procedures, and knowledge of technology and IT-personnel have some similarity to the remote consultation measure education and level of education). The teleradiology measure 'connect all the department's workstations' has some similarity to what has been found previously for remote consultations (Aas, 2002), i.e. easily available equipment plays a role for the volume of remote consultations.

Generally, close to half of the collaboration measures for teleradiology and remote consultations are either similar or have some similarity. Performing work by telecommunications can create some similarity in needed collaboration measures. The differences in collaboration measures can be due to differences in the nature of the services (radiology and clinical medical consultations represent different work processes) and their synchronous and asynchronous nature.

Learning in Telemedicine Dependent on Collaboration Measures

Obtaining benefits from telemedicine is dependent on a well functioning collaboration. Learning is a leading benefit of telemedicine. Obtaining the learning benefit from telemedicine is dependent on implementing collaboration measures. Few other studies (than those cited here) deal with collaboration in telemedicine, but in rehabilitation the finding of efficient videoconferences was explained by factors such as clear roles for all participants, active involvement of all and presence of clear leader (Careau et al. 2008). These factors have a similarity to the measures in tables two and three.

WHAT ORGANIZATIONS CAN DO

Why should organizations in health care collaborate? The explanation can be found in very basic health care issues: quality, needs, and costs. Likewise, telemedicine collaboration is motivated by the benefits, both for patients and organizations. So far, learning has been given limited attention in the telemedicine community. Not at least the potential significance of learning taken into consideration.

Involvement in Change Process

When telemedicine is planned, the entire organization should be receptive to change (Jennet et al. 2003), but changing organizations is not just easy. Involvement of management is required. Telemedicine often means inter-organizational collaboration and inter-organizational collaboration always requires management involvement (even involvement of top management). For implementation of telemedicine, management at different levels should be involved and key stakeholders from both clinical and administration spheres should be coordinated (Fortin et al. 2002). Cooperation between organizations may be more easily obtained at operational level. At strategic level, cooperation is more problematic (Gils, 1984). Such problems could be related to fear of loss of power and control. Telemedicine can be of importance for policy issues and, when so, policymakers should be involved. Responsibility for telemedicine can be allocated to a telemedicine working group, procedures and guidelines for use can be published in a form available for all. Such working groups can be cross-professional. In cross-professional groups, we find different professions' knowledge and knowledge of their different working methods. Cross-professional working groups can more easily find solutions working for all to be involved in telemedicine.

Selection of Telemedicine Participants

For participation in telemedicine networks, it can be necessary to perform a conscious selection of individuals and organizational partners. Participants must be motivated for telemedicine and the job to be done. This applies both at team level and for organizations to be included. It can be wise to limit the number of partners from each organization to reduce the complexity of the communication process (it can be more difficult to agree with many than few) and to obtain a situation of control for monitoring. Profiling practitioners according to personality to obtain best teams may be of help (Brown et al., 2002), but then the question comes up of which personalality traits are advantageous for participation in telemedicine? Selection of organizational partners can be done on the basis of complementarity of resources, alignment of their objectives, similarity in values and culture, and relative strength and size (Schilling, 2005). Organizational self-interest is an obvious motivator for network participation (Gregg & Moscovice, 2003). For individual organizations considering joining a network some questions are central: 1) What can the organization achieve by joining the network? 2) By joining the network all wishes cannot be fulfilled, but which compromises with the other organizations are acceptable? 3) Are other solutions, than joining a network, better to achieve goals?

Strategy for Change

Little telemedicine means a mismatch between actual activity and level of activity that can bring greater gains. When organizations want to obtain the learning benefits of telemedicine, a job must be done concerning collaboration. A strategy for the change process should be developed. It is recommended that managers lead change processes in their organizations to fully realize the telemedicine learning potential. Measures for improved collaboration should be put in place. If organizations starting with telemedicine struggle to make it work, the answer can be to take advantage of the experiences of others. The present chapter makes it possible not needing to start from scratch. The most obvious collaboration measures for consideration are the 17 described for teleradiology and the 10 for telemedicine remote consultations. The organizations should then find out which telemedicine applications are best to cover own needs, including learning needs. With the positive aspects of learning in mind, it could be possible to persuade organizations to transform own learning strategy into a more technology based learning strategy. The organizations may then ask the question of what the next step is. Adapting organizations in the direction of learning organizations and including the right organizations in telemedicine networks are the next steps.

FUTURE RESEARCH DIRECTIONS

Implementing telemedicine obviously has organizational and management aspects, but even in the international telemedicine research community people with such competence have been little involved. The diffusion problems may, in part, be due to this. Competence is required to do research in organizational aspects of telemedicine, to understand research already done and to transform research based knowledge into change strategy for own organization. More communication concerning organizational problems for telemedicine could develop improved understanding.

(a) Little research has been done on learning in telemedicine (with associated aspects: team organization, learning organizations, network organization), but future research should have more focus on this.
(b) For the future of telemedicine, it is considered important that research includes investigations on collaboration for other telemedicine applications than the two described here. A knowledge pool could be developed with information about which collaboration measures different applications require. The results for collaboration in the present chapter are based on empirical research. It is thinkable that other research methods will produce other results than those of the present chapter.

CONCLUSION

Telemedicine's greatest problem is not to make the technology work. Many can make software and hardware work. More focus should be given to the humanware. It is organizations and humans in organizations who will decide the future of telemedicine. Organizations consist of humans in interaction and around electronic networks organizations and humans must interact.

Telecommunications have potential to play a more significant role for learning in health care by taking the advantage of: a) increased volume of telemedicine collaboration, b) teamwork thinking, c) the concept of learning organizations, and d) aspects of network organization. The present chapter shows that such thinking may well be important for the future of telemedicine and health care organizations. Grid technology's lack of centralized control and use of open, general-purpose protocols and interfaces may be advantageous. Not at least so when a top-down process cannot be expected. The development may occur in a decentralized way.

Organizations planning larger volumes of telemedicine have a job to do, but none of the problems with collaboration seem large enough to prevent effective collaboration. Communication technology does not represent an insurmountable barrier for good collaboration. Implementing collaboration measures of the kind described here may well be crucial to obtain a higher volume of telemedicine. With the slow diffusion of telemedicine in mind, new thinking is necessary. In health care, learning is a word with positive associations. Promotion of eLearning could be wise. The next steps are considering teamwork, learning organizations and network organization.

REFERENCES

Aas, I. H. M. (1997). Organizational change: decentralization in hospitals. *The International Journal of Health Planning and Management*, *12*, 103–114. doi:10.1002/(SICI)1099-1751(199704)12:2<103::AID-HPM461>3.0.CO;2-5

Aas, I. H. M. (2001). Telemedical work and cooperation. *Journal of Telemedicine and Telecare*, *7*, 212–218. doi:10.1258/1357633011936426

Aas, I. H. M. (2002). Learning in organizations working with telemedicine. *Journal of Telemedicine and Telecare*, *8*, 107–111. doi:10.1258/1357633021937569

Aas, I. H. M. (2005). Organizational cooperation in teleradiology. *Journal of Telemedicine and Telecare*, *11*, 45–50. doi:10.1258/1357633053430449

Aas, I. H. M. (2006a). Organizational centralization in radiology. *Journal of Telemedicine and Telecare*, *12*, 27–32. doi:10.1258/135763306775321344

Aas, I. H. M. (2006b). Organizational decentralization in radiology. *Journal of Telemedicine and Telecare*, *12*(Suppl. 1), 1–3. doi:10.1258/135763306777978524

Aas, I. H. M. (2007). The organizational challenge for health care from telemedicine and e-health. Oslo, The Work Research Institute. Retrieved November 20, 2008, from http://www.afi.no/stream_file.asp?iEntityId=2088

Abrahamian, H., Schueller, A., Mauler, H., Prager, R., & Irsigler, K. (2002). Transfer of knowledge from the specialist to the generalist by videoconferencing: effect on diabetes care. *Journal of Telemedicine and Telecare*, *8*, 350–355. doi:10.1258/135763302320939248

Anderson, R. J., & Boumbulian, P. J. (1997). Beyond the safety net in Dallas. *Health Affairs*, *16*, 27–29. doi:10.1377/hlthaff.16.4.27

Axelsson, R., & Axelsson, S. B. (2006). Integration and collaboration in public health - a conceptual framework. *The International Journal of Health Planning and Management*, *21*, 75–88. doi:10.1002/hpm.826

Bee, P. E., Bower, P., Lovell, K., Gilbody, S., Richards, D., Gask, L., & Roach, P. (2008). Psychotherapy mediated by remote communication technologies: a meta-analytic review. *BMC Psychiatry*, *8*, 60. doi:10.1186/1471-244X-8-60

Biggs, S. (1997). Interprofessional collaboration: Problems and prospects. In Ovretveit, J., Mathias, P., & Thomson, T. (Eds.), *Interprofessional working for health and social care* (pp. 186–200). Houndsmills, UK: MacMillan Press Ltd.

Binder, B., Hofman-Wellenhof, R., & Salmhofer, W. (1511-1514). Okcu, A., Kerl, H. & Soyer, H.P. (2007). Teledermatological monitoring of leg ulcers in cooperation with home care nurses. *Archives of Dermatology*, 143.

Blum, A., Hofman-Wellenhof, R., Luedtke, H., Ellwanger, U., Steins, A., & Roehm, S. (2004). Value of the clinical history for different users of dermoscopy compared with results of digital image analysis. *European Academy of Dermatology and Venerology*, *18*, 665–669. doi:10.1111/j.1468-3083.2004.01044.x

Brown, H. G., Poole, M. S., & Walsum, K. V. (2002). Trust, trait theory, and collaboration in telemedicine: a circumplex perspective. In *Proc 36th Hawaii International Conference on System Sciences (HICSS'03)*. Washington DC: IEEE Computer Society.

Burduli, A., Sheklashvili, G., & Kldiashvili, E. (2008). The application of medical databases for elearning. *Ukr Z Telemed Med Telemat*, *6*, 275–277.

Buunk, B. P. Jonge. de J., Ybema, J.F, & Wolff, de C.J. (1998). Psychosocial aspects of occupational stress. In P. J. D. Drenth, H. Thierry, & C.J. de Wolff (eds.), *Handbook of work and organizational psychology. Volume 2: Work Psychology*, (2nd ed., pp. 145-182). East Sussex, UK: Psychology Press Ltd.

Buxton, P. J. (1999). Teleradiology – practical aspects and lessons learnt. *European Journal of Radiology*, *32*, 116–118. doi:10.1016/S0720-048X(99)00136-9

Careau, E., Vincent, C., & Noreau, L. (2008). Assessing interprofessional teamwork in a videoconference-based telerehabilitation setting. *Journal of Telemedicine and Telecare*, *14*, 427–434. doi:10.1258/jtt.2008.080415

Cascio, W. F. (1999). Virtual workplaces: Implications for organizational behaviour. In C.L. Cooper & D.M. Rousseau (eds.), *Trends in organizational behaviour. Volume 6. The virtual organization*. (pp. 1-14). Chichester, UK: John Wiley & Sons Ltd.

Chanlat, J.-F. (1997). Conflict and politics. In Sorge, A., & Warner, M. (Eds.), *The IEBM Handbook of Organizational Behaviour* (pp. 472–480). London: International Thomson Business Press.

Chen, F., Romano, N. C., Nunamaker, J. F., & Briggs, R. O. (2002). A collaborative project management architecture. In *Proc 36th Hawaii International Conference on System Sciences (HICSS'04)*. Washington, DC: IEEE Computer Society.

Chisholm, R. F. (Ed.). (1998). *Developing network organizations: Learning from practice and theory*. Reading, MA: Addison-Wesley.

Cohen, S. G., & Mankin, D. (1999). Collaboration in the virtual organization. In C.L. Cooper & D.M. Rousseau (Eds.), *Trends in organizational behaviour. Volume 6. The virtual organization* (pp. 105-120). Chichester, UK: John Wiley & Sons Ltd.

Cuevas, de C., Arredondo, T., Cabrera M.F., Sulzenbacher, H. & Meise, U. (2006). Randomized clinical trial of telepsychiatry through videoconference versus face-to-face conventional psychiatric treatment. *Telemedicine and e-Health*, *12*, 341-350.

Detmer, D. E. (2000). Information technology for quality health care: a summary of United Kingdom and United States experiences. *Quality in Health Care*, *9*, 181–189. doi:10.1136/qhc.9.3.181

Dhar, V., & Olson, M. H. (1989). Assumptions underlying systems that support work group collaboration. In Olson, M. H. (Ed.), *Technological support for work group collaboration* (pp. 33–50). Hillsdale, NJ: Lawrence Erlbaum Associates Publishers.

Ekeland, A. G. (1999). Teleradiologi - virkemiddel for solidarisk helsepolitikk? *Tidsskrift for Den Norske Laegeforening*, *119*, 4345–4347.

English, T. (1997). Personal paper: medicine in the 1990s needs a team approach. *British Medical Journal*, *314*, 661.

Finch, T., May, C., Mair, F., Mort, M., & Gask, L. (2003). Integrating service development with evaluation in telehealthcare: an ethnographic study. *British Medical Journal*, *327*, 1205–1209. doi:10.1136/bmj.327.7425.1205

Fortin, J.-P., Gagnon, M.-P., Cloutier, A., & Labbé, F. (2002). Evaluation of a telemedicine demonstration project in the Magdalene Islands. *Journal of Telemedicine and Telecare*, *9*, 89–94. doi:10.1258/1357633033321327948

Foster, I. (2002). *What is the grid? A three point checklist. Argonne National Library & University of Chicago*. Retrieved November 10, 2008, from http://www-fp.mcs.anl.gov/~foster/Articles/WhatIsTheGrid.pdf

Gerrard, L., Grant, A. M., & Maclean, J. R. (1999). Factors that may influence the implementation of nurse-centred telemedicine services. *Journal of Telemedicine and Telecare*, *5*, 231–236. doi:10.1258/1357633991933765

Gils, van M.R. (1984). Interorganizational relations and networks. In P.J.D. Drenth, H. Thierry, P.J. Willems & C.J. de Wolff de (Eds.), *Handbook of work and organizational psychology*, (Vol. 2, pp. 1073-1100). Chichester, UK: John Wiley & Sons Ltd.

Goodfellow, T., Bali, R. G., Wickramasinghe, N., & Naguib, R. N. G. (2008). From data to decisions: introducing knowledge management to effect superior operations in a radiology department. *Int J Biomedical Engineering and Technology*, *1*, 259–272. doi:10.1504/IJBET.2008.016960

Gortiz, L.G., Karnabatidis, D., Siabatidis, D. & Nikifordis, G. (2006). Clinical-oriented collaboration over the Web during interventional radiology procedures. *Telemedicine and e-Health*, *12*, 448-456.

Greenhalgh, T., Glenn, R., Bate, P., Macfarlane, F., & Kyriakidou, O. (2004). Diffusion of innovations in service organisations: systematic review and recommendations. *The Milbank Quarterly*, *82*, 581–629. doi:10.1111/j.0887-378X.2004.00325.x

Gregg, W., & Moscovice, I. (2003). The evolution of rural health networks: implications for health care managers. *Health Care Management Review*, *28*, 161–178.

Grimshaw, D., Willmott, H., & Rubery, J. (2005). Inter-organizational networks: Trust, power, and the employment relationship. In Marchington, M., Grimshaw, D., & Rubery, J. (Eds.), *Fragmenting work: blurring organizational boundaries and disordering hierarchies* (pp. 34–61). Oxford, UK: Oxford University Press.

Hagedoorn, J., & Duysters, J. (2002). Learning in dynamic inter-firm networks: The efficacy of multiple contacts. *Organization Studies*, *23*, 525–548. doi:10.1177/0170840602234002

Harrison, R., Clayton, W., & Wallace, P. (1996). Can telemedicine be used to improve communication between primary and secondary care? *British Medical Journal*, *313*, 1377–1380.

Haythorntwaite, C. *(2005). Knowledge flow in interdisciplinary teams. In* Proc 38th Hawaii International Conference on System Sciences (HICSS'05). *Washington DC: IEEE Computer Society.*

Hebert, M.A., Jansen, j.J., Brant, R., & Hailey, D. & Pol, van M. (2004). Successes and challenges in a filed-based, multi-method study of home telehealth. *Journal of Telemedicine and Telecare*, *10*(suppl. 1), 41–44. doi:10.1258/1357633042614348

Hertog, den F., & Tolner, T. (1997). Groups and teams. In A. Sorge & M. Warner M (Eds.), *The IEBM Handbook of organizational behaviour*, (pp. 492-501). London: International Thomson Business Press.

Hjelm, N. M., Wootton, R., & Staines, D. (2003). Social capital, gold for telemedicine? *World Hospitals and Health Services*, *39*(3), 11–12, 42, 44.

Jennet, P., Yeo, M., Pauls, M., & Graham, J. (2003). Organizational readiness for telemedicine: implications for success and failure. *Journal of Telemedicine and Telecare*, *9*(suppl 2), 27–30. doi:10.1258/135763303322596183

Lindberg, I., Öhrling, K., & Christenson, K. (2007). Midwives' experience of using videoconferencing to support parents who were discharged early after childbirth. *Journal of Telemedicine and Telecare*, *13*, 202–205. doi:10.1258/135763307780908102

Mars, M., & Dlova, N. (2008). Teledermatology by videoconference: experience of a pilot project. *South African Family Practice*, *50*, 70–70d.

May, C., Harrison, R., Finch, T., MacFarlane, A., Mair, F., & Wallace, P. (2003). Understanding the normalization of telemedicine services through qualitative evaluation. *Journal of the American Medical Informatics Association*, *10*, 596–604. doi:10.1197/jamia.M1145

Modal, I., Jabarin, M., Kurs, R., Barak, P., Hanan, I. & Kitain, L. (2006). Cost effectiveness, safety, and satisfaction with video telepsychiatry versus face-to-face care in ambulatory settings. *Telemedicine and e-Health, 12*, 515-520.

Mohrman, S. A., Cohen, S. G., & Mohrman, A. M. (Eds.). (1995). *Designing team-based organizations: New forms for knowledge work.* San Francisco: Jossey-Bass Publishers.

Monnier, J., Knapp, R. G., & Frueh, B. C. (2003). Recent advances in telepscyhiatry: An updated review. *Psychiatric Services (Washington, D.C.)*, *54*, 1604–1609. doi:10.1176/appi.ps.54.12.1604

Myers, K. M., Valentine, J. M., & Melzer, S. M. (2007). Feasibility, acceptability, and sustainability of telepsychiatry for children and adolescents. *Psychatric Services*, *58*, 1493–1496. doi:10.1176/appi.ps.58.11.1493

Nikula, R. E. (1999). Organisational learning within health care organisations. *International Journal of Medical Informatics*, *56*, 61–66. doi:10.1016/S1386-5056(99)00039-8

Nilsen, L. L., & Moen, A. (2008). Teleconsultation – a collaborative work and opportunities for learning across organizational boundaries. *Journal of Telemedicine and Telecare*, *14*, 377–380. doi:10.1258/jtt.2008.007012

Nordhaug, O. (Ed.). (1993). *Human capital in organizations. Competence, training, and learning*. Oslo, Norway: Scandinavian University Press.

O'Reilly, R., Bishop, J., Maddox, K., Hutchinson, L., Fisman, M., & Takhar, J. (2007). Is telepsychiatry equivalent to face-to-face psychiatry? Results from a randomized controlled equivalence trial. *Psychatric Services*, *58*, 836–843. doi:10.1176/appi.ps.58.6.836

Ogasawara, K., Endoch, A., & Sakurai, T. (2001). What do radiographers think about teleradiology in Japan. *Journal of Telemedicine and Telecare*, *7*, 161–166. doi:10.1258/1357633011936327

Ovretveit, J. (Ed.). (1993). *Coordinating community care. Multidisciplinary teams and care management.* Buckingham, UK: Open University Press.

Ovretveit, J. (1996). Five ways to describe a multidisciplinary team. *Journal of Interprofessional Care*, *10*, 163–171. doi:10.3109/13561829609034099

Ovretveit, J. (1997). Planning and managing interprofessional working and teams. In Ovretveit, J., Mathias, P., & Thomson, T. (Eds.), *Interprofessional working for health and social care* (pp. 34–52). London: Macmillan Press Ltd.

Paul, D. L. (2005). Collaborative activities in virtual settings: Case studies of telemedicine. In *Proc 38th Hawaii International Conference on System Sciences (HICSS'04)*. Washington, DC: IEEE Computer Society.

Plaszczak, P., & Wellner, R. (Eds.). (2006). *Grid computing: The savvy manager's guide*. San Francisco: Morgan Kaufman Publishers.

Powell, W. W. (1990). Neither market nor hierarchy: network forms of organization. *Research in Organizational Behavior, 12*, 295–336.

Puskeppeleit, M. (2008). Improving telemedicine onboard Norwegian ships and drilling platforms – A study of intersectorial co-operation in maritime medicine. [Göteborg: Nordic School of Public Health.]. *MPH, 2008*, 13.

Rice, R. E., Grant, A. E., Schmitz, J., & Torobin, J. (1990). Individual and network influences on the adoption and perceived outcomes of electronic messaging. *Social Networks, 12*, 27–55. doi:10.1016/0378-8733(90)90021-Z

Rogers, E. M. *(2003).* Diffusion of innovations, (5th, Ed.). *New York: Free Press.*

Sandkuhl, K., & Fuchs-Kittowski, F. (1999). Telecooperation in decentralized organizations: conclusions based on empirical research. *Behaviour & Information Technology, 18*, 339–347. doi:10.1080/014492999118922

Schilling, M. A. (2005). *Strategic management of technological innovation*. New York: McGraw-Hill Irwin.

Schrader, T., & Kldiashvili, E. (2008). Virtual health care center in Georgia. *Diagnostic Pathology, 3*(suppl 1), S4. .doi:10.1186/1746-1596-3-S1-S4

Senge, P. M., Kleiner, A., Roberts, C., Ross, R. B., & Smith, B. J. (Eds.). (1994). *The fifth discipline fieldbook. Strategies and tools for building a learning organization*. New York: Doubleday.

Shannon, G., Nesbitt, T., Bakalar, R., Kratochwill, E., Kvedar, J., & Vargas, L. (2002). Organizational models of telemedicine and regional telemedicine networks. *Telemedicine Journal and e-Health, 8*, 61–70. doi:10.1089/15305620252933400

Shershneva, M., & Olson, C. A. (2005). Education through telemedicine networks: setting quality standards. *Journal of Telemedicine and Telecare, 11*, 127–134. doi:10.1258/1357633053688732

Shulman, A. D. (1996). Putting group information technology in its place: Communication and good work group performance. In Clegg, S. R., Hardy, C., & Nord, W. R. (Eds.), *Handbook of Organization studies* (pp. 357–374). London: Sage Publications.

Sjøvold, E. (Ed.). (2006). *Teamet. Utvikling, effektivitet og endring i grupper* [The team. Development, efficiency and change in groups]. Oslo, Norway: Universitetsforlaget.

Snow, C. C., Lipnack, J., & Stamps, J. (1999). The virtual organization: Promises and payoffs, large and small. In C.L. Cooper, D.M. Rousseau, (Eds.), *Trends in organizational behaviour, Volume 6, The virtual organization* (pp. 15-30). Chichester, UK: John Wiley & Sons Ltd.

Stead, W. W. (1998). The networked health enterprise: A vision for 2008. *Journal of the American Medical Informatics Association, 5*, 412–415.

Voss, H. (2009). *Telepsykiatri i Danmark – hvad ved vi fra udlandet? Udenlandske erfaringer med anvendelse af videokonference i psykiatrien. DSI projekt nr. 2654*. København, Denmark: Dansk Sundhedsinstitut.

Vuonovirta, T., Timonen, M., Keinänen-Kiukaaniemi, S., Timonen, O., Ylitalo, K., Kantse, O., & Tanila, A. (2009). The attitudes of multiprofessional teams to telehealth adoption in northern Finland health centres. *Journal of Telemedicine and Telecare, 15*, 290–296. doi:10.1258/jtt.2009.090108

Wagner, E. H. (2000). The role of patient care teams in chronic disease management. *British Medical Journal*, *320*, 569–572. doi:10.1136/bmj.320.7234.569

Walther, J. B., Bunz, U., & Bazarova, N. N. *(2005). The rules of virtual groups. In* Proc 38th Hawaii International Conference on System Sciences (HICSS'04). *Washington, DC: IEEE Computer Society.*

Weinstein, R. S., Dunn, B. E., & Graham, A. R. (1997). Telepathology networks as models of telemedical services by cybercorps. *Nature Medicine*, *1*, 235–241.

Welch, G., Sonnenwald, D. H., Fichs, H., Cairns, B., Mayer-Patel, K., & Söderholm, H. M. (2009). 3D medical collaboration technology to enhance emergency healthcare. *Journal of Biomedical Discovery and Collaboration*, *4*(4).

Welsh, T., & Pringle, M. (2001). Social capital. *British Medical Journal*, *323*, 177–178. doi:10.1136/bmj.323.7306.177

Werner, P. (2004). Willingness to use telemedicine for psychiatric care. *Telemedicine and e-Health, 10*, 286-293.

Whitten, P., & Kuwahara, E. (2004). A multi-phase telepsychiatry programme in Michigan: organizational factors affecting utilization and user perceptions. *Journal of Telemedicine and Telecare, 10*, 254–261. doi:10.1258/1357633042026378

Chapter 3
Health and Health Care Grid Services and Delivery Integrating eHealth and Telemedicine

Thomas Clark
Global Telemed Limited, UK

ABSTRACT

Health Grids offer new solutions and alternatives to existing models for the delivery of Healthcare Services to diverse Populations across dissimilar Geographical and Political Regions. Incorporating new medical science, legal systems, systems and networks, financing, technologies, processes, procedures, business and government participation, competitive, cost-effective integration with existing, experimental and competing delivery models is a basic requirement. Integration is likely to be performed locally and may be required to avoid the disruption of existing models, e.g., Patient, Practitioner and Payer choice. This chapter addresses a selection of issues that have been encountered in other high-technology integrations. Less-complex and more limited-in-scope than Health Grids they indicate a need for adaptability and multiple solutions. Choice and options will be important. The ability for Users to personalize, and re-structure as needed or desired, a Health Grid will be paramount.

OVERVIEW

Many historical Health-related writings have failed to resolve the Mind-Body dualism in Western Cultures (The Mind and the Body are the Same Thing, 2010); Eastern Cultures have not adopted this Dualism and hence consider the Mind and Body as one. Immediately there is conflict since there is a strong, provable interaction between Mental and Medical Health.

This Chapter addresses Personal Health and the application of Grids to deliver Services. eHealth and Telemedicine Services are emphasized. To begin it must be stated that the networking of Healthcare Services has existed for many years, long before the Internet, and retains traditional forms at this time, e.g., rural areas in many Countries.

DOI: 10.4018/978-1-61692-010-4.ch003

Modern Western evolutions have resulted in centralized and specialized Services, e.g., the City Hospitals. Future evolutions are expected to come in the form of additional and increased specializations within the established Healthcare Services Infrastructure.

The Internet is available in most modern Cities and their complement of modern City Hospitals. The underlying Infrastructures having been developed and deployed over many years. Access available to all and to Healthcare-related Services remains major issues.

Whether existing Infrastructures constitute 'good candidates' for Grid applications must at least be determined locally since local Infrastructures have development and deployment histories. For example, local infrastructures are mostly developed and deployed in response to local demands and resources; hence current state, capacity, performance and scalability may even be unique; a locality servicing an economy based upon agriculture is likely to be radically different than one based upon finance.

Rural areas generally are not 'good candidates' since infrastructure are missing or incapable of sufficient and sustained capacity, performance and scalability.

If a Health-related Grid is to be successful the Market must be shrunk to modern Cities and their complement of modern City Hospitals. Starting from this point one must estimate the actual Market for Health-related Grid Services.

Many modern City Hospitals currently support Internet access to internal Organizations, Services and Personal Records. There must be advantages and additional Services that would cause the typical Patient to consider Grid Services. Immediately the concern arises as to Grid Services becoming a replacement for, an extension of, a source of additional, beneficial Health Services, or some combination thereof.

An underlying, pervasive requirement is the satisfaction of significant, healthcare-oriented, personal goals and objective for all Patients. A proposed Healthcare Grid must be both cost-effective relative to Services provided and competitive relative to currently-available Services.

The current organization of Healthcare Services is based upon Community-resident General Practitioners and Primary Care adjuncts, with specialized equipment, facilities and Specialists located in the modern City Hospitals and Clinics. In short, Primary Care in the Neighborhoods; Specialist Care in the Hospitals and Clinics.

The concern for years has been funding increased specialization in the modern City Hospitals and Clinics. Primary Care in the City Neighborhoods and Rural Health Care have advanced little in some developed Countries; others have and enviable record of achievements; under-developed Countries remain mostly lacking.

The obvious questions that jump to the foreground are:

Even if one Engineers a Health-related Grid, What will it cost? Who will buy it ? and to What applications can it be applied?

Before proceeding one must briefly consider competitive and complementary technologies. As mentioned earlier, cost-effective, competitive Healthcare Grid-based Services would be requirements. Consider the modern Patient in a modern City. Why and How would they choose to associate with a Healthcare Grid?

The modern Resident of a modern City is mobile and connected and expected to evolve further in the future. Major opportunities for associated Healthcare Services exist. At the same time modern Residents expect greater access to advanced medical devices that are mobile, non-invasive, and present in the environment, e.g., Patient Monitoring.

Portable Medical Devices have been available for many years. Size has been reduced and functionality increased. They are now Personal, Portable Medical Devices and the resultant data is available to the Patient and the Practitioner. Embedded Medical Systems and Networks represent another significant market for Healthcare Services.

Data created and controlled by Health Care Providers is regulated, sequestered and isolated, unavailable to Patients unless the Jurisdiction has Legislation granting Patient access. Personal Medical Devices are regulated for accuracy, precision, quality and safety. When privately owned the data generated is privately owned.

Where is Health Care Grid Services to be Applied?

Developers are actively supported by multiple Vendors of embedded Systems and Networks many of which support their products with common Operating Systems, Networks and Applications. From there the Developer is responsible for Application Development. There is little 'Cookbook' or 'How-To' documentation; development experience is helpful.

Synopsis

Health, Health Care Services, the deployment of these Services, their associated quality and effectiveness, and the acceptance and support of the Beneficiaries are subject to change; minor/major, noticeable/silent, acceptable/objectionable, positive/negative, legal/questionable. The root causes of changes may be less important than the potential for future changes.

The need to write this Chapter arose because of demands to integrate the popularization of Computing Grids formerly and almost exclusively a tool of High Energy and Particle Physics Researchers.

First exposure to these branches of Physics occurred at Argonne National Laboratory, North Chicago, Illinois in connection with data reduction processing on a 13.5 BEV Proton Synchrotron, typically using the George Machine. The need to 'connect' remote Physicists and their work was obvious and essential. Computing Grids have become highly successful.

This spawned efforts to replicate Computing Grids within non-Physics Communities for applications that could benefit from Resource-Sharing Computing (RSC). Some notable successes have been achieved. RSC, however, requires availability, co-operation and commitment in advance.

Significant Goals and Objectives involved are typically not personal, e.g., remote strangers are unlikely to share resources. Furthermore, it is unlikely that remote strangers would be willing to share resources to support personal Electronic Health Records (EHRs). This may change in the presence of a commercial benefit.

Beside a very large gap in the Goals and Objectives, constraints, limitations and requirements may intervene to prohibit use of RSC in the handling of personal EHRs or other Health, Health Care and personal data and information. The Health Care Industry, for example, is typically highly regulated.

As a regulated Industry it is subject to a Legislature, Administration, Judiciary and Regulatory Enforcement Body. Going forward a main issue is: The integration of relevant Grid-based technology within the Health Care Industry? Significant changes to RSC are expected.

The concept of a Grid within the Health Care Industry is similar to the architecture of existing Clustered Systems and distributed Services. Before proceeding it is helpful to recall that the Health Care Industry is replete with software systems and applications, proprietary and open-source, that are in wide use with committed User Communities.

Embarking upon a Grid-based new product development should be proceeded by a Market Analysis directed at identifying the Services and applications that must be modified or replaced.

This should be followed by a Market Analysis of the various Participants, i.e., Patients, Practitioners, Providers, Public Health and Epidemiology, and Government Agencies. Patients are the Consumers, all others are Suppliers and Regulators.

The Health Care Industry is in a migration within the models for Health Care Delivery, the three majors model currently being: (1)Traditional, (2)Patient-Centric, aka Outcome-Determinative, and (3)Personalized Medicine. Together they indicate a major shift in demand for increased and sophisticated data and information Services from Practitioners, Providers, Payers and Patients.

Future demand from Patients is expected to be very substantial since Patient-Centric and Personalized Medicine require the Patient to assume greater responsibility for the Management and Control of their Health and Health Care Services. This future demand is likely to drive the development of various Grids for Health and Health Care Services.

Related development issues are:

- Integrated Health and Health Care Services
- the modification of existing infrastructures, organizations and Facilities
- training and re-direction of Practitioners and Providers
- new mechanisms, processes, procedures and sources of funding
- evolutions within the Legislative, Administrative, Judicial and Regulatory Government Bodies and Agencies
- real performance, scalability and cost improvements
- global co-operation, research, development and participation in Health, Health Care, the practice of Medicine and the tools of the trade, e.g., pharmaceuticals
- recognition of an Individual's right to adequate and competent Health care
- provisioning of Health, Health Care, Mental and Medical Services based upon a Patient's need for such Services
- equal treatment of all medicinal systems to the extent that they are beneficial, productive, cost-effective for the individual Patient
- transparency.

Caveat: There are other issues to be considered that are Jurisdiction-related. Consult records for a prior successful project to capture the relevant data and information.

Presumptions

The following presumptions apply:

- The Reader has an understanding and knowledge of:
  1. Medical and Mental Health
  2. Health Psychology
  3. the Practice of Medicine and Specialist Care
  4. Health Care Services plus their current and future models for delivery
  5. Pharmaceuticals, their applications and use
  6. eHealth and Telemedicine
  7. Information Technology
  8. Enterprise Level Computing
  9. Grid Technologies
  10. Patient Populations, their categories (e.g., by condition) and classifications (e.g., computer literate)
  11. local Business, Cultural, Government and Political attitudes, Law, Regulations, rules, sensitivities and traditions.
- A prior decision has been made to study and/or develop a Grid-based replacement for an existing infrastructure that supports Health and Health Care Services including Telemedicine and eHealth.
- A detailed, extensive Study, with a wide, inclusive membership, has been completed successfully showing conclusively that further activity is warranted and will be supported.
- No current, pending or suggested Law, Rule, Regulation, Judicial Decision or Proposition is in conflict, thereby subjecting the Project to Legislative and/or Judicial Process.

WHO Definition of Health

"Health is a state of complete physical, mental and social well-being and not merely the absence of disease or infirmity".

General

Health and Health Care Grids require an in-depth analysis of the structure, organizations, workflows and personnel in the target environment, e.g.,

- Health and Health Care Practitioner, Patient, Provider and Payer Communities
- Medical and Mental Health Research, Development and Support Communities
- Health and Health Care IT, Computing, Networking and Support Communities
- Relevant Education, Training, Standards, Licensing and Regulatory Bodies
- Administrative, Accounting and Management Bodies
- Governmental Bodies including the Judiciary
- Established Bodies of Relevant Law, In-Country and Cross-Border
- Established International Law

Caution is advisable at this point since the goals, objectives and plans of the proposed Grid-based infrastructure must include those of the existing infrastructure(s), e.g., Business, Cultural, Government and Political, but not conflict with them.

Before addressing issues related to the integration and/or upgrading of existing operational infrastructure with such Grids, detailed and extensive plans, procedures, simulations and alternatives must be prepared.

The development and operation of a 'parallel' development system until such time as the Grid-based System is fully operational, at desired performance and scalability, can reduce overall risk of failure, ensure High Availability and Recovery, verify performance and scalability, and support required education and training.

At a minimum there must be a very favorable cost-benefit projected outcome and substantial financing available. A detailed and thorough, approved, Business Plan is required. This Plan must include provisions for satisfactory completions and achievements plus appropriate Exit Plans.

Efforts directed at introducing these Grids into existing infrastructure must include at least the following:

- competent knowledge and appreciation of the applications supported and relevant Participants
- in-depth knowledge of and training on the existing infrastructure
- acquisition of detailed performance, scalability and cost data and information on the existing infrastructure
- prior experience and training on similar infrastructures including personnel management
- in-depth knowledge of the personnel management, policies, rules and regulations covering the current infrastructure
- detailed information on the technical and operational deficiencies and short-comings of the current infrastructure
- extensive knowledge of the costs associated with the design, development, integration and operation of the proposed infrastructure
- concrete, unwavering data and information on Managements' relevant goals and objectives, favorable and unfavorable.

Especially important to the success of a Grid-based development is support from the existing Health and Health Care Practitioner Communities. A caveat concerns the promotion of Grid-Based development at the expense of existing Health care Services. In all cases the existing Health and

Health Care Practitioner Communities must be involved, included and committed.

The Practice of Medicine is 'enabled' by advanced technologies such as eHealth and Telemedicine. Common ground includes sensors, data, measurements, analysis, diagnosis and treatments. Practicing with more and better data from more and better sensors is common ground a Grid-based development can rely upon.

After common ground a viable Business Plan can develop real interest and co-operation.

Going forward in this document the major focus is upon 'DELIVERY'. The Delivery of Health and Health Care Services is in fact the single most crucial, overriding issue. Some Services may receive special attention at time but they tend to be grouped together in Practice.

DELIVERY

General

The Delivery of Health and Health Care Services is a continuing issue. What constitutes 'Delivery' is equally perplexing. Telemedicine and eHealth share similar issues with other Services.

In many Legal Jurisdictions 'Telemedicine' and 'eHealth' are relatively new concepts within the Law and hence may have unintended consequences as written into the Law. It must be kept in mind that current law is the product of multiple, interacting groups many of which are political in nature.

All Services are subject to the Law, its Judicial Interpretation and its Administration. It remains the responsibility of the population-at-large to know and understand the relevant Law and to effect change when and where required. The rationale is simple: Patients are the ultimate Beneficiaries of Health and Health Care Services.

Here this task must cover Telemedicine and eHealth. It is possible to adopt a position that a major component of eHealth is to pursue this task continually for all Health and Health Care Services.

Delivering Services from a Health-Related Grid

Overlooking for a moment the Originators, Sustainers, Developers and initial Beneficiaries of a specific Grid-based Service, the following issues establish and initial boundary for the Service:

- What Legal Entity controls the Grid and the Service?
- Who has access to the Service and at what priority?
- What is the cost associated with Maintenance and Access?
- What structure and/or Organization controls, updates and otherwise changes the Service?
- Does access imply equality?
- Is there a System for Resolutions and Remedies?
- Is this substantially different from a traditional, local, non-Grid-based Health Care Service?

Meaningful responses to these issues can be provided by Participants having and maintaining access to the Service, and those unable to obtain access. Managing such a Services is a very complex set of tasks well beyond the current scope.

Delivering Grid Services to Professionals from a Health-Related Grid

HealthGrid 2009 Conference

"... The HealthGrid conference is the premier conference on the transformation of biomedical research, education and medical care through the application of Grid technologies. HealthGrid is dedicated to:

- *Enhancing biomedical research and healthcare delivery*
- *Creating an open collaborative virtual community*
- *Communicating the collective knowledge of the HealthGrid community*

HealthGrid is an interdisciplinary community of computer scientists, physicians, medical educators and students, epidemiologists, bioinformatics and medical informatics experts, military medicine specialists, security and policy makers, economists and futurists.

The conference program will include a number of high-profile keynote presentations, complemented by a set of refereed papers, which will be selected through the present call for papers. ...” (http://berlin2009.healthgrid.org/)

This is a typical Professional Conference responding to the wishes of a small select Community with specific interests. From a Health Care Practice viewpoint this may be of limited value.

Professionals in Practice

Commercial Grid-based solutions for professionals in Practice are available.

Grid Computing From IBM

“... Highlights

- *Improve patient care by ensuring fast, on demand access to medical images in-house, cross campus or across the country*
- *Eliminate data silos and reduce costs by optimizing storage utilization*
- *Ensure business continuity and address regulatory disaster recovery considerations*
- *Lower total cost of ownership with solutions that deliver cost-effective file sharing across multicampus sites, and seamlessly inter-operate with installed technologies*
- *Support infrastructure resiliency with end to end Storage virtualization tools that enable a more dynamic organization*

The IBM Healthcare and Life Science’s Grid Medical Archive Solution (GMAS) employs an unparalleled combination of features to cost-effectively deliver enterprise-wide medical image access with real-time business continuity.

...

The solution can help you securely store and efficiently transmit diagnostic images and documents within your enterprise or across multisite facilities. It combines the power of grid computing with intelligent information lifecycle management to optimize the storage of large volumes of fixed-content data. Further, it complements and extends existing assets by providing interoperability between high-performance grid-based storage and existing PACS. The end result is an ability to deliver patient images wherever they’re needed-at the moment they’re needed-which can lead to improved diagnosis and treatment.

...

For small to medium healthcare and life sciences businesses, GMAS is delivered in pre-priced packaged GMAS Bundles beginning with a capacity of 6TB and that can scale to 32TBs, supporting affordable entry into the solution with investment protection as complexity of Disaster Recovery plans expand and exponential image retention requirements develop. For all configurations available, minimal onsite integration means a simple installation and a manageable low cost entry point that can easily scale to additional sites as organizational needs change....” (http://www-03.ibm.com/linux/grid/medical_archive_solution.shtml)

This set of solutions illustrates what is available today in the Business Communities.

Delivering Services to Patients from a Health-Related Grid

An immediate and primary issue at hand is: Should a Patient know about the availability of Grid Services and if so, what Services would be made available?

This rapidly becomes a moot issue since current models for the delivery of Health Care Services are requiring that the patient assume additional responsibility for the management and control over their own Health and Health Care Services. Forcing the assumption of additional responsibility requires immediate and in-depth participation of the Patient in all matters except those directly linked to the practice of Medicine.

Added to this is the additional complications surrounding Patient Privacy and Security. In many Legal Jurisdictions ownership of Electronic Records has been transferred to the Patient, thereby giving the Patient special interests in and rights to the Electronic Records.

Payment for Grid-Based Services

As Consumer of multiple, varied Services, over time, the realization that Services become and remain available upon payment translates into an expectation that Services require payments. New Members of the Work Force may initially be quite disappointed at this arrangement.

Health Care Services are available when there is a Payer. Grid-based Services are no different. Health and Health Care Grids, Telemedicine and eHealth all provide payment-based Services. Cost-effectiveness becomes a major factor in their design, development, deployment and operation.

With this enhanced knowledge comes Population-based, Conditional Acceptance, a Quid Pro Quo ("something-for-something"). Legal Communities, e.g., Contracts and Remedies, are quite familiar with the Term; Shopkeepers are familiar as well. Purveyors of Grid-based Services are closely associated.

The Selection of Grid-Based Health and Health Care Services

Now that Conditional Acceptance has been introduced, the focus can be redirected to the Services offered to a Consumer (Patient) that would overcome their reluctance to become involved. This is a 'trading' environment involving at least individuals, Communities, history and current Services, e.g., current bad Services typically mitigate against any agreement.

The selection of Services is well-beyond the current scope as is the resolutions of issues, conflicts and remedies.

Alternatives to Grid-Based Health and Health Care Services

The selection of Grid-based Services may involve the offering of Alternatives where Conditional Acceptance has been negative. Detours on the Road to achieving Acceptance of Grid-based Services may be necessary.

Management and Control of Grid-Based Health and Health Care Services

Self-management and control are rarely attributes of such Services. Unless performed well continually, Conditional Acceptance may turn to Rejection and hence Failure.

Failed Grid-Based Health and Health Care Services

Before initial deployment Exit Strategies must be defined and in place to remove failed Services. This is good Management Practice.

NEW TECHNOLOGIES

General

There is often associated with new technologies sufficient mystic that Conditional Acceptance is granted based upon presumptions, often misconceived, that 'new' must be better than 'old', or this time someone 'got it right'. New Technologies often present new Risks without competent Risk Management Tools and Techniques.

Competent Risk Management is necessary well-before the initial deployment. If Risk Management is insufficient, incorrect or ineffective the Exit Strategy must include removal.

Embedded Medical Systems and Networks

The Industrial Process Control Industry predates many of the current embedded systems and networks used to design, develop and implement Embedded Medical Systems and Networks. Although Industrial Process Control Industry continues to make significant advances in Embedded Systems and Networks, the Embedded Medical Systems and Networks Industry continues to establish significant records ((*Embedded System*, n.d.), (Vahid & Givargis, 2002), (*Application for Medical Diagnostics*, 2008), (Konieczny, 2010) (Jafari, 2006)).

Digital Libraries

"... a Library in which collections are stored in digital formats ... and accessible by computers. The digital content may be stored locally, or accessed remotely via computer networks. ... an online collection of information must be managed by and made accessible to a community of users ... A digital library can be built around specific repository software..." (Digital Library, 2010).

A suitable example of a Digital Library used in Health and Medicine is found in ((Digital Librarian: a librarian's choice of the best of the Web, Health & Medicine, 2009), (Health and Medicine Digital Library – Online Medical Library – Academic Info, 2010)).

"...Linking the electronic health record to the digital library is a Web-era reformulation of the long-standing informatics goal of seamless integration of automated clinical data and relevant knowledge-based information to support informed decisions. The spread of the Internet, the development of the World Wide Web, and converging format standards for electronic health data and digital publications make effective linking increasingly feasible. Some existing systems link electronic health data and knowledge-based information in limited settings or limited ways.

...

The idea of linking automated clinical data and knowledge-based information to support health care, research, and education gained prominence in the early 1980s when the vision of Integrated Advanced Information Management Systems (IAIMS) was first articulated.1 The National Library of Medicine's Unified Medical Language System (UMLS) project was initiated in 1986 to facilitate the development of IAIMS systems capable of linking and integrating different types of machine-readable biomedical information, including patient records, the biomedical literature, factual databanks, and expert systems

...

As expected by those involved with IAIMS, UMLS, or both, the amount of useful patient data, clinical information, and biomedical knowledge in electronic form has increased dramatically since the 1980s. Also as anticipated, computers have continued to decrease in cost and size while in-

creasing in speed, functionality, and ease of use. Not so generally predicted, but even more critical for the integration of the electronic health record and the digital library, the spread of the Internet and the development of the World Wide Web have simultaneously:

- *Reduced the technical complexity of integrating access to disparate legacy systems developed on different technical platforms*
- *Provided de facto technical standards to which new electronic resources can be designed*
- *Made it possible for researchers, health professionals, and patients both to retrieve and to create information at home as well as in the library, office, clinic, and hospital*
- *Increased the perceived benefit of having a computer and an Internet connection*

These developments make integrated access to computer-based health records and related knowledge-based information increasingly feasible. The rise of Web technology has also contributed to expansive definitions of both the electronic health record and the digital library. In fact, these two concepts now meet at the edges..." (Electronic Health Record Meets Digital Library, n.d.).

This design and development altered the practice of Medicine for practitioners. The boundary between Practitioners and Patients has in many areas been breached and the developed Technologies are being applied in Patient Communities.

A significant caveat exists however. The Patient Communities have limited organization, goals, objectives, constraints and limitations when compared with the Health and Healthcare Professional Communities. Adaptations of future systems and networks to specific Communities may be very common.

Social Networking

"... made of individuals (or organizations) called "nodes," which are tied (connected) by one or more specific types of interdependency, such as friendship kinship, financial exchange, dislike, sexual relationships, or relationships of beliefs, knowledge or prestige...." (Social Networking, n.d.)

Personal Health and Healthcare Services are suitable candidates for the basic reason that individual have and seek personal Support Groups.

"... several recent scientific studies have found that real-life social networks are quite relevant to health. Indeed, a study published earlier this year in the New England Journal of Medicine evaluated a large social network of over 12,000 people over 32 years to assess the person-to-person spread of obesity ... friends, siblings and spouses have an even greater effect on a person's risk of obesity than genetics..." (Jessen, 2007)

"...A study to examine the inherited characteristics of social networks using Add Health data appeared in Harvard Science. The research was conducted by James Fowler and Christopher Dawes of UC San Diego and Nicholas Christakis of Harvard.

...

Researchers found that popularity, or the number of times an individual was named as a friend, and the likelihood that those friends know one another, were both strongly heritable. Additionally, location within the network, or the tendency to be at the center or on the edges of the group, was also genetically linked. However, the researchers were surprised to learn that the number of people named as a friend by an individual did not appear to be inherited

...

One of the things that the study tells us is that social networks are likely to be a fundamental part of our genetic heritage..." (Add Health, n.d.)

"...The findings also illuminate a previously unknown limitation of existing social network models, which had assumed that all members behave as interchangeable cogs.

...

To address these intrinsic differences in human beings that contribute to the formation of social networks, the researchers have created a new mathematical model, called the "attract and introduce" model

...

Because both health behaviors and germs spread through social networks, understanding how contagions flow through social networks has the potential to improve strategies for addressing public health concerns such as obesity or the flu.

...

"I think that going forward, we are going to find that social networks are a critical conduit between our genes and important health outcomes," says Fowler. Fowler and Christakis have also published on other aspects of social networks, such as the spread of obesity, smoking, and happiness...." (Lavoie, 2006)

Social Networking appears to be an ideal framework upon which to build Health and Healthcare Services Grid-based applications. It is a good example for many Community-based applications. It does not, however, appear to be a good basis upon which to build Personal Health and Healthcare Services Grid-based applications.

The genetic-based research indicates that other approaches, e.g., allowing the Patient to form, join, dissolve, modify Personal applications may be more suitable with less identified impacts to Patients.

Patient-controlled Frameworks for the development of Personal Health and Healthcare Services applications are proposed.

Wide-Area Internet Access Supports Telemedicine and eHealth

Background wide-area Internet access enables Telemedicine and eHealth by supporting resident and remote applications for Health and Healthcare Services. A requirement would be that a Patient or a Practitioner would be able to initiate and monitor ongoing activities.

This process has been verified within Poznan, Poland using a 'blueconnect' device and supporting software (*Polska Telefonia Cyfro Has HSDPA Across Entire 3G Network*, 2006, About ERA, 2010).

Coupled with commercially-available embedded systems and networks, sophisticated Telemedicine and eHealth applications can be continuously supported.

Upon this base can be developed a Country-wide network of Grid-like Health and Healthcare Services applications.

Such Country-wide applications are likely to evolve and be accepted more readily than similar classes global applications. Existing Healthcare Systems and Networks, Social Networking, languages, custom and history are likely to be major factors, and at times obstacles.

Grids for Embedded Medical Systems and Networks

The References provided should compel a conclusion that the basic components required by User-Level Grids are present in Embedded Systems and networks. There is one major difference.

Where the User-Level Grids require additional resource allocated by Administrators and Managers, the Embedded Systems and Networks are often dedicated to specific Task Sets. Hence the Embedded Grid would serve this Task Set well.

Medical Systems and Networks are by regulations and requirements strictly controlled within restricted applications. Hence the Embedded Medical Grids are application restricted. Within their Application Task Sets they can be significantly productive.

A Potential Application

The European Institute for Telesurgery (European Institute of Telesurgery,n.d.) performs a highly constructive and productive set of applications using currently available Computing Systems and Networks. Within this Application Task Set there are multiple potential applications for Embedded Medical Grids, both locally and at remote sites.

REPORTING RESULTS

General

This can be described as ***Effective Communications***. Recall that Patients are encouraged to assume additional responsibility for the Management and Control of their own Health and Health Care Services. Effective Communications is therefore mandatory.

In the Health and Healthcare Industries reports are daily handled in traditional ways but standard equipments. Can Embedded Grids modify this situation?

Embedded Medical and Non-Medical Reporting Grids

Medical Reporting is highly regulated and restricted; non-Medical Reporting is not. Embedded Systems and Networks are easily structured to accept and handle both types.

This takes on added significance when considering that massive amount of data and information (medical and non-medical) reside upon collections of very large storage subsystems. Migrating, accessing and creating this data and information are major, costly tasks.

Embedded Systems and Networks cover Storage Subsystems and Networks. Hence data and information can be both stored, transmitted and processed therein.

An interesting Project would be building an Embedded System with re-configurable structure to serve specific tasks, short- and long-term. Perhaps a Load-Balancing or a 'Fast-Transfer' application that takes advantage of the structure imposed by 'embedding', e.g., Bridging the 'User-Level' and 'Embedded' worlds.

THE DISCLOSURE OF DATA AND INFORMATION

General

The full disclosure of data and information to a Patient, or their Support Groups may not be advisable. It may be prudent for the Physician to review what data and information is disclosed, however, preventing a disclosure is also neither advisable nor warranted. A suitable Representative for such disclosures should be chosen early to avoid negative implications and accomplish adequate disclosure.

INTEGRATIONS

General

The Basic Services of a Health or Health Care Grid should be deployed, tested, measured for Performance and Scalability before additional Services are integrated. This approach will insure that the Basic Services are performing as required and that should integrations develop difficulties they can immediately segmented and removed, restoring the Grid to a known good state.

eHealth

A personal preference is an integration of eHealth-related Services first. This will make available immediately a large amount of Health-related data and information to Patients. Presuming that the eHealth Service contains full documentation for all Services, a Patient should have adequate information in advance for all operations, Health and Health Care services.

Telemedicine

A Patient may choose to 'opt-out' of Telemedicine or may be unable to, or choose not to, fully participate in this Service. The 'character' and 'function' of the Grid may be in conflict with the operation of a Telemedicine-based Service, e.g., and Emergency Services or Intensive Care Department on a dedicated Grid.

Patient Data Grid

As Patient assume more responsibility for the Management and Control over their own Health and Health Care Services, they may produce large amounts of relevant data that does not necessarily need to be analyzed immediately by a Physician or a Specialist. It may have value to the Patient only.

The Patient Data Grid can securely accumulate this data for the Patient and permit them to retrieve, edit and modify the stored content.

This data may also be very significant, e.g., daily recordings of a Diabetes Patient with a second condition. The Patient is in control of the accumulated data; the grid supplies a Service to the Patient.

Equipment Grids

Medical Facilities acquire a large number of equipments that require supervision and control to ensure proper working conditions, data on operations performed, and life cycle data that indicates major repairs. A Grid for a single, large Facility is realistic; one for a Medical more so, and one for a Region absolutely necessary.

Justifications for such Grids is simple, i.e., good Health Care requires properly maintained, documented and used equipment.

SUMMARY

This Chapter has addressed Health and Healthcare Grid Services and Delivery, integrating eHealth and Telemedicine. The presentation covers two diverse Communities: Practitioners and Patients. Practitioner Communities have integrated and are using Grid-like systems and networks developed over many years. Patient Communities are essential newcomers. Developing Grid-like Applications for Telemedicine and eHealth for Patient Communities must accommodate unique associated attributes.

The following major factors associated with potential Grid-like Applications are significant:

- Grids can be composed of existing computer systems and networks resources and components
- Health and Health Care Grids are supplemental to existing Health and Health Care Services
- Conditional Acceptance of the Health and Health Care Grids is a major factor in success or failure
- Telemedicine and eHealth can be integrated into or grafted upon a successful Health and Health Care Services Grid

- the various disciplines of Telemedicine and health utilize a common pool of computing resources.

The following major factors associated with Patient Communities are significant:

- Legal Jurisdictions, Law, Regulations
- Social Mores and Folkways
- Language, custom, ethnicity, history
- Existing Health and Healthcare Systems and networks
- Current Social Networks
- Health and Healthcare Services Social Networking
- Personalization
- Wide-area Internet Access
- Current Research into Patient-Centric Health and Healthcare Services, e.g., genetic predispositions

Frameworks and Tools for Developers and Choice, adaptability, personal social networking and support (medical and mental) for individual Patients are needed. 'One size fits all' approach is unlikely to prove suitable.

CONCLUSION

In conclusion, there are serious concerns that need to be dealt with before healthcare providers and patients embrace a health grid system. In particular, healthcare providers need more incentive to adopt a health grid system, because the current system in place gives them no incentive to do so. In addition, they need protection from liabilities that can be introduced by the health grid, particularly increased malpractice lawsuit costs.

Also, healthcare providers need to implement a record system to ensure that no unauthorized access to patient data is taking place, and that all patient data being accessed is for strictly medical purposes only.

Patients need their data to be secure on the grid – both doing transmission and on arrival, and the freedom to choose what data goes on the grid, and what doesn't.

In addition, both groups need to have the choice to be completely off the grid if they so choose. However, both groups must also recognize the huge benefits offered by a health grid.

ACKNOWLEDGMENT

This research was funded by a grant from the National Science Foundation, and was supported by the University of Connecticut and Dr. Chun-Hsi Huang (http://www.cse.uconn.edu/~huang/REU_08/Reports/Bardiya_Vaziri.pdf).

Apendix A is a working document on the processing of personal data relating to Health in electronic health records (EHRs), Adopted on 15 February 2007

REFERENCES

About, E. R. *A*. (2010). Retrieved from http://www.era.pl/en/home/company/ptc

Application for Medical Diagnostics. (2008). Retrieved from http://www.sblsoftware.com/embedded-medical.aspx

Beowulf.org. *The Beowulf Cluster Site*. (2009). Retrieved from http://www.beowulf.org/

Bosch-Sijtsema, P. (n.d.). *Virtual organisations and knowledge development: A Case of Expectations*. University of Groningen, Groningen, The Netherlands. Retrieved from http://www.uni-hildesheim.de/~chlehn/isko2001/abstracts/bosch_petra.html

Cluster Computing Info Centre. (2010). Retrieved from http://www.gridbus.org/~raj/cluster/

Da Silveira, M., & Guelfi, N. (2009). The Concept of a Platform for Remote Monitoring Patient's Health State. In Jordanova, M., & Lievens, F. (Eds.), *Global Telemedicine and eHealth Updates: Knowledge Resources* (*Vol. 2*, pp. 278–282). Luxembourg: Luxexpo.

Digital Library. (2010). *Wikipedia*. Retrieved from http://en.wikipedia.org/wiki/Digital_library

Electronic Health Record Meets Digital Library. (n.d). Retrieved from http://www.pubmedcentral.nih.gov/articlerender.fcgi?artid=79039

Embedded System. (n.d.). *Wikipedia*. Retrieved from http://en.wikipedia.org/wiki/Embedded_system

European Institute of Telesurgery. (n.d.). Retrieved from http://www.eits.fr/

Ganguly, P., & Ray, P. (1998). *Telemedicine over Enterprise-wide Networks: A Case Study.* IEEE Global Telecommunications Conference (GLOBECOM98), Sydney, November. Retrieved from http://www.apuhc.org/pradeep

Health, A. (n.d.). *Add Health research on genetic influence in social networks is featured in HarvardScience*. Retrieved from http://www.cpc.unc.edu/projects/addhealth/news/add-health-research-on-genetic-influence-in-social-networks-is-featured-in-harvardscience

Health and Medicine Digital Library – Online Medical Library – Academic Info. (2010). Retrieved from http://www.academicinfo.net/medlibrary.html

Jafari, R. (2006). *Medical Embedded Systems.* Doctoral Dissertation, University of California, Los Angles, CA. Retrieved from http://www.utdallas.edu/~rjafari/publications/JAFARI_Dissertation.pdf

Jessen, W. (2007, December 4). Social Networks and Health. Posted to *Highlight HEALTH: Discover the Science of Health*. Retrieved from http://www.highlighthealth.com/highlight-health-web-site/social-networks-and-health-the-research-and-the-reviews/

Konieczny, E. (2010). *Embedded Medical Innovations*. Retrieved from http://www.embeddedintel.com/technology_applications.php?article=1065

Kopper, K. (2005). *The LINUX ENTERPRISE CLUSTER*. San Francisco, CA: No Starch Press. Retrieved from http://books.google.com/books?id=wiCGoCq8n4oC&dq=cluster%2Bcomputing&printsec=frontcover&source=bl&ots=NoUyFCqT3s&sig=Rx054L-cBDPbybnU0ClS2_zAZ0&hl=en&ei=bb7PSaK1FaectAOMm8ygAw&sa=X&oi=book_result&resnum=8&ct=result#PPP1,M1

KUB. *Virtual Organisation*. (n.d.). Retrieved from http://www.strategyforbusiness.co.uk/html/virtual_organisation.html

Lavoie, A. (2006, January 26th). The genes in your congeniality: Researchers identify genetic influence in social networks. *Harvard Science.* Retrieved from http://www.harvardscience.harvard.edu/culture-society/articles/the-genes-your-congeniality

Librarian, D. *a librarian's choice of the best of the Web, Health & Medicine*. (2009). Retrieved from http://www.digital-librarian.com/health.html

Löhr, H., & Ramasamy, H. Sadeghi, A-R., Schulz, S., Schunter, M. & Stüble, C. (2006). *Enhancing Grid Security Using Trusted Virtualization*. Paper accepted for 1st Benelux Workshop on Information and System Security, November 8-9, Antwerpen, Belgium. Retrieved from https://www.cosic.esat.kuleuven.be/wissec2006/papers/12.pdf

Networking, S. (n.d.). *Wikipedia*. Retrieved from http://en.wikipedia.org/wiki/Social_network

NIEeS GridInfo. *Virtuial Organisation.* (2006, March 12). Retrieved from http://gridinfo.niees.ac.uk/index.php/Virtual_Organisation

Polska Telefonia Cyfro Has HSDPA Across Entire 3G Network. (2006, October 30th). Retrieved from http://www.3g.co.uk/PR/October2006/3834.htm

The Mind and the Body are the Same Thing. (2010). Retrieved from http://mentalhealth.about.com/gi/o.htm?zi=1/XJ&zTi=1&sdn=mentalhealth&cdn=health&tm=15&gps=37_59_882_523&f=00&su=p284.9.336.ip_p736.8.336.ip_&tt=2&bt=1&bts=1&zu=http%3A//serendip.brynmawr.edu/exhibitions/Mind/Descartes.html

Vahid, F., & Givargis, T. (2002). *Embedded System Design, A Unified Hardware/Software Approach.* Chichester, UK: John Wiley & Sons. Retrieved from http://esd.cs.ucr.edu/

APPENDIX

Appendix A: Executive Summary

Provides guidance on the interpretation of the applicable data protection legal framework for EHR systems and explains some of the general principles.

...

also gives indications on the data protection requirements for setting up EHR systems, as well as the applicable safeguards

...

examines the general legal data protection framework for EHR systems ... recalls the general prohibition of the processing of personal data concerning health of Article 8 (1) of the Data Protection Directive 95/46/EC, and then discusses the possible application of the derogations in Article 8 (2), (3) and (4) of the Directive in the context of EHR systems by stressing the need for interpreting such derogations in a narrow fashion.

...

also reflects on a suitable legal framework for EHR systems and provides recommendations on eleven topics where special safeguards within EHR systems seem particularly necessary in order to guarantee the data protection rights of patients and individuals. These topics are:

1. *Respecting self determination*
2. *Identification and authentication of patients and health care professionals*
3. *Authorization for accessing EHR in order to read and write in EHR*
4. *Use of EHR for other purposes*
5. *Organisational structure of an EHR system*
6. *Categories of data stored in EHR and modes of their presentation*
7. *International transfer of medical records*
8. *Data security*
9. *Transparency*
10. *Liability issues*
11. *Control mechanisms for processing data in EHR*

...

invites the medical profession, all health care professionals, all involved persons and institutions as well as the general public to comment on this Working Document.

(http://ec.europa.eu/justice_home/fsj/privacy/docs/wpdocs/2007/wp131_en.pdf)

These references are included to demonstrate the complexity of Legal issues and their resolutions.

Appendix B: The Delivery of Health Care Services

General

An existing infrastructure that supports Health and Health Care Services, including Telemedicine and eHealth, will impact many people even though contact may be infrequent and possibly limited. Changes to the infrastructure will elicit responses from those affected. The responses must be well-managed.

Health and Health Care Grids are unlike Scientific Computing Grids that seek to share resources and enable very large-scale processing. They are affected with both Personal and Public Legal interests, e.g., Patient Privacy and Security, Electronic Health, Health Care, Medical and Patient Records, plus Quality and Medical Errors. Activities, Records and Participants may cross National Boundaries thereby raising additional issues, e.g., a Practitioner may be participating in a cross-border procedure but licensed only in one Jurisdiction.

Additional issues may arise due to the goals, objectives and planned operations of the proposed Grid, e.g., the Grid is planned to operate in six Jurisdictions whereas the current infrastructure operates in two.

The Delivery of Health and Health Care Services must improve. Remaining the same is likely to be viewed negatively by Participants.

Available Resources

This is a reminder that modifications and/or new developments require necessary and sufficient amounts of available resources. A proposal for any modification, expansion or new development must properly address and report on available resource.

Participants

Health Care Services Participants and other affected Parties must be included with the Group of Participants that will be monitoring and actively participating in comments and review of Grid development- and operations-related activities.

Multiple Groups may evolve and their lifetime and involvement may be lengthy and detailed. The introduction of such Grids will result in major changes and adaptations, e.g., work-flow and Communities.

Requirements, Goals, Objectives, Evaluations and Performance

New Design and Development activities require Benchmarks against which progress is measured. These Benchmarks may migrate into the operations environment where they will be joined by more definitive operations-oriented Benchmarks.

Ideally the operations Benchmarks will become standards governing ongoing, and automatic, processes, procedures, performance, scalability, integration, project management, testing, maintenance and repair.

Concentrations of Services

General

Health and Health Care Services are concentrated in areas where:

- demand and utilization are very high
- costs are moderate-to-low
- Patient-to-Practitioner ratios are high
- moderate travel is required of outlying, but close-in, Areas, e.g., Satellite Cities and Towns.

Areas that do not fall within this scheme are labeled Rural Areas and addressed separately.

Hospitals

The greatest concentrations of Services typically occur in Hospitals and Hospital Groups. These are routinely chosen as design and development sites for Health and Health Care Grids. Specialization does occur thereby limiting activities to specific Disciplines.

Hospitals can provide:

- Primary Health Care Services
- Emergency Health Care Services
- Specialty Services
- In-Patient and Out-Patient Services
- Patient Monitoring and Support
- Telemedicine and eHealth Support
- Electronic Health, Health Care and Patient Records Storage and Access
- Health Care Grid Access and Applications

Hospital Grids can therefore reflect a mosaic of Hospital Services but not necessarily all-inclusive. The configuration of such a Grid at any time may be heavily influenced by the resident Health Care Providers and Payers. Gaps in coverage may occur.

Clinics

Clinics can provide:

- Primary Health Care Services
- Selected Specialty Services
- Patient Monitoring and Support
- Telemedicine and eHealth Support
- Electronic Health, Health Care and Patient Records Storage and Access
- Health Care Grid Access and Applications

Attachment to Health and Health Care Grids within Clinics may be limited to support of Practitioners, with Grid-based data and information available to Patients on a request basis. This limitation is likely to be due to the perceived availability provided to Patients.

Patients and Their Support Groups

Telemedicine and eHealth have been well-received by Patient Communities, e.g., Patient Monitoring and Home Care. Access to Internet-connected Computers and Networks is common in many developed Countries and is increasing. Health and Health Care Grids are conceivable in both Metropolitan and Rural Communities.

The basic requirements of high performance data transmission facilities, e.g., Broadband communications, and associated Internet Services are being satisfied in both Communities rapidly. When completed in an area, Internet Services follow quickly.

Presuming a range of services suitable for Patients, deployment of Health and Health Care Grids could follow soon.

Providing Grid Services directly to Patients would be very expensive and problematic due principally to the very large number of attachments to individuals that would be required.

An Alternative is configuring the Grid so that Patients can access it with relative ease and economy. Internet Services provide Internet Access Points to Individuals. Grid Access Points could be managed in Parallel. This may be a minimalist solution in that the Legislation, Regulations, Certifications and Licensing for Internet Services could be simply extended.

Emergency Services

Telemedicine and eHealth have been successfully extended to Emergency Services. An issue is whether Health and Health Care Grids can be extended to Emergency Services.

Access to Electronic Health, Health Care and Patient Records can be crucial and life-saving. Telemedicine and eHealth can provide access to Practitioners; the Grids can provide access to the records and pre-analyzed Patient Summaries. Bundled together, the Practitioners receiving the Patient from Emergency Services may have a sufficient Knowledge Base on the Patient to continue Care.

For Emergency Services issues may address how to connect Emergency Services to available, relevant Grids.

Service Gaps

Gaps in coverage and gaps in available services are major issues for such Grids. Effectiveness requires that sufficient Redundancy be provided so that most gaps can be overcome. High Availability is a major requirement and it may be joined in some applications by Fault Tolerance.

An expectation that Fault Tolerance and High Availability is a major, crucial requirements for Hospitals and Clinics is justifiable.

Appendix C: Availability and Access to Grid Services

Payers

Health Care Services are available to Participants when financing is available, i.e., when one or more Payers provide the necessary funding to make them available. Payments for such Services may be direct or indirect or some combination thereof. The financing of Health Care Services is beyond the scope here but remains a major issue and requirement.

Health Care Insurance

Various forms of Payment-for-Services can be covered by Health Care Insurance. Patients often are required to participate in covered payments for Health Care Services.

Payment for Health and Health Care Grid Services presents additional complex issues. Privacy and Security will remain key issues. Whether Grid Services can be covered by Insurance remains an issue for future resolution.

Metropolitan Services

Metropolitan Area Health Care Services (**MAHCS**) are typically organized to service the prevailing Communities within the Area. **MAHCS** can, therefore, diverge substantially with respect to provided Health Care Services, e.g., Heavy Industrial Manufacturing Metropolitan Areas (lower average Wage Scales) tend to diverge from Areas that are predominately Financial Services (higher average Wage Scales).

Medical and Mental Practitioner Communities within a **MAHCS** must focus on the prevailing and anticipated demands for Services. The Communities will quickly adapt to Local Requirements and changes therein. Advances in Medicine and changing demands may result in changes in the Communities or the appearance of new Communities.

Support for Health and Health Care Information Technology and Informatics (**HHCITI**) is dependent upon these Local Requirements. Financing must be made available if support translates into implementations and operations. External Financing may be required.

Implementations and related operations in Metropolitan Areas can be very expensive, e.g., they often are dependent upon existing infrastructures and related costs but can be deprived of existing infrastructures and forced to develop new infrastructures and new costs.

Where Telemedicine and eHealth can initially build upon existing Internet Services, up to a point where additional loading adversely impacts performance and scalability, additional costs for implementations and operations can be incremental.

Associated Metropolitan Area Grid Services are likely to require different operations models. Standard Services with Patient-specific, secure data and information would be typical. Other optional Services may be available. These may also be available as Standard Services with Patient-specific, secure data, information and functions.

Suburban Services

Suburban Communities are often distinguished from City-Centre Communities by life style, environment and available Services. The availability of Health and Health Care Services differs as well.

At some point variances in Grid Services available in different Communities can, unfortunately, rise to the level of a major issue. This is more likely to happen where significant variance occurs.

Design and Development Teams must ensure that equality in Services among the various Communities is established and maintained.

Rural Community Services

Rural Communities are a major challenge. There are significant differences among the various Communities and their surrounding areas. In many areas Internet Service is not available, i.e., there is no Data Transmission Services, and hence, neither is Telemedicine and eHealth.

Without adequate Data Transmission Services, Internet Services, Telemedicine and eHealth Services, the deployment of Health and Health Care Grid Services is inappropriate.

In those Rural Communities where adequate Data Transmission Services, Internet Services, Telemedicine and eHealth Services exist, the deployment of Health and Health Care Grid Services should proceed.

Regional Services

The configuration of Health and Health Care Services across a Region may not be uniform and maybe highly selective, e.g., one Centre for Health Care Services. This is likely to be the manifestation of an acute lack of resources to cover the region adequately.

Redistributions of resources is likely to be strongly opposed and simple not realistic.

Where this configuration of resources exists, Internet Services, Telemedicine, eHealth plus Health and Health Care Grid Services become critical resources throughout the region.

Appendix D: Services

General

The number of potential Services that could be offered by a Hospital is very large; the actual number offered by a specific Hospital can be selective and much smaller. Additionally, the Services offered, in some cases, can be limited by time and resources. At a specific geographic location, during all time periods, it may be very difficult to discover what Services are readily available.

This deficiency can be alleviated in part through very-accessible applications. Such applications would provide this type of real-time data and information through data communications mediums, e.g., telephonic and Internet-based services.

Grid Services may assist in data and information acquisition and dissemination but their participation is neither necessary nor sufficient. Suitable infrastructures exist.

Services discussed here are dependent in some way on Grid-based Services.

Hospitals

Hospitals are configured to suit Departments, Work-flows, and Local requirements. IT infrastructure is modified according to current and future demands.

IT backbones, e.g., Optical Networks, as high-performance, large capacity data routing and transfer Facilities are poorly suited to internal infrastructure and hence, attach to appropriate intermediate performance interfaces that perform internal data routing and transmission tasks. Work-station and work-group networks and sub-nets attach to this internal infrastructure.

Hospital Groups may support Optical Networks that interconnect Member Hospitals, thereby configuring an appropriate internal network and subnets spanning individual Hospitals.

Hospital Groups may develop and support 'internal' Health Grids that remain within the 'Close' of the Hospital Group. Admittedly this is an optimal approach since the Hospital Group has control over most parameters and variables.

In this case an internal Health Care Grid is likely to approximate a Campus Area Network (CAN) with specialty sub-nets. Major issues such as privacy and security remain, however, but they remain within the Hospital Group.

Because they are internal to a Health Care Organization that can exercise total control over them, they are beyond the scope of this Chapter. This is not the case with a Hospital Group that utilizes Public Service Health Care Grids. All issues in some sense directly impact a public service.

In the following the discussion is limited to those Grids that provide a public service.

Clinics

Clinics can be categorized by the Services they provide, their Staff and their Supporters. Support for Health Care Grids within each Category can vary significantly.

Services

Individual Clinics can focus upon some number of services that they have chosen to provide, have developed a reputation or competence in, or due to necessity or organization have participated in.

Health and Health Care Grids may or may not contribute significantly to the performance of the Clinics Services. The Services provided by the Clinic may be self-limiting. Where some Service could benefit substantially from participation in a Grid, the Clinic may become involved where the Cost-Benefit-Performance is substantial or necessary.

Staff

Where Principal Staff Members of a Clinic strongly support participation in a Grid, the Clinic may become involved where the Cost-Benefit-Performance is substantial.

Supporters

Clinics can be heavily influenced by Supporters, e.g. Financial Contributors. Participation in a Grid can initiated due to external influences.

Impacts

Clinics tend to provide focused Health Care Services. Large Clinics provide highly specialized Services or many specialized Services may participate in Grid Services.

Most Clinics can benefit from Telemedicine and eHealth Services since those Services are focused mainly on Patient-Practitioner interactions.

Patients and Their Support Groups

General

The Traditional Model for the Delivery of Health Care Services requires that a Patient be fully dependent and reliant upon Practitioners, Providers and Payers. To resolve some major problems with this model another Team- and Output-Oriented model has been developed. A third model has been proposed that is compatible with the new fields of Personalized Medicine.

All models provide Services, however, each model may not provide one or more Services required by an individual Patient. Furthermore, Payers may tend to restrict the number and types of Services available to Patients.

As Patients and their Support Groups attempt to navigate available future Health and Health Care Services they will by necessity assume the responsibility for certain services. Electronic Records are likely candidates.

Patients Plus Health and Health Care Grid Systems

Large-scale Scientific Computing Grids have expanded beyond the Research Facilities so that Computing Grids are available to a much large set of Research-oriented Communities. In this expansion the structure of these Grids has not changed substantially and does not present a substitution for main-line, Enterprise-level Computing Systems and Networks.

Grid Computing has, however, found a niche in the Enterprise-level Computing Market.

"... IBM introduced its Grid Medical Archive System (GMAS)—an industry-specific grid offering based on its Grid Access Manager ... it extends an industry-specific grid program

...

GMAS is based on a grid storage technology

...

GMAS' strongest selling point is its virtualized storage capability, which makes it easier for health-care providers and life-sciences researchers to grapple with the storage resource management (SRM) problems posed by rapidly-expanding data volumes.

...

storage grids are decentralized by design

...

the decentralized nature of storage grids that allows storage administrators to think of managing their environments in very different ways

...

[P]patient-care facilities are increasingly doing their medical imaging such as X-rays and MRIs directly to digital formats rather than analog film

...

These files alone, when taken in aggregate, can consume hundreds of terabytes of storage, depending on the size and average age of the patient population served. Add to that the growth in the level of resolution and detail of these scans, as well as the growth of other types of patient files [such as]

...

documents, audio, video, invoices

...

[that are] also increasingly being committed to digital formats..."

(IBM, Sun Prove Why Grid Computing is Alive and Well, http://esj.com/articles/2007/06/19/ibm-sun-prove-why-grid-computing-is-alive-and-well.aspx)

As the growth in stored digital data increases, the cost of Health Care increases, with increased demand by Patients for guarantees of Privacy and Security, and the willingness of Patients to assume additional management and control over their own Health and Health Care Services, ownership over an increasing percentage of the available stored digital data will pass to the Patient and their Support Groups.

Partial, or complete, availability to selected Practitioners, and possibly Payers, will occur. Retention, analysis, collation, reporting and structuring are likely to be performed consistent with the Patients and their Support Groups requirements.

Legal Issues and Representation

Current Health and Health Care Systems are unable to properly manage current and projected Services, their cost, complexity and requirements, regulation, population growth, Patient awareness, interest and competency, inadequate staffing, Quality issues plus Security at all levels.

Change is required. It will occur in all areas and will result in major changes in the Legal environment. Current explorations must be continued. The Conclusion of the following report by:

Bardiya Shadmehr
University of Texas at Dallas
800 West Campbell Road, Richardson, TX 75080-3021

Appendix E: Computing Systems

Cluster Computing

Cluster Computing is quite common in Enterprise Computing and hence, is present in those Computing Centres and Systems that support the Health Care Industry. Availability, Performance, Scalability and Security are major requirements.Enterprise-Level Computing that will integrate Grids.

*"... **Cluster** is a widely-used term meaning independent computers combined into a unified system through software and networking. At the most fundamental level, when two or more computers are used together to solve a problem, it is considered a cluster. Clusters are typically used for **High Availability (HA)** for greater reliability or **High Performance Computing (HPC)** to provide greater computational power than a single computer can provide. ..." (Cluster Computing Info Centre, 2010), (Kopper, 2005).*

Beowulf Clusters

"... **Beowulf Clusters** *are scalable performance clusters based on commodity hardware, on a private system network, with open source software (Linux) infrastructure. The designer can improve performance proportionally with added machines. The commodity hardware can be any of a number of mass-market, stand-alone compute nodes as simple as two networked computers each running Linux and sharing a file system or as complex as 1024 nodes with a high-speed, low-latency network. ...*" (*Beowulf.org, The Beowulf Cluster Site*, 2009)

Grid Computing

Grid computing (or the use of a computational grid) is the application of several computers to a single problem at the same time – usually to a scientific or technical problem that requires a great number of computer processing cycles or access to large amounts of data.

Grid computing depends on software to divide and apportion pieces of a program among several computers, sometimes up to many thousands.

Grid computing can also be thought of as distributed and large-scale cluster computing, as well as a form of network-distributed parallel processing. It can be small -- confined to a network of computer workstations within a corporation, for example -- or it can be a large, public collaboration across many companies or networks.

It is a form of distributed computing whereby a "super and virtual computer" is composed of a cluster of networked, loosely coupled computers, acting in concert to perform very large tasks. This technology has been applied to computationally intensive scientific, mathematical, and academic problems through volunteer computing, and it is used in commercial enterprises for such diverse applications as drug discovery, economic forecasting, seismic analysis, and back-office data processing in support of e-commerce and Web services.

What distinguishes grid computing from conventional cluster computing systems is that grids tend to be more loosely coupled, heterogeneous, and geographically dispersed. Also, while a computing grid may be dedicated to a specialized application, it is often constructed with the aid of general-purpose grid software libraries and middleware.

Virtual Organisations

The following definition of a Virtual Organisation is definite and appropriate for a Business (*KUB: Virtual Organisation*, n.d.).

A discussion on a Grid Project Virtual Organisation is less definite but appropriate for a Grid-based Project (*NIEeS GridInfo: Virtuial Organisation*, 2006). As a matter of choice, both are suitable.

Expectation Management

Within a Virtual Organisation the expectations of the Members can vary significantly. The variance can at times become unproductive. The following is an Abstract for a three-year Study of a "research virtual organisation" in Sweden.

"... The virtual organisation (VO) is viewed as an organisation consisting of independent partners, who try to combine their strengths, skills, resources, risks and finances in order to produce ideas or a product. Members of the VO are often geographically dispersed and communicate with help of information technology.

The VO is a popular organisation structure, but ***it is also known that the VO is difficult to manage****. Members work rather individual and there is* ***hardly any control****. Some problems of the VO are that it is* ***difficult to motivate*** *its members, members suffer from* ***social loafing and absenteeism****.*

...

On the other hand it is ***unclear how such an organisation can reach a synergetic or learning effect by co-operating with each others core competencies****. Learning is inhibited by several organisational boundaries of a VO. These boundaries are within time, space, structure, diversity and distribution of results and information.*

...

Current literature on learning, does not often take into account the ***geographical dispersion and fluctuating workforce of a VO****, although some do take into account learning between organisational partners (Hamel 1991, Nonaka 1995).*

In Sweden a research virtual organisation was followed for three years, where the main question was: ***how is knowledge developed in a VO****. Important aspects were to* ***investigate boundaries and enablers of knowledge development*** *in a VO, the* ***role of management and the role of IT*** *in this development process. The data was collected with help of* ***interviews, observations and questionnaires****.*

...

It was found in the research VO, that besides a high use of e-mail for communication and information distribution, ***rich modes of communication were important*** *(e.g., telephone and face-to-face). However, due to several reasons the* ***information system was not often used****.*

...

Furthermore, it was found that the ***expectations of members were of importance for the success of the organisation****. The expectations of members are* ***based on past experiences, personal values, professional specialization and the role in hierarchy*** *(Ring & Van de Ven, 1994).*

...

Depending on expectations of members, a match or mismatch with the content of the work, the role of members, the development process of the organisation, the way information and results were distributed and the role of the autonomous partners could be seen.

...

A difference in expectations could be viewed between project leaders and project members, where project leaders had a low to moderate vague expectation, while project members often had a high to moderate expectation*, which was more detailed described.*

...

For the development of knowledge in a VO, it ***might be important, that management could harmonize the expectations of its members****. Expectation management is proposed as stimulating, maintaining and creating expectations within a VO, in order to overcome the earlier mentioned problems of a VO. ..." (Bosch-Sijtsema, n.d.)* ***(Emphasis Added)****.*

Appendix F: Grid Security

Trusted Visualization

"... Grid applications have increasingly sophisticated functional and security requirements. However, current techniques mostly protect only the resource provider from attacks by the user, while leaving the user comparatively dependent on the well-behavior of the resource provider.

...

In this paper, we take the first steps towards addressing the trust asymmetry by using a combination of trusted computing and virtualization technologies. We present the key components for a trustworthy Grid architecture and propose an implementation.

...

By providing multilateral security, i.e., security for both the Grid user and the Grid provider, our architecture increases the confidence that can be placed on the correctness of a Grid computation and on the protection of user-provided assets.

...

In order to maintain important scalability and performance aspects, our proposal aims to minimize overhead. Towards this end, we propose a scalable off line attestation protocol, which allows selection of partners in the Grid with minimal overhead. ..." (Löhr, Ramasamy, Sadeghi, Schulz, Schunter & Stüble, 2006).

Chapter 4
The Teams of Leaders (ToL) Concept:
The Grid, the Mesh, and the People in the World of Information and Knowledge-Based Global Healthcare

Dag von Lubitz
MedSMART, Inc., USA & Bieda Poco Dargante Institute, Denmark

ABSTRACT

The revolution in computer, information, and telecommunication sciences facilitated revolution in "the way we do business." Despite the wealth of new actionable information and actionable knowledge that this revolution created in healthcare, it was not enough to break the barriers of thought, bureaucracy, and politics. Thus, although the knowledge and professional expertise that are required to avert the threatening collapse of global healthcare are readily available, they remain locked in isolated pools separated by historical barriers, increasing intra- and interdisciplinary specialization, and by stiflingly narrow perception of healthcare complexity. Based on maximum integration of CT, IT, IM, KM, and multidimensional human expertise, the concept of "Teams of Leaders" (ToL) has been employed with rapidly growing success. Implementation of ToL leads to the development of "actionable understanding" that converts highly capable but isolated islands of creative power, into unified mission and task oriented "swarms" endowed with a vastly expanded, collective expertise and operational capabilities. With its roots deep in the advanced technologies of IT/IM/KM, Teams of Leaders transcend bureaucracies and politics, and the collaborative outputs generated through ToL-based operations may constitute one of the pivotal elements of the desperately needed healthcare restructuring.

DOI: 10.4018/978-1-61692-010-4.ch004

Multae manus onus levant

GLOBAL HEALTHCARE IN CRISIS

Thomas Barnett divided the world into two entities – the functioning core and the non-integrating gap (Barnett, 2004) - where the functioning core represents either the Western societies or those fully embracing Western sets of values. The non-integrating gap consists, on the other hand, of states in social or economical disarray or disintegration. Although Barnett's division may be viewed as a Westerner's condescending view of the impoverished and struggling nations, it is also true. The chasm separating the core and the gap is seen with particular clarity in the access to one of the most basic human rights – health and its maintenance (WHO, 1946).

While the Western nations (e.g., European Union, USA) make giant steps toward the widest access to highest possible quality of healthcare to all citizens (European Institute of Medicine, 2003; National Coalition on Healthcare, 2004), within the "gap" even rudimentary services are often non-existent (Akhtar, 1991; Gesler, 1983). Thus, in 1983, among the developed countries (such as US, UK, France, Japan, etc.) there were, on the average, 19 physicians per 10.000 people. In Mexico, the number fell to seven, while in Tunisia there were only 3 physicians serving the population of 10,000 people (Gesler, 1983). Statistically, in several African countries the number is less than one (Gesler, 1983). Most importantly, twenty years later, the situation has not improved (Chen et al., 2004; Scheffler et al., 2008).

Per capita expenditure on healthcare is not the best indicator of money spent on actual maintenance of health. The average expenditure in the EU is about 50% less than in the US, yet, compared to their US counterparts, the Europeans appear to receive equal if not better quality of care (World Health Organization Report, 2000; 2004). However, the differences in the healthcare expenditure between the richest countries and the rest of the world may still provide a striking measure of the existing disparities in the level of healthcare available to citizens of individual countries of the globe: in 2001 the United States spent nearly $ 4,900 per person while Mexico spent only $ 370. Mali could afford only $ 12. (World Health Organization Report, 2004, see also Abel Smith, 1989). In the end, there are only so many syringes or typhus vaccines that can be obtained for 12 instead nearly 5.000 dollars!

The significance of these figures becomes alarming when seen in the context of mortality rates caused by "common illnesses" such as cardiovascular diseases (CVD). For a very long time the latter have been associated with the affluent lifestyle of Western societies. Yet, a recent study showed that in India and South Africa (countries approximately at the middle of the healthcare expenditure list – see WHO, 2004) CVD-mortality rates are vastly higher than in the West, and nearly identical to those seen in the US thirty years ago, i.e., prior to the development of effective means of treatment (Leeder et al., 2004). Hart's observation (1995) that increasing demand for healthcare is accompanied by proportionately fewer resources available to provide such care becomes increasingly ominous since rapidly growing evidence indicates that diseases affect nations not only by forcing them to spend money on their elimination, but also by reducing productivity, i.e., their gross national product (World Health Organization Report, 2004; Leeder et al., 2007; Hart, 1995). Countries belonging to the "Gap." Feel this impact most strongly.

Recent outbreaks of potentially pandemic diseases such as SARS, or avian and swine influenza demonstrated that diseases other than AIDS, malaria, or tuberculosis may have devastating economical consequences across the world globe (Lee et al, 2003; Lee and McKibbin, 2003; Economist, 2003). Unsurprisingly, the members of the World Economic Forum stressed that health will not only have a major impact on the future of business but also on global security (World Economic forum, 2002; Evans, 1993). However, the threat is far greater than the regional destabilization and the related social unrest posed by, for example, HIV/AIDS. Many of the diseases currently seen as major candidates for bioterrorism applications are endemic in the countries of the "non-integrating gap" (Barnett (2004) characterized by the combination of poverty, poor healthcare, and politico/economical instability. That combination of socio-economic factors also serves as the natural breeding substrate for political attitudes and sentiments that ultimately manifest in regional conflicts and global terrorism (Barnett, 2004). In other words, addressing problems posed by inadequacy of global healthcare becomes the issue of survival rather than the subject of largely inefficient and rather sentimental philanthropic attitudes projected traditionally by the Western countries at the impoverished world.

THE MEDICI EFFECT

In 2006 Frans Johansson published "The Medici Effect," a book in which he described the inspiring effect created by the confluence of several outwardly independent developments – the point of intersection of ideas – from which new, often path-breaking concepts emerge and cause dramatic changes both in our perception of the surrounding world, and the manner we interact with it (Johansson, 2006).

In healthcare, a number of originally widely disparate ideas entered the confluence stage at the transition of the 20th and 21st centuries. First to arrive was the inescapable realization that global healthcare entered the crisis state. To counterbalance the mounting and seemingly unsolvable problems associated with the rapidly approaching catastrophe, it has been proposed that a comprehensive "systems approach" be used as the foundation for any realistic solution. Importantly, the proposed approach offered the opportunity for a comprehensive approach to the wide range of present and future healthcare issues rather than, as it has been done so far, the intense concentration of effort on the consequences created by a specific illness at the expense of all other equally critical concerns (Akhtar, 1991). Ultimately, the governments and political bodies of both European Union and of the United States came to view the "systems approach" as the only viable option (National Coalition on Healthcare, 2004; European Institute of Medicine, 2003; Kyprianou, 2005). Unfortunately, one of the primary consequences of the emphasis on the systems approach to healthcare was not the readily perceptible improvement of healthcare in either region. Instead, there was an unprecedented expansion of healthcare-related industries whose growth was stimulated by the immense intricacy and range of tasks demanded by the selected approach (Frost & Sullivan, 2004; Plunkett, 2004; OECD, 2004).

As a measure of both addressing these tasks, and also in order to contain the explosive escalation of fiscal demands posed by the enhanced tempo of healthcare operations, growing emphasis has been placed on information, computer, and communication technologies (IC^2T) as the most effective means to reduce costs and increase operational efficiency (e.g., European Institute of Medicine, 2003; National Coalition on Healthcare, 2004). Consequently, the second half of the 1990ies witnessed the unparalleled emergence of completely new concepts based on the widely available access to the Internet and the World-Wide-Web. E-commerce, banking, and governmental operations became readily recognizable, "household" terms whose enthusiastic practical implementation resulted in the exceptional growth of individual and organizational wealth. Globalization became an inescapable fact of daily life (Rifkin, 2001). The reliable, accessible, and continuously improving IC^2T operations necessitated by the outburst of e-world provided the second element of the emerging confluence (von Lubitz et al., 2002).

The third element has been furnished by the dramatic changes in biomedical research, the majority of which has been greatly stimulated by the advances in molecular biology, pharmacology, and the new insights into pathological processes consequent to the Human Genome Project (e.g., Rifkin, 1998; Shostak, 1999; Collins and McKusick, 2001). New fields of medical research emerged (e.g., genomics, proteomics, molecular drug design, etc.), and the need to analyze the vast numbers of data generated by these disciplines created demand for new computing techniques. By the beginning of the 21st century, grid computing entered the healthcare intersection point as the only viable means of addressing the increasingly larger computational requirements made by the revolution in biomedicine (Braverman, 2004).

GRID COMPUTING IN HEALTHCARE OPERATIONS

The European Project SHARE (Olive et al. 2008a) defines grid as "A fully distributed, dynamically reconfigurable, and autonomous infrastructure to provide location independent, pervasive, reliable, secure and efficient access to a coordinated set of services encapsulating and virtualising resources" (Olive et al, 2008a, p. 31). In essence, the computer grid is thus nothing else but a complex technology platform which "offers rapid computation, large scale data storage and flexible collaboration by harnessing together the large number of computers or clusters of other basic machines. The grid was devised for use in scientific fields, such as particle physics and bioinformatics, in which large volumes of data, or very rapid processing, or both, are necessary" (Olive et al., 2008, p.9; see also Olive et al., 2007). It is also envisioned that grid computing will rapidly expand beyond computationally-heavy arenas of physics and biomedicine, and find intense applications throughout the entire range of healthcare – from molecular biomedicine to epidemiology at the level of world-wide populations (The Healthgrid White Paper, 2005; Hernandez and Blanquer, 2005.)

Although successfully used in several disciplines (e.g., Foster and Kesselman, 2003, see also Table 1), the uses of grid computing remain largely experimental, and, in the context of healthcare applications, continue to be considered predominantly in the context of computationally-intense fields such as bioinformatics, bio-system modeling, molecular pharmacology and drug discovery (e.g., Claus and Johnson, 2008; Coveney and Fowler, 2005;; Gillet et al., 2004). Moreover, and in similarity to other pathbreaking concepts in information technology (e.g., virtual reality), a certain degree of confusion exists among a wide range of commercial users as to what *really* constitutes grid computing (Gillet et al., 2004).

In the realm of science, grid computing is the equivalent of clustered computing (as, for example presented by the European EEGE Enabling Grids for EsciencE, (see http://project.eu-egee.org/index.php?id=104). Outside the world of scientific applications, the definitions vary from the one provided above to a synonym for utility computing in which individual results generated by individual machines are pooled into a comprehensive and comprehendible body of information at the output stage of the process.

The very broad span of existing perceptions on the nature of grid computing may have a very significant bearing on the equally wide range of its healthcare applications: the meaning and significance of the concept may be entirely different to a molecular scientist and to a health insurance executive. Thus, despite the belief that grid computing provides a very powerful technology permitting interdisciplinary efficiency withhin the *obvious* territory of healthcare (Olive et al., 2007), the diverging views of what grid computing is, and what it is capable of, may also provide significant barrier to establishing wide ranging collaborative efforts within the "*domain of domains*" of healthcare comprising several widely disparate domains

Table 1. Currently prevailing applications of grid computing

Field	Application
Healthcare and medical sciences	Genomics and proteomics Molecular modeling Drug discovery Disease modeling Physiological modeling Complex visualization and medical imagery Epidemiology and public health Education Financial forecasting
Science and Engineering	Biotechnology (non-medical) Geology Physics Astronomy Complex modeling (e.g. biosystems) Chemisty Collaborative engineering CAD/CAM design Aerospace Education
Business	Financial analysis and modeling Financial services Large scale insurance operations Management of complex enterprises Supply chains management Data/information/knowledge sharing Worldwide distribution and logistics operations
Military	Resource allocation Intelligence operations Human-robotics interaction Command and control

and their individual sub-fields and disciplines (von Lubitz and Wickramasinghe, 2006a).

Interdisciplinary collaboration that grid computing is expected to facilitate is greatly complicated by the current incompatibility of the numerous individual databases and analytical methods even within individual disciplines, and also by the absence of broadly accepted standards (Galperin, 2005; 2008). In 2006, Radetzki et al. stressed the urgent need for "adapters, shims, and glue" as the solution to interoperability difficulties that affect biomedical experiments involving grid-derived techniques and manipulation.

The magnitude of the already felt setbacks poised by standardization increases significantly when several disciplines must be put together "under the same roof" to act as a concerted entity generating universally valid, and operationally useful and reliable outputs. E-health represents the perfect example of such "transboundary complexity" (Bescos et al., 2005; Hernandez and Blanquer, 2005; see also Blanquer et al., 2008). Unsurprisingly, with the promise held by grid computing in biomedical research (and research in other domains as well), solutions to problems of interoperability are sought very actively (e.g., Oliveira et al, 2005; Radetzky et al., 2006; Benkner et al., 2007; Saltz et al., 2008; BioMoby Consortium, 2008; Oster et al., 2008). Yet, because a number of different approaches have been proposed, it remains to be seen whether one will be selected as a fairly universal standard or, as it happened in the past, individual healthcare sub-fields will choose standards that are most suitable only to the demands and peculiarities of each individual discipline and without further attention to the need for inter-disciplinary collaboration. The latter choice continues to be the bane of the relatively uncomplicated issue of the electronic patient issue that continues to delay widespread implementation of this and similar healthcare tools (von Lubitz and Wickramasinghe, 2006a).

Several authors continue to draw attention to the persistently retarding impact of missing universal standards on the implementation of cross-domain grid computing as a tool in collaborative, broad-scope approaches to national and international healthcare (Hubbard, 2002; Karasavvas et al., 2004; Bartocci et al., 2007). With the problems of integration and standardization growing in importance, it appears that the implementation of grid computing in healthcare arrived at the crossroads of either following the hide-bound traditional approaches that proved to be ineffective, or seeking a dramatic departure from the old mentality of mundane, task-specific applications of extraordinarily powerful technologies. In order to make such departure, a much greater degree of inter- and trans-disciplinary cooperation and collaboration is needed.

However, if worst comes to worst, and the choice of discipline-specific standards prevails again despite the growing need for integration and collaboration, a new set of middleware linking individual domains will need to be developed. Problems of reliability, adaptability, and conformity of such middleware with both future and legacy platforms are certain to emerge. In the end, considering the prevailing, commercially driven "platform-centric" mentality of healthcare (von Lubitz and Wickramasinghe, 2006a), the ensuing difficulties will add another layer of complexity to the already tangled field. In the subsequent fray, the beneficiaries of loudly touted technologies will not be the patients, but vendors supplying "untangling technologies" and the costs of healthcare will continue to creep upwards.

Probably the least recognized yet very significant concern associated with grid computing is the user's level of comfort among ground-level healthcare practitioner/providers. Commonly endowed with only average degree of computer literacy, personnel involved in delivery of healthcare may have major difficulties in interacting with the increasingly complex operational environment of the grid (Kalawsky et. al, 2005; Shefter SM, 2006; Ward et al., 2008). Although implementation of user-transparent portals has been proposed (Andronico et al., 2005; Aloisio et al., 2005; Ichikawa et al., 2005; see also Neerincx and Leunissen, 2005), the continuing problems with higher level computer literacy and skills among healthcare personnel both in the UK and US (Devitt and Murphy, 2004; Lacher et al., 2000), the intimacy between healthcare practitioners and "the grid" may still be quite far away. As an interim remedy, a new class of professionals – the human "grid-user interfaces" – may need to be created. Neither the problem nor its solution are without precedent in medicine where the analysis and interpretation of complex clinical trials relies heavily on professional statisticians. However, even in the most advanced countries, the need to educate a new generation of specialists familiar with both grid computing and a considerable range of healthcare-related disciplines will slow down the emergence of grid computing as an inter-domain collaborative platform even further.

With healthcare plight most intense among Less Developed Countries (LDCs), the problem of wide availability of healthcare-relevant grid computing within a foreseeable future becomes near-unsolvable. The problem is exacerbated by the fact that among most LDCs computer literacy becomes a secondary issue to the banal, and yet still unaddressed issue of computer availability (Blignaut, 1999; Bello et al., 2004; Callen et al., 2007; Eddirippulige et al., 2007). An interesting, even if only partial solution to the dilemma has been offered by Kalawsky et al. (2005), who proposed a PDA interface as the entry point into the grid. The combination of a relatively simple PDA, ASP (Application Software Provider) philosophy with wireless access to the Internet may be of particular interest in the remote/underdeveloped regions where, even with continuing "computer starvation," the presence of reliable wireless networks rapidly increases (von Lubitz and Patricelli, 2006,2008; von Lubitz et al., 2006).

Regardless of numerous and often quite spainful problems, there is no doubt that grid computing opened new and exciting horizons in several domains of science, and that biomedical research (particularly bioinformatics) is among the principal beneficiaries (von Lubitz and Wickramasinghe, 2006b). The combination of immersive virtual reality (VR), agent-based modeling (ABM), and grid computing necessary to handle very large volumes of data required by high quality real time visual outputs have been proposed as the ideal technology envelopes in neurological disease modeling, and as complex disease management and skills training systems already in the mid-nineties (Griffiths et al., 2000). Few years later, a pioneering project combining simultaneous application of grid computing, VR, ABM, and human patient simulation has been implemented in a practical *in silico* approach to pathophysiology studies of extensive burns, development of novel forms of treatment, and at providing an advanced clinical decision making and skills training platform for the acute management of such burns (von Lubitz et al., 2001, see also Beier et al., 2001). Recently, several authors suggested grid computing as a sole-platform driver (without simultaneous integration with other methods and technologies such as VR, IM/KM tools, etc.) of simulation training systems that will develop and enhance management skills of HIV infections, and cardiac and cerebrovascular disorders (Alonso et al., 2008; Sloot et al., 2008; Sadiq et al., 2008).

Despite extraordinarily broad scope of current and potential uses, one must bear in mind that grid computing represents a *technology platform*. As such, and in similarity to all other technology platforms, grid computing is associated with a number of already mentioned limitations (e.g., interoperability, standardization, and integration).

Paradoxically, the extreme application flexibility of grid computing constitutes another limiting factor. It is because of that flexibility that the present applications of grid computing are both very wide-ranging and highly domain-specific (e.g., particle physics, bioinformatics, drug discovery). Hence, the development of grid computing as a practical tool is at its most vigorous in specific areas where the need for rapid computational analysis of vast data sets is essential. Consequently, despite the best intentions most of even collaborative endeavours based on grid computing are still discipline-centered, while much of the information of significance to a broader healthcare community continues to be disseminated in the traditional form of publications, lectures, and university level training. At the moment, from the perspective of healthcare as a "*domain of domains*" (which is emphatically different from healthcare-relevant *discipline* perspective), grid computing is an extraordinarily powerful information management (IM), but only a relatively weak (at best) knowledge management tool (KM).

Finally, and that will surely change with time, grid computing of today is best described by the part of its own name – "grid." It is essentially a two dimensional, highly capable and potent IM platform (Figure 1) which allows execution of tasks that have been hitherto either impossible or unrealistically time consuming, and whose outputs generate new *germane knowledge* (von Lubitz and Wickramasinghe, 2006c; Wickramasinghe and von Lubitz, 2007) at the *intra-domain* level. As an inter-domain tool, grid computing offers rich and significant *actionable information* outputs, but only a very limited *inter-domain* content of *actionable knowledge* (von Lubitz et al., 2008a). Moreover, as currently practiced, grid computing does not allow the development of *real time operational awareness*. Its primary targets are semi-static environments characterized by vast amounts of raw data whose processing and analysis need not be performed *while the data are generated*, and the outputs of such analyses need *not* be concurrently correlated with outputs of simultaneous analyses of several other, disparate data sets generated in parallel to all other ongoing processes. *Yet, it must be remembered that many major healthcare-related events (e.g., disaster and humanitarian operations, bioterrorism, pandemics) center on situations that require simultaneous analysis, correlation, and synthesis of physically much smaller but numerous, largely unrelated, and rapidly changing and heterogenous data/information sets and subsets into a single, coherent stream of actionable knowledge of frequently critical importance for the overall success of the mission* (von Lubitz 2008, von Lubitz and Wickramasinghe, 2006c; von Lubitz et al., 2008a,b).

In response to these problems, the concept of network-centric healthcare operations has been proposed (von Lubitz and Wickramasinghe, 2006a) and elaborated in a series of subsequent papers (von Lubitz and Wickramasinghe, 2006b,c.d; von Lubitz et al., 2006; von Lubitz and Patricelli, 2006, 2008; von Lubitz et al., 2008a,b,c)

NETWORKCENTRIC OPERATIONS

The notion of networks as the informational backbone for complex, time-dependent operations performed in unpredictably evolving environments is not new. The brain-child of the late Vice Admiral Cebrowski, USN, the concept of network-centric warfare was created and developed several years ago by a group of scientists at the US Department of Defense (DoD; see Alberts et al., 2000, 2001), rapidly becoming one of the cornerstones of the transformation philosophy embraced by the US DoD (Garstka, 2004) and a number of military establishments in Europe and Asia (Boyd et al., 2005; Haine, 2005; Jonas 2005).

The civilian applications of network-centricity differ in several important aspects from the original concept developed and presented by Admiral Cebrowski in the late 90ies (Cebrowski and Garstka, 1998). The definition of civilian network-centric operations has been provided nearly a decade after the concept has been extensively implemented by the armed forces of the US and NATO (von Lubitz and Wickramasinghe, 2006a). Accordingly to that definition, network-centric healthcare operations allow timely, unfettered sharing of data, information, and knowledge among applications, platforms, and users that is independent of time, technology, and user boundaries and distance, and that results in improved situational awareness, significant reduction of decision-making cycles, and increased operational efficiency.

The concept of network-centricity evolved into two parallel approaches: the *Doctrine of Network-centric Warfare* (DNW, e.g., Wilson C, 2004, also known as *Network-centric Warfare*, or NCW) and *Network Enabled Capability* (NEC, see NATO, 2005). The differences between the two approaches are quite significant (Table 2), and provide insight in the way network-centricity is deployed operationally.

Contrary to the overall "driving" role of the network-centric doctrine, NEC (also known as Network Enabled Operations - NEO) constitutes the *enabler* of effects-based operations both at the level of command and control, and at the level of operational capability. The NEC concept may be, therefore, more adaptable to the specific conditions of large scale national, international, and multinational healthcare (and other civilian activities) in which a multitude of frequently uncoordinated and disorganized governmental, nongovernmental, private, and academic actors must collaborate within the same operational environment.

Prodrome: the period of routine operations prior to the critical event

Figure 1. Schematic representation of a computing grid. Accessible through increasingly "user-friendly" portals, and consisting of a wide array of computing and information management resources which can be simultaneously engaged in addressing a single, computationally exceptionally complex or time-critical task, the grid offers a platform allowing rapid execution of missions that, until recently, posed nearly insurmountable challenges in several disciplines (e.g., bioinformatics, particle physics, complex real time modeling and visualization.) However, the actionable knowledge generated through the application of computing grids is directed predominantly into the grid-associated knowledge management resource systems. "Mission-critical" for the disciplines that employ grid computing routinely (e.g., bioinformatics.), the generated actionable knowledge for the most part inaccessible to disciplines less dependent on grid computing (e.g., clinical aspects of healthcare.) The problem is the consequence of either extreme specialization (e.g., genome analysis) or discipline isolation (e.g., fiscal operations vs. clinical delivery of healthcare). However, it must be remembered that actionable information resulting from applications of grid computing in disciplines such as drug discovery or genome analysis represents an increasingly important downstream input in a wide variety of healthcare operations.

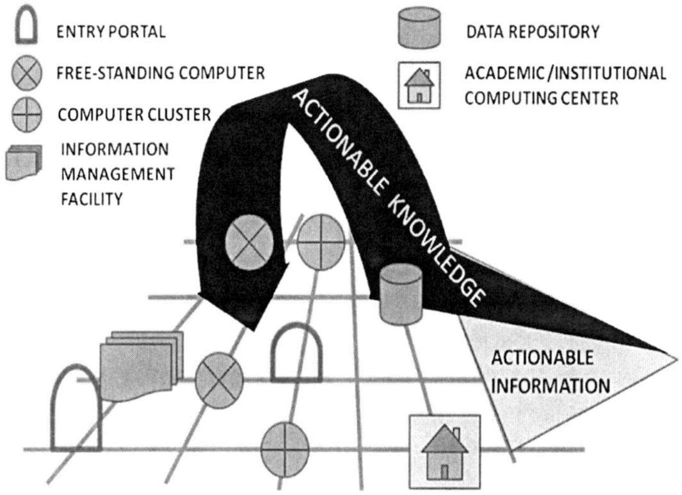

Table 2. differences between the doctrine of network-centric warfare and network enabled capability concepts (after von Lubitz et al., 2008b)

ELEMENT	NCW	NFC
PHILOSOPHY	Doctrine	Gradual improvement of effectiveness among actor aggregates
NETWORK	Primary driver	Enable
RESOURCE ROLE	Resource driven	Resource dependent
DEVELOPMENT	Planned, structured *de-novo* development of required technologies	Networking existing, constituent operational entities into a "super system"
APPLICABILITY	Warfare only	National, International, and Multinational Healthcare operations; Operations Other Than War (OOTW), disaster management; complex multidisciplinary research; civilian business and logistics

Critical event: Triggering episode (incident) whose consequences affect the entire spectrum of operations.

Recovery: the period after the critical event during which the intensity of all operations returns to their prodrome level

*) Event has a benign nature, and its consequences evolve over a longer period of time, e.g., policy changes, emergence of new morbidity and mortality trends, etc. Threat represents a significantly destabilizing event whose rapid evolution may result in catastrophic consequences (e.g., a pandemic disease, approach of a major hurricane, bioterrorism incident, or unforeseen highly adverse side effects of a newly released drug.)

**) During a critical event stage, NEC may assist in accelerated detection and elimination of threats secondary to the main event

***) While NEC will not be useful in detecting the criticality (magnitude) of an earthquake that will take place within reasonable future and, hence, in will not be useful to determine the associated demand for healthcare services, it may assist in developing responses appropriate and adequate to counter the consequences of an earthquake of any magnitude. However, NEC may be instrumental in reducing the potential threat of, for example, a pandemic disease by assisting the development of processes that enhancing surveillance, containment, and response measures.

By providing integrated retrieval, assessment, management, and distribution of data, information, and knowledge (von Lubitz and Wickramasinghe, 2006d) NEC becomes an essential tool in detection of potential threats and vulnerabilities (NATO, 2005; Jonas, 2005; von Lubitz et al., 2008a,b)

Major, particularly international and multinational, healthcare operations involving a wide range of actors, policies, and needs are conducted in the atmosphere largely incompatible strategies based on incompatible operational principles and plans, the latter resulting from frequently divergent or conflicting interests, non-integrated data/information sharing mechanisms, and disparate telecommunication platforms. The operational implementation of NEC reduces friction by offering is associated with a series of distinct preventive, detection, and correction measures (Table 3).that difficult to attain through application of other technological platforms.

The existence of robust information/knowledge management operations and telecommunication systems providing the backbone of business operations in the rapidly evolving "knowledge-based economy" provides the essential building blocks for the development of healthcare-centered NEC. In practical application, NEC consists of a mesh of grids (Boyd et al., 2005, see also Figure 2), each associated with a number of information collecting/processing/and disseminating nodes (von Lubitz and Wickramasinghe, 2006a; von

Table 3. Operational advantages of NEC in large-scale healthcare operations (after von Lubitz et al., 2008b)

ACTION TYPE	PRODROME	CRITICAL EVENT	RECOVERY
Risk Avoidance	Major impact	Some impact	Minimal impact
Event/threat detection*)	Major impact	Some impact**)	No impact
Reduction of event/threat/occurrence/intensity	Major impact	Some impact	Minimal impact
Reduction of vulnerability	Major impact	Some impact	Significant impact
Asset allocation/logistics	Major impact	Major impact	Major impact
Reduction of criticality	Contextual***)	Contextual	No impact
Recovery	Major impact	No impact	Major Impact

Lubitz and Patricelli, 2006, 2008) capable of integrating intra-domain information with the relevant information derived from inter-domain, and even seemingly mission-unrelated sources (Boyd 1987, von Lubitz and Wickramasinghe, 2006a).

Walmart, Inc. was the first civilian US organization to pioneer practical applications of network-centric principles (Cebrowski and Garstka, 1998). Unfortunately, like with many other pathbreaking ideas (including grid-computing), acceptance of network-centricity by the world of business led almost inevitably to its rapid trivialization. The meaningless slogan that emerged conveys nothing but a pedestrian and common-sense driven collaborative use of the already well-functioning information and knowledge management network systems (e.g., Chang, 2007). There is nothing new in such approach: the Europeans have been extensively and successfully employing the combined information and data networks for well over a decade (Rifkin, 2005).

As originally intended by the creators of the concept (e.g., Cebrowski and Garstka, 1998), the output of network-centric activities is aimed at improving coherent and coordinated operational command and control of very complex activities addressing time and space critical problems. The *actionable knowledge* generated through network-centric activities is based on mission-specific

Figure 2. Schematic representation of the network-centric mesh. The mesh consists of several intra- and interdisciplinary, closely coupled non-hierarchical networks (A,B,C,D) each associated with wide range of nodes. A node can be an individual as much as a team of task-centered individuals, or an organization. The node provides data/information/knowledge inputs into the mesh, perform analyses of data and information (e.g., a computing grid), and/or deliver actionable knowledge based on such analyses. Access portal can also constitute a node (see von Lubitz and Wickramasinghe, 2006d). Note that one of the nodes in the figure contains its own virtual organization (VO). Net-centricity assures unfettered, multidirectional flow of information and tacit, explicit, and germane knowledge (arrows within the mesh) and provides multidirectional outputs available to all users (for a detailed analysis of the civilian network-centric concept and network-enabled capabilities see von Lubitz and Wickramasinghe 2006a, and von Lubitz at al. 2008a,b).

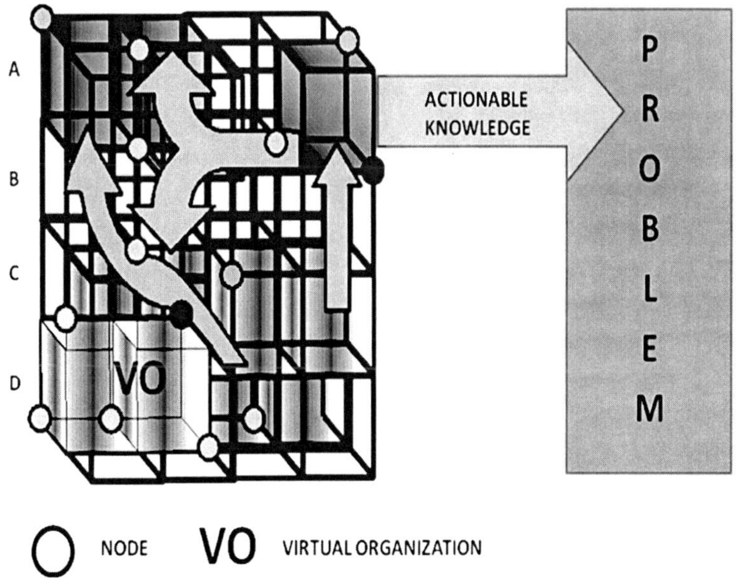

(information and knowledge) and mission-related (directly and indirectly).outputs generated by all individual sub-components of the network. The collaborative action of intra- and inter-domain links reduce "information granularity" (e.g., ESRI; von Lubitz et al., 2008b) by enhancing the quality and reliability of the generated actionable knowledge. The principal *functional* attribute of network-centricity is therefore the nature of output *which is directed at specific operations* rather than at the generation of *strategy*. It is, however, the latter that defines the nature, scope, sequence, and execution (often concurrent) of *all* operations whose successful implementation leads, in turn, to the attainment of the sought objective.

In similarity to implementation of the Doctrine of Network-centric Warfare (DNW) within national defense establishments, introduction of NEC in healthcare will require significant changes in the current culture of operations and their administration at practically all levels. At present, extensive fragmentation of functions and procedures both within the same agency (e.g., US Department of Health and Human Services or the European Directorate General for Health and Consumers) and among several agencies of the US Federal and State Administration (or, in the case of EU – member state bureaucracies) combine with intra and inter-agency rivalries for political and operational significance, Such fragmentation of roles and missions may be among the principal underlying causes for the spectacular inefficiency in preparation for major disasters and their subsequent consequence management (Rosenthal et al., 1995; Cooper and Block, 2006; Rubin, 2008). Hence, NEC-based operations may provide an important tool in the transition from hierarchical to adaptive management philosophy needed to assure collaborative and flexible responses to the present and forthcoming healthcare challenges, major disasters, etc. (Wiese, 2006; see also Rifkin, 2005).

In summary, when considered from the perspective of the definition of network-centric (or network enabled) operations, grid computing constitutes a very important sub-component of a much larger conceptual entity. The actions of the latter are enabled by the intense cross-platform and cross-discipline/domain links based on unhindered up-, down, and lateral exchanges of data, information, and knowledge (von Lubitz and Wickramasinghe, 2006d) supported by a redundant, disruption-resilient, and platform-independent telecommunication framework (von Lubitz et al., 2006b; von Lubitz and Patricelli, 2008).

Contrary to the original definition by the authors of the concept (e.g., Cebrowski and Garstka, 1998), civilian network-centric operations are based on a system of systems, a mesh of tightly collaborating, multi-platform and multi-domain grids, rather than a stack of relatively loosely interconnected hierarchical grids. The mesh facilitates maximum flexibility and maximum actionable knowledge generation (von Lubitz et al., 2008a,b) that is required by a particular mission or a set of missions.

Under ideal circumstances, all actors embedded in the mesh have equal status and equal access to all inputs and outputs generated by the assembly of all nodes within the mesh (Figure 2). In reality, however, network-centric operations emerged as a hierarchical system of grids in which information is passed in a bottom-up flow, converted at the topmost layers into actionable knowledge, then distributed in form of standard operational practices, doctrines, rules, and regulations in a top-bottom direction. Moreover, in the current practice, network-centric operations continue to be domain-related. Unsurprisingly, the generated actionable knowledge affects only those at whom it is directly aimed. Those for whom such knowledge would be *pertinent and germane* (von Lubitz and Wickramasinghe, 2006e) but who are outside output distribution of the network remain unaware that such knowledge exists. As the costly brush with SARS showed, in the increasingly complex and volatile environment of global healthcare, such lack of awareness may lead to catastrophic downstream consequences that will affect practically all other activities (e.g., Day et al., 2004).

Despite all deficiencies, network-centricity offers an important advantage during operations conducted in dynamic environments characterized by high complexity and unpredictability, potentially rapid evolution cycles, and large number of hierarchic and non-hierarchic actors. Healthcare unquestionably belongs in such category. Consequently, the fast pace of the conducted activities demands that in order to be efficient the rate of OODA Loop revolutions of each participating actor is suitable elevated (von Lubitz and Wickramasinghe 2006a, von Lubitz et al., 2008b).

THE OODA LOOP

Since its development over twenty years ago (Boyd, 1987), OODA Loop has been used as the quintessential "common sense" cognitive approach in medicine, business, warfighting, and crisis management (Wickramasinghe and von Lubitz, 2007). It provides the essential framework for information and knowledge-based, multidimensional critical thinking, and for rapid decision-making in complex, rapidly and unpredictably changing environments. Successful in such environments demands real time decisions followed by precise, focused actions whose execution. The latter may subsequently determine the future course and evolution of the entire environment within which all actions are are conducted (Richards, 2004). Hence, the quality of decisions made has paramount importance.

The concept of OODA Loop is based on a cycle (Loop) of four consecutive stages of Observation, Orientation, Decision, and Action (Figure 3)

During the *Observation Stage* information gathering takes place. Information is collected from all sources both *inside* and *outside* the operational environment. The *inside* inputs are based on pertinent, historical knowledge, and represent the "static" foundation of the Observation Stage. The inputs provided by the *unfolding circumstances* represent the latest, *real time* information. Information from *outside* sources represents all pertinent but *not necessarily immediately relevant* facts that need to be incorporated in order to produce a complete picture of the environment. The latter two types of information *must* be included into the decision-making process to make it situation-relevant. In essence, at the Observation Stage raw information is extracted from the operational environment then correlated with the historical knowledge and the ongoing stream of

Figure 3. The OODA Loop Sequence (Boyd, 1987; courtesy of the Estate of COL. John Boyd, USAF)

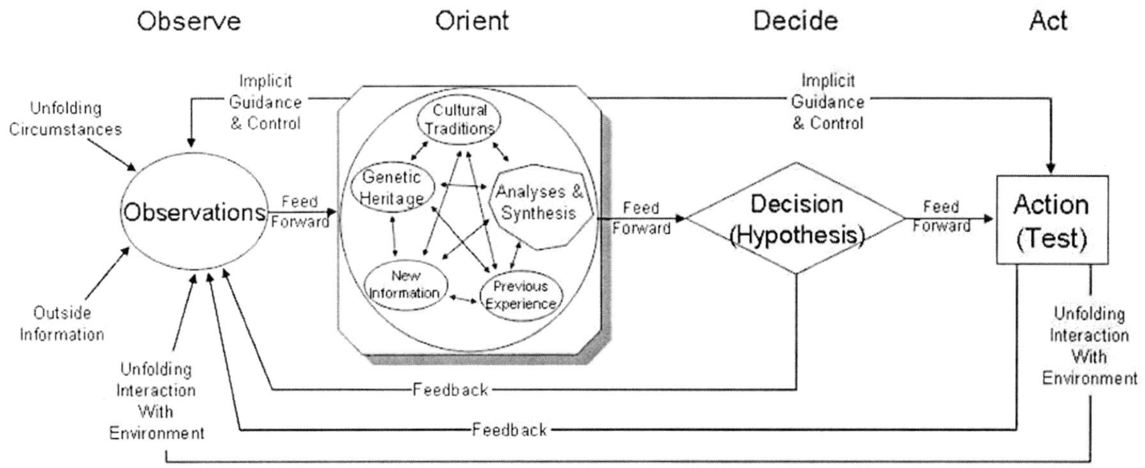

data. The analysis of information gathered at the Observation Stage provides *real time* characterization of the operational environment and contains all *current* events and actions taking place within that environment.

It is essential to remember that the breadth of information and knowledge gathered at the Observation stage is critical. Frequently, what appears unrelated or irrelevant may in reality be the crucial element that determines success or failure of all subsequent actions. Broad-based knowledge of several fields is therefore of utmost importance for a senior decision-makers and leaders (von Lubitz et al., 2005, 2008a)

Orientation Stage of the Loop is probably the most important: it shapes the course of the subsequent steps. At the Orientation Stage, information and knowledge gathered during the Observation step of the Loop are subject to final analysis. Grouping individual elements into coherent and cohesive blocks helps to precisely define larger volumes of the operational environment. Such definition allows accurate determination of the extent to which the contents of these blocks impact evolution of the entire environment. The purpose of the Orientation Stage is to establish *situational awareness* or *clarification* when the disorganized information pieces characterizing the environment are transformed into cohesive, easily recognizable elements, realigned, and transformed from prior chaos into a structure of increasingly greater familiarity. It is at that time the "center of thrust" (or "center of gravity") is determined. The center represents the point at which maximum effort needs to concentrate in order to assure maximum efficiency and effect of these efforts.

As Figure 3 indicates, the Observation Stage is affected by a number of intangible factors: experience, cultural background and heritage, analytical capability, etc., play a significant role. Objective and open-minded approach to all processes involved in the Orientation Stage is, therefore, critical to the success of all subsequent stages. Prejudice, disdain, narrow-mindedness, inflexibility, or perception of reality based on one's own subjective criteria can wreak havoc with one's strategy (Rosenthal et al., 2005; Lagadec, 2007).

Determination Stage defines action that is to be taken: its nature and form are firmly determined, the type of resources and their required concentration at the center of thrust (gravity) is established, and the resources are then allocated, and deployed. The Determination Stage defines the level of preparedness: *the availability (prepositioning) of all resources, both human and physical, necessary for the management of, or the consequences of, a specific event or event complex* (von Lubitz, 2008). At the Determination Stage, the preponderance of cognitive processes involved in the preceding stages is substituted by predominantly physical activities consisting of logistic preparation, reorientation and redistribution of physical resources and personnel, and the final, pre-action assessment of the operational environment. It is at this stage that the definitive *work-flow pattern* is finally constructed.

Action Stage concludes the full revolution of the Loop. At this stage the planned- and prepared-for action is executed. The execution must be swift, unwavering, and focused on the center of gravity. The rule of "*economy of force*" is dominant: *overwhelming* resources must be applied at the target of the main thrust. All other potential distracting elements or threats are countered by using minimum means necessary to contain them at the *status quo* level (the rule of *economy of force*.) Dissipation of strength at this stage may have catastrophic consequences on the sought outcome, and employment of limited and inadequate resources at the center of gravity is the most common reason for the subsequent failure (Gray, 2006)

The next revolution of the Loop starts with the termination of the Action phase: the Observation Stage of the following revolution begins. At this time, the consequences of all activities and actions performed during the preceding revolution are determined, correlated with whatever new information might be forthcoming, and the environment is described and characterized based on the totality of information now at hand. As can be seen, each preceding stage of the Loop has a direct bearing on the subsequent one until the final Action Stage is reached, action executed, and all activity aimed at the attainment of a specific task ("mission") ceases.

A common error made in the interpretation of the Loop is the assumption of its linearity. In fact, the Loop does not merely "roll" along the time axis - the stages within the Loop are simultaneous, delicately intertwined, and balanced. Action does not interrupt Observation, nor does Decision halt Orientation. The Loop is multidimensional, embraces not only time but all constituents of the environment. However, "shortening the Loop," i.e., reduction of time required to execute individual Stages is rewarded by a "tighter" Loop: its revolution rate increases. By the virtue of tightening the radius and enhancing the revolution rate one imposes *the tempo* of action necessary to retain initiative and dominance. The actor enhances his *control* of action and, therefore, of the environment in which this action is executed as well. Enhanced predictability and stability of the environment follow and the attainment of the pre-set goal becomes progressively easier and more assured.

Importantly, proper implementation of the Loop enhances the state of readiness: *the instantaneous ability to respond to a suddenly arising major crisis based on the immediately and locally available/ un-prepositioned and un-mobilized countermeasure resources* (von Lubitz, 2008). As such, Loop-based thinking provides the framework of particular importance in the development of *resilience*: the ability to predict, contain, and manage crises with speed and efficiency.

The Loop constitutes the cognitive work flow pattern, and as such represents the essential "human control" ingredient in both grid computing and in the "grid of grids" (or "mesh") of network-centric operations. It would appear, therefore, that the combined application of OODA Loop-based operational "work flows" and IM and KM based on the described technology platforms may offer an exceptionally powerful and near-universal methodology to address virtually every aspect of the increasingly ailing healthcare. After all, grid computing may offer unprecedented advantages in shortening both the Observation and Orientation segments of the Loop, while "mesh-based" operations will enhance the sampling within the operational environment. Theoretically at least, the result of such combination would be a substantial increase in the revolution rate and enhancement of the operational volume "encompassed" by the Loop.

Trivial as it sounds, the concept of "healthcare" does not represent a monolithic block, but serves as a loose descriptor of a vast range of disciplines ranging from molecular biology to politics whose joint output, the "effector pathway," is expected to offer and assure the benefit of the universal right upon which practically all nations of the globe agreed - the right to health. However, the complexity of tasks involved in converting this near-Nirvanatic vision into a reality demands participation of a vast number of actors – from individual scientists, healthcare providers, and administrators, to private and governmental organizations, their international associations, and global political bodies which, today, all act within their own domains, and, for the most part, not only independently of others but also without much mutual coordination (Frenk et al, 1997; Coulter and Ham, 2002). Unsurprisingly, actionable knowledge derived from the combined output of computing grids, network-centric operations, and OODA Loop-based activities is often *not even domain oriented* (e.g., facilitation of drug discovery process through application of grid computing) but *agency oriented* (e.g., individual laboratory, healthcare provider/insurance group, industry, regulatory agency, etc.) What follows is rather astounding: due to the significantly improved state of *actor-oriented actionable knowledge*, the efficiency of individual actors involved in healthcare hyper-domain may actually *decrease*. An example of this situation is provided by the paradox of increased drug discovery rate stimulated by the new insights offered by the combination of genome sciences and bioinformatics (Drews, 2000; Evans and McLeod, 2003) accompanied the corresponding decrease in the number of regulatory approvals for the clinical use of new drugs. The lower approval rate is caused to large degree by the enhanced awareness of the real and potential side effects resulting from the improved understanding of biological systems in turn facilitated by the very same technologies that helped to discover the new drugs in the first place (Associated Press 2007; FDA, 2004; Kola and Landis, 2004). Equally incongruously, the wealth of *discipline-specific* actionable knowledge has the potential for introducing *interdisciplinary* disconnect (Lindsay, 2005; Sams-Dodd, 2005) or even chaos – example from large scale healthcare operations associated with humanitarian and disaster relief provide probably the starkest example of the latter (Brennan and Nandy, 2001; Maresko, 2008; Silenas et al., 2008).

The preceding arguments point out a disturbing fact: despite the exponential growth in both power and capability of IM and KM, the "stove-pipe effect" that historically isolated individual disciplines from each other not only persists but may actually be on the increase. Despite our belief that technology may solve the issues of collaboration and cooperation, the existing evidence contradicts this belief particularly when very complex issues involving a large array of diverging disciplines or even domains are at stake. In the end, the creation of- and access to actionable knowledge appears not to be enough, and: in some situations it may be the source of additional discord or even chaos.

The trinity of "technology, processes, and people" has been the cornerstone of modern business thought for quite a long time (e.g., Littler et al., 1998; Fogg, 2003, Wickramasinghe and von Lubitz, 2007). Yet, as the preceding discussion indicates, even the most advanced healthcare-relevant technologies and processes appear to be wanting in several respects.

What about people then, and the need, possibly a desperate one, for the attainment of *actionable understanding* as the foundation for everything else? After all, the intended actions are to be performed in the "hyper-rich" and "hyper-turbulent" environment that is uniquely founded on the rapidly growing global need, and which is characterized by the simultaneous presence of a multitude of often incompatible local, national and international actors defined by disparate agendas, and subject to often conflicting rules, procedures, and professional, organizational or even national cultures. Is it then conceivable that that any measure of success through the development and implementation of meaningful and effective solutions to the current and forthcoming healthcare problems can be attained only through the closest cooperative effort of the involved people rather than even the most impressive technological *tour de force*?

TOL

Bradford and Brown (2008) introduced "actionable knowledge" as the final output of actions executed in the "Teams of Leaders" (ToL) environment. The origins of ToL can be traced to the entirely new demands faced by the US Army following the end of the Cold War. The expanded range and character of missions demanded a completely new readiness model which emphasized flexibility and deployment readiness, and incorporated the new realization that within the enlarged mission spectrum the performance of an individual soldier could lead to strategic consequences. Decisions made by the "man on the spot" had the potential to influence the fate of nations

To satisfy such unprecedented demands a new breed of soldier-leaders was needed: flexible, adaptable, versatile, and comfortable within the complex setting of Joint Interagency, Inter-government, Multinational (JIIM) operations (Bradford and Brown, 2008). In several aspects, the problems that affected the US Army are similar to the difficulties influencing large-scale healthcare operations of today. Organizational complexity, wide mission spectrum, the need for mission-centered cooperation of numerous local, national, and international agencies emphasize the need to change in order to address the mounting host of rapidly diversifying issues, while continuing simultaneous engagement in routine operations. The *status quo*.of the past ceased to serve in the "new" world torn by increasing disparities of economy, social unrest, and the ever growing threat of infectious diseases against which either limited or no defensive measures exist.

Conceptually, ToL is deceptively simple: centered on the active fusion of three elements consisting of advanced IM, KM and High Performing Leader Teams (HPLT, see Figure 4), it can be readily mistaken for a specialized social network serving a group of select professionals. The cardinal difference between such network and ToL, and one that also constitutes the prerequisite for the development of HPLT, is the shared foundation of *skills, knowledge, and attitudes* (SKA) which is, in turn, based on previously acquired appropriate and universally high-quality level of professional preparation of individual team members trained to *task, condition, and standard* (TCS), and able to demonstrate their mastery in practice and without prior warning.

In the case of the US Army, the training and performance proficiency requirements are developed and set by the Army's Training and Doctrine Command (TRADOC). In the civilian world of healthcare, similar standards are developed by schools of medicine and nursing, universities, research organizations, etc. These are, in turn, subject to identical or nearly identical accreditation requirements, peer reviews, and adherence to national and international standards of service (e.g., World Federation on Medical Education, 1998, 2000). Professions ancillary to healthcare are governed by rules that are practically indistinguishable from those governing the world of medicine and elaborated by the ongoing efforts Bologna and European Commissions aimed at defining universal standards of qualifications, quality of education and training (Bologna Declaration, 1999, European Commission, 2007), and of professional performance based on these.

Rigorous training that satisfies a defined set of metrics-based performance standards assures general uniformity of outcomes and of professional capability of the participants. It also assures the development of shared confidence in mutual professionalism and ability to act appropriately under a wide range of conditions. However, individual training is not sufficient during the process of Leader team development As indicated by several studies ((Gokhale, 1995; Cavalier and Klein, 1998; Lou, 2001), it must be supported by active and collaborative learning which promotes significantly improved critical thinking and task performance compared to the more traditional individual learning methods.

Team learning/training is not new to medicine (e.g., Salmoni and Gonzales, 2008; Wiecha and Barrie, 2002; Curran et al. 2008; see also Kyle and Murray, 2008). To assure

the required task performance to a predetermined task/condition/standard, the learning process is experiential rather than didactic, and involves routine exposure to sudden changes ("confounders") that assists in the development of appropriate flexibility and adaptability both by individuals and by the entire team (Brown 2002; Bradford and Brown, 2008; Kyle and Murray, 2008). The process has been pioneered and traditionally used as one of the cornerstones of professional education in medicine, nursing, etc. (e.g., Wong JG, 1996; Kyle and Murray, 2008), and results in the mastery of essential skills, knowledge, and the related mental and physical attributes that allow competent practical performance as much under the most routine

Figure 4. A High Performing Leader Team (HPLTs) may consist of individuals (I), organizations (O), and virtual organizations (VO). The latter may be created ad hoc by the team members as the means of addressing specialized aspects of the mission, or enter HPLT as already formed entities. The foundations of an HPLT are shared Skills, Knowledge, and Attitudes (SKAs) based on shared trust, vision, competence, and confidence. Competence is attained through rigorous education and training. Fully collaborative, purpose-oriented, and meaningful interactions among Team members are based on/facilitated by the extensive and platform-independent use of all available IT/IM/KM resources (depicted as three network-centric meshes) and lead to the rapid development of the final aspects of HPLT foundation: shared vision, and the rapidly generated, empowering sense of mutual trust and confidence. SKAs are necessary for the conversion of actionable knowledge possessed by individual team members into mission-oriented actionable understanding shared by all members of the team. In the process of that conversion, new pertinent knowledge is generated (von Lubitz and Wickramasinghe, 2006e) and fed back (bottom-up) into the world of network-centric meshes. There, it is converted into tacit and/or explicit knowledge, then distributed (top-bottom) either as such or as actionable information within the HPLT "universe." The entire process constitutes a closed loop of continuous, real time interactions and exchanges that are made possible only through the advent of powerful IT/IM/KM tools. The wide variety of high-level expertise characterizing HPLTs serves as the principal facilitator in access to, acquisition, and transformation of multi-domain information and knowledge into a unified, mission-relevant body of knowledge that supports generation of mission-oriented actionable understanding. The latter is the culminating output of the team.

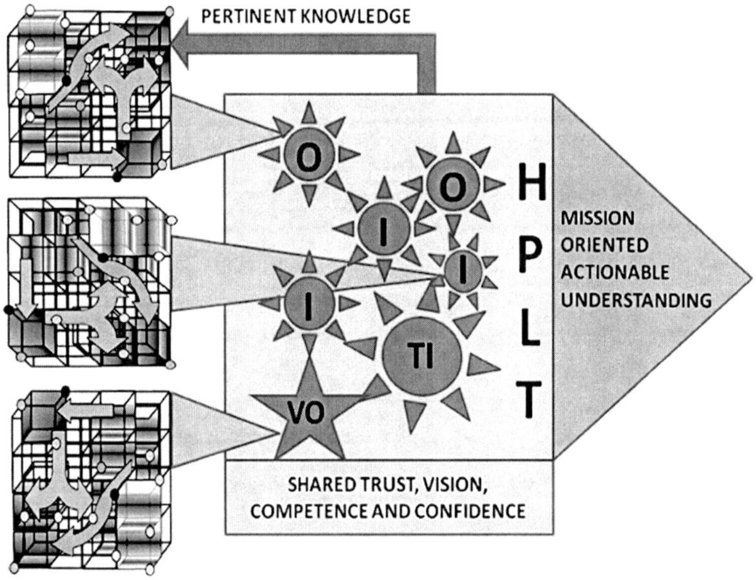

circumstances as under conditions of maximum stress, uncertainty, and speed of events.

Performance assessment under rigorous and highly demanding conditions constitutes the essential part of High Performing Leader Team development. Consequently, training turns into self-evaluation and evaluation promotes further training, a process through which teams attain pitch operational efficiency. Due to the standardized approach used in HPLT development, they can be inserted as "modular elements" whenever and wherever required. The "value added" component of such approach is the tacit "quality assurance": organizations, whether real or virtual, which co-opt HPLTs as part of their operational profile will have full confidence and trust in their deployed capabilities. The latter is of the greatest significance in the development of unit cohesion and effectiveness that serve in turn as the efficiency lubricant in multi-organizational efforts. It has been demonstrated on several occasions (e.g., McEntire, 1999; van Rooyen et al., 2001; Buck et al., 2006; Perry 2006) that absence of such trust and acceptance are among the primary reasons for several failures during complex humanitarian relief operations in which healthcare activities nearly always play a major role (van Rooyen et al., 2001; Noji, 2005; Silenas et al, 2008).

As noted above, the current applications of network-centric concept promote top-to-bottom distribution of knowledge (but see von Lubitz et al., 2008b) accompanied by the reverse direction of information flow. While accepted in hierarchically organized systems (e.g., the military or civilian governmental institutions), the approach impedes the development of new, actionable knowledge and may result in "stove-piping." The ToL concept circumvents the problem through the wide-ranging "horizontal spread" conducted via platform-independent peer-to-peer exchanges, social and professional networks, text- and visual blogs, avatars, etc., all of which are supported and expanded by the rapid maturation of Web 2.0 (Anderson, 2007).

Combined with the ready access to the primary information and knowledge sources such as WebMD, BMJ Portal, MDChoice, or CDC Portal and the web-based professional fora (e.g., NetDoc, DocGuide, or GlobalMedNet, see Table 4), the pervasive, system-wide use of IT promotes generation of *ad hoc* collaborative entities (teams). Such multi-talented teams are uniquely capable of addressing common problems, development of "just-in-time" solutions, and fostering creation of new knowledge and best practices. Their creativity is promoted by the fact that they operate in the environment free of constraints of time, space, organizational/inter-organizational cultures, and – most importantly – status and rank. The approach is based on the already well proven methods and techniques implemented by the US Army, the organization of great complexity, involved in a rapidly growing range of highly diversified missions (of which active combat constitutes only a comparatively small part). The success of these missions is contingent on cooperative interactions with other, equally complex civilian organizations at nationally, international, and global, multinational levels (e.g., EU, UN, WHO, see Dixon et al., 2005; Bradford and Brown, 2008))

The extensive use of IT, IM, and KM as the means of sharing information and knowledge has proven to be a powerful promoter of rapid development of shared vision, competence, confidence, and trust (Bradford and Brown, 2008, see Fig. 5), and the attainment of these attributes by members of the collaborating leader teams transforms those into High Performing Leader Teams. It is the activity of the latter that converts the previously top-down structure into a bottom-up/lateral knowledge and "best practices" generator. In the process of that conversion, the pervasive nature of the generated exchanges demolishes organizational barriers, promotes socialization, and fosters mutual confidence and trust among members of individual leader teams. As the cumulative result, Teams of Leaders emerge: the previously physically and/or organizationally isolated individuals and groups convert into "swarms" (Figure 5) which converge accordingly to the requirements of task and mission at hand. Operations of such swarms are increasingly recognized as essential for addressing problems affecting performance at the level of "domain of domains." Healthcare is one of those.

Throughout the course of transition from HPLT to ToL a less tangible but critical advantage emerges: people who previously had no knowledge of each other, who might have been separated by distance, institutional or specialty barriers begin

Table 4. Examples of international professional and general medical knowledge access portal

LANGUAGE	PROFESSIONAL	GENERAL
English	MedScape/WebMD http://www.medscape.com/medsapetoday Center for Disease Control http://www.cdc.gov National Institutes of Health http://nih.gov The Merck Manuals http://merck.com/mmpe/index.html MedicineOnline http://www.medicineonline.com	http://www.drkoop.com Wrong Diagnosis http://www.wrongdiagnosis.com Yahoo Health http://health.yahoo.com HealthCentral http://healthcentral.com CarleHealthgate http://carle.com/HealthGate/default.asp?id=Conditions HealthForum http://www.healthforum.org
French	Haute Autorité de Santé http://www.has-sante.fr/portail/jcms/j_5/ sitemap CISMeF http://www.chu-rouen.fr/cismefp/ Cadusee.net http://www.caducee.net L'association médicale franco-britannique http://www.anglofrenchmedical.org/ IRDES http://www.irdes.fr/ INSERM http://www.inserm.fr/fr/home.html Public Health Agency of Canada http://www.phac-aspc.gc.ca/chn-rcs/index- eng.php	CISMeF http://www.chu-rouen.fr/cismefp/ Heart and Stroke http://www.fmcoeur.com/ Haute Autorité de Santé http://www.has-sante.fr/portail/jcms/c_5071/grand- public?cid=c_5071 Guide Santé http://www.guidesante.gouv.qc.ca/fr/index.shtml
German	MedKnowledge http://www.medknowledge.de/	Gesundheit.com http://www.gesundheit.com/ Patienten-information.com http://www.patienten-information.de/ Medicine Worldwide http://www.onmeda.de/
Spanish	MedLinePlus http://medlineplus.gov/esp/ Merck Manual http://www.msd.es/publicaciones/ mmerck_ hogar/index.html AHRQ http://www.ahrq.gov/consumer/es- panoix.htm	Familydoxtor.org http://familydoctor.org/online/famdoces/ home.html Healthfinder.gov http://www.healthfinder.gov/espanol/

to rapidly form a network of close social relationships. Consequently, the development of collaborative spirit that often characterizes interactions between the local ambulance company and the emergency department of a county hospital can now emerge between, for example, emergency physicians and rescue personnel residing in two different parts of the country or in different countries. Actionable knowledge generated through network-centric activities that might have been shared between the two isolated groups (von Lubitz et al., 2008a) transforms through ToL-based interaction into "*actionable understanding*" (Bradford and Brown, 2008; Figure 6). The latter constitutes the essential prerogative for operational efficiency in the environments of uncertainty and rapid, unpredictable change characterizing responses to major disasters or rapidly escalating healthcare threats presented by pandemics or bioterrorism-related events (von Lubitz and

Figure 5. The Teams of Leaders concept (ToL). Individual, multi-, inter-, and trans-disciplinary HPLTs join into mission-oriented "swarms." Intense interactions both within and among individual HPLTs generate mutually shared actionable understanding – the foundation for the development of a joint strategy and the subsequent implementation of precise, focused ("effect-oriented"), and simultaneous operations. The goal of the latter (for which the state of actionable understanding is critical) is the comprehensive, stable, and long-range solution to problems affecting the "domain of domains" environment. Note that some of these solutions can be attained through direct application of actionable knowledge (topmost arrow, see von Lubitz et al., 2008 a,b).

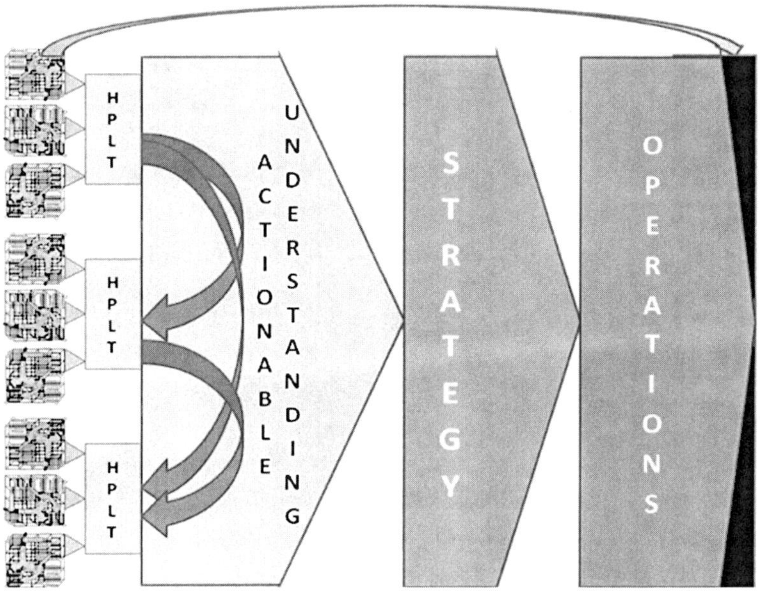

Wickramasinghe, 2006a; von Lubitz and Beakley in press). Circumstantial evidence indicates solid reasons to contend that the lack of such understanding was among the chief sources of errors in the response of national healthcare systems to, for example, the European heat wave of 2003 or Hurricane Katrina in 2005 (Bouchama, 2003; Ballester et al., 2003; Michelon et al., 2005; Cooper and Block, 2006).

As indicated above, the essential conceptual and structural elements such as the basic IT infrastructure, and information and knowledge bases required for the development of ToL already exist Others tools, such as robust, damage resilient IT infrastructure needed to accommodate both open and secure communications among individual subcomponents of healthcare operations are under intensive development (von Lubitz et al., 2006; von Lubitz and Patricelli, 2006; 2008). However, the widely dispersed nature of the existing knowledge repositories ancillary to the narrowly defined arena of healthcare (e.g., sociology, economics, security, military affairs, etc.) will require development of a consistent, "user friendly" format that is both standardized and integrated into the overall pool consistent with what is currently understood as "healthcare-relevant knowledge base." The new format will also need to allow for the intensive employment of decision support systems (DSS) and executive decision support (EDS) tools required for unhindered fusion of ancillary disciplines with the strictly healthcare-related ones (von Lubitz and Patricelli, 2006, 2008; Wickramasinghe and von Lubitz, 2007).

Figure 6. The maximum use of all IT/IM/KM resources combines with the intrinsic qualities of an HPLT and its intense interactions both within its internal environment and with the outside world of knowledge and expertise. The process generates unprecedented level of collaborative spirit and leads to generation of actionable understanding that plays the pivotal role in addressing fundamental problems emerging in highly complex and conflicted "domain of domains" environments such as healthcare. Effective solutions to highly specific "concept-centric" issues such as the development of drugs against specific disorders, (indicated in the figure by the bottom and top horizontal arrows) can be frequently solved by implementation of collaborative technology platforms.

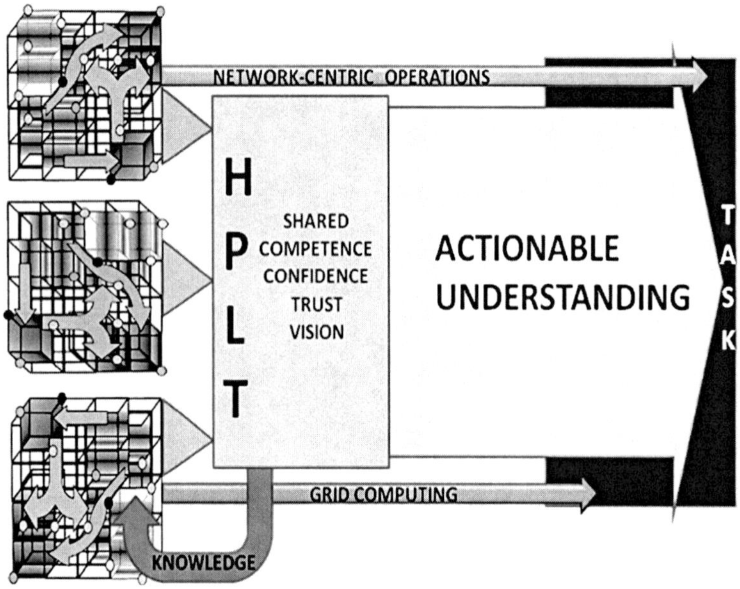

None of the required infrastructure modifications and improvements need to be either capital-heavy or labor intensive. Suitable "best practice" systems are either already in operations (e.g., Wickramasinghe and von Lubitz, 2007) or can be acquired at a significantly lesser cost than that associated with *de novo* development using national or international agency mechanisms (as seen in during implementing network-centricity by the US Department of Defense, e.g., Dianic, 2006). Most, importantly, even at the existing IT/IM/KM capacity, the implementation and practice of ToL concept in healthcare can be readily achieved due to the rapidly spreading use of the computing grids and network-enabled capabilities that employ with increasing efficiency the available data, information, and knowledge bases, and whose operations are supported by the essential social network platforms and reliable telecommunication backbones. Continuing advances in distributed learning and collaborative research suchas cloud computing and easily accessible avatar-based and virtual collaborative space environments make such introduction even easier (Redfern and Naughton, 2002; Kamel Boulos and Wheeler, 2007; Kamel Boulos et al., 2007; Martin and Hoover, 2008). On the non-technical side, standards of learning and of training evaluation similar to those currently practiced by the medical community will need to be developed for non-medical personnel. However, the principles of the existing medical model can be readily modified and adapted throughout the entire global healthcare system (Davis, 1998; ASME 2008; Ruiz et al., 2006)

The gains emerging from implementing ToL (Table 5) throughout the entire spectrum of

Table 5. Organizational and personal impact of ToL-based activities

TYPE	IMPACT
OPERATIONS	Generates actionable understanding Promotes mission definition Promotes actor cooperation and collaboration across disciplines and domains Speeds OODA Loop cycles Increases OODA Loop operational space and reach Promotes extraction and analysis of mission-relevant intelligence Promotes generation of alternative approaches ("workarounds") Serves as force multiplier Maximizes mission support through the employment of shared skills, knowledge and attitudes
RESOURCES	Promotes mission-centered, parallel use of intellectual and material resources Maximizes optimal resource exploitation Utilizes legacy and future IT/IM/KM platforms Maximizes resource deployment speed Promotes mission-relevant resource concentration Maximizes utilization of platform independent CT/IT/IM/KM resources
ORGANIZATION	Promotes creation of collaborative actor grids Promotes ad hoc creation of collaborative virtual organizations and communities of pf practice Maximizes mission-centered utilization of actionable information and actionable knowledge Supports hierarchical and peer-to-peer interaction Maximizes information and knowledge sharing among all actors of the mission grid Generates bottom-up actionable knowledge generation and top-bottom actionable information flows Promotes interdisciplinary and interdomain information and knowl-edge distribution and use
SOCIAL	Maximizes generation of trust and understanding among all actors Enhances mentoring Maximizes personal contacts Enhances personal knowledge and competence beyond boundaries of own discipline/specialization (promotes "generalist" education) Maximizes development of shared skills, knowledge, and attitudes

healthcare operations will be both immediate and long-lasting. Information and knowledge sharing at peer-to-peer level of interaction promotes lateral spread of knowledge extending beyond one's own professional specialty. Likewise, ToL supports *downward* migration of knowledge from more experienced/senior professionals within teams to the more junior ones. The immediate advantage of such spread is the enhancement of *distributed* socialization *across unrelated but mutually relevant intra and inter-domain professional specialties* that hitherto has been unattainable. Finally, as in other professions, broad on-line "communities of practice" will rapidly develop and facilitate/amplify innovation, and further lateral and vertical dissemination of knowledge. Emergence of such ToL-based communities will foster energetic development of new evidence-based approaches and methods to issues transcending (even if frequently incorporating) purely medical practice (Seely Brown and Duguid, 1991; Weneger, 2000; McLure et al., 2000). The essential value of evidence-based methodologies in routine practice has been has been repetitively demonstrated in the healthcare setting (e.g., Kersten et al, 2008, Nash and Quigley, 2008; Seers, 2007), and has been recently emphasized by auf der Heide (2006) in the context of disaster planning.

There is the final, and hitherto unobserved, advantage of ToL: acceleration of the OODA Loop (Figure 7). The overall effect is not only the increased precision of actions performed during each stage of the Loop that will in turn provide higher quality inputs to the following one, but also the shortening of time required for the completion of that stage. Also, ToL facilitates "inter-stage shortcuts" by allowing more activities to be performed simultaneously. The result of such parallel operations may allow bypassing individual segments of the Loop and the reduction of time necessary for the completion of each individual revolution of the Loop. The overall outcome is a dramatic increase in the progression of the Loop both in time and space (von Lubitz and Wickramasinghe, 2006c).

Several major practical consequences ensue from the application of ToL to OODA Loop-based activities: the mission scope can be expanded without undue increase in overall complexity (several multidisciplinary HPLTs working concurrently rather than sequentially provide a *force multiplier*), the overall time-frame of mission execution is significantly shortened, and the precision of execution is greatly increased due to the enhanced cooperation of all participants within each stage of the Loop. In summary, implementation of ToL as the OODA Loop driver represents probably the maximum attainable level of combined, collaborative, and multidisciplinary use of all advantages offered by grid computing and network-centricity within complex missions conducted in highly dynamic and unpredictable environments.

TOL AND HEALTHCARE: WHY?

The preceding sections provide a highly stylized, general outline of ToL (for details the concept and its implementation see Bradford and Brown (2008), Lipnack et al., in press, and the recently published Teams of Leaders Coaching Guide published by EUCOM).. But even a brief look at the concept leads to several salient observations. First of all, medicine is not a stranger to the ToL concept, and one might contend that physicians were its first, albeit intuitive, practitioners.

From the very early days of the profession, its practice relied heavily on tools that served as the equivalent of modern IM and KM: the written *consilia* (information), and networks of personal contacts (knowledge). Even today, in technologically disadvantaged regions identical tools continue to be implemented on a daily basis (e.g., Callen et al., 2007). Furthermore, physicians were among the first to share formally their specific skills, knowledge, and attitudes (whose most important tenets are contained within the Hippocratic Oath). Finally, the medical council, where several physicians debated the best course of treatment, often doing so at great distances by means of letters or even messengers, can be readily compared to the High Performance Leader Team of ToL. Personal contacts and the thorough awareness of shared skills, knowledge, and the fundamental attitudes characterizing the entire profession were the source of mutual confidence and trust. As the result, actionable understanding emerged on which, in turn, the practice of medicine was based. Medical knowledge was generated at the level of practitioners – the "bottom" – and was shared freely within the profession (peer-to-peer). It also flowed *down* from the most senior and respected practitioners: Paracelsus, Avicenna, and Galen are probably the best known examples of early physicians whose work greatly influenced the entire profession for several centuries (Porter, 1997; 2006). Also, whenever necessary (e.g., during the XV century European plagues) knowledge

Figure 7. Consequent, practical implementation of the OODA Loop facilitates greatly all interactions with the operational environment (Boyd, 1987; Richards, 2004; von Lubitz at al., 2008a) and may play the essential role in assuring eventual success of the conducted operation. However, the Loop revolving at constant speed (upper part of the figure) may be too slow to anticipate very sudden changes within the operational environment (e.g., sudden explosion of a pandemic, economical crisis, military conflict, etc.) Implementation of ToL at each stage of the Loop shortens significantly the time needed complete that stage. Hence, the overall revolutions speed of the Loop is greatly increased (V_{delta}). As all activities performed within the ToL environment are, by definition, inter-, trans-, and multi-domain, the volume of the operational environment sample that is analyzed, and ultimately responded to during each individual revolution of the Loop is also greatly enhanced (lower part of the figure.) The overall effect of ToL employed concurrently with the Loop is the increased tempo and precision of actions, enhanced responsiveness to sudden and unpredictable changes within the operational environment, enhanced precision of operational prognoses, and significantly decreased time to goal accomplishment

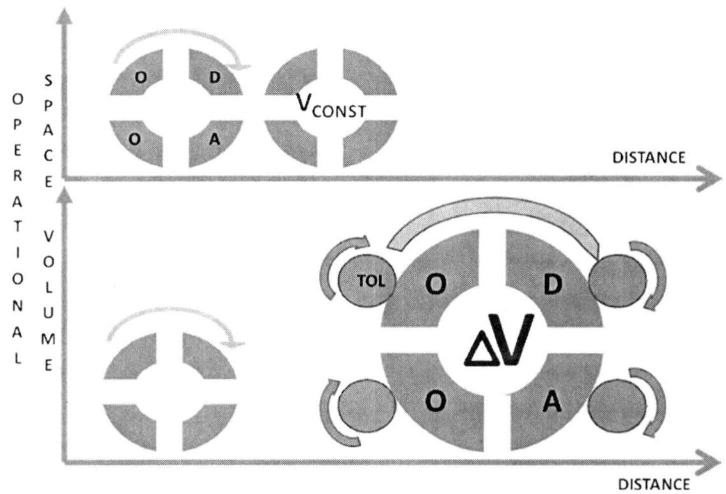

was passed to the administrative "top" – the municipal and royal bureaucracies – converted into "actionable information" of regulatory decrees, and distributed among the populace (e.g., Byrne, 2006).

Many, if not all of these aspects still remain in place. The advent of advanced IT, IM, and KM technologies merely increases speed and efficiency of distribution, access, and sharing of information and knowledge, making it all vastly more universal. Physicians continue to swear the Hippocratic Oath, and "do no harm" continues as the pivot of their shared attitudes. What changed is the nature of healthcare.

Global population growth, increasing poverty, large scale migrations, increased percentage of elderly among the wealthy nations and raising child mortality in the underdeveloped ones, all pose their own healthcare problems and risks whose solution (or absence}may influence the stability of nations, regions, and even the entire globe (Garrett, 1994; von Lubitz et al., 2002; Lewis, 2006). These are the issues that cannot be solved either by merely increasing *per capita* number of healthcare workers, improved immunization programs, or by development of new retirement facilities. Today, healthcare became tightly intertwined with economy, politics, urban development, climate change, and military operations. Suddenly, it became the integral part of the global societal mesh, and from a simple concept of assuring health to a manageable number of patients, healthcare became one of the cornerstones of nearly everything we do. In truth, the efficiency of global healthcare network may determine the future of the human race: an uncontained outbreak of a pandemic disease will have a worldwide, destabilizing impact whose consequences are both and entirely unpredictable (Garrett, 1994; The Economist, 2003; Osterholm and Branswell, 2005; PandemicfluGov; Vallat, 2007).

It is almost trivial to state that modern healthcare became a "domain of domains," a transboundary arena of unprecedented significance, complexity, and multi disciplinary richness than encompasses professions until recently considered entirely unrelated to healthcare (e.g., military operations or advanced computer technologies and methods, see Silenas et al., 2009; Kun, 2001; Kulkarni et al., 2005). Today, healthcare represents probably the only field outside military operations where success of missions (particularly when conducted on a national, international, or global scale) *demands* extraordinarily close cooperation of vast numbers of individuals, agencies, and nations.

All realize the need for such cooperation. Yet, operational costs increase at a staggering rate, the access gap widens alarmingly, and the uncontrollable *human* bioincursion into new habitats enhances chances of the exposure to pathogens for which we are entirely unprepared. AIDS and may be the best known examples of the "exotic threats" but several other equally deadly diseases have been described in the past decade alone (Garrett, 1994; GAO, 2004).

If that were not enough, since September 2001 the world lives under the constant shadow of bioterrorism, while disasters like Tsunami of 2004, Hurricane Katrina, or Myanmar Cyclone of 2008 indicate pointedly that neither national nor international healthcare organizations are capable of dealing adequately with catastrophic events. At present, the entire healthcare system of the world labours painfully, inefficiently, and very expensively under constrains imposed by the conflicting bureaucracies, politics, national interests and philosophies, that combine with often shocking indifference and common greed that hide under the coat of political correctness and sentimentality (Fernandez, 2002; von Lubitz et al., 2002).

The absence of a clearly defined "global perspective" and foresight among the Western nations, and our failure to incorporate into the future plans anything beyond the most obvious, are not typical of healthcare alone. The inability of the West to detect, analyze, and counteract the growing dissatisfaction with its policies is among the principal causes underlying the explosive emergence of anti-Western sentiment, religious extremism, and – ultimately – international terrorism as the sole means available to the populations of the "gap" to attain emotional if not economical "parity" with the developed countries (Barnett, 2004; Onen, 2004).

The political destabilization that typically accompanies the extreme forms of protest against social injustice weakens the economies of the underdeveloped regions, promotes escalation of poverty, and leads to an even greater decline of their already meager (or practically nonexistent) healthcare systems (Akhtar, 1991). Consequently, despite substantial funds provided by the multinational Western sources (e.g., US Mission to the UN Release, 2002; Li et al., 2003), attempts to establish comprehensive solutions to healthcare needs of the developing and underdeveloped world continue to fail (Zupen, 2003; Pal and Mittal, 2004; Afford, 2003; Attran, 2004). In the end, the units of predominantly US, NATO, and allied armed forces are dispatched with the expectation to serve as the collective policeman, school and road builder, teacher, and the local nurse and family doctor (Brown and Bradford, 2008; Richards, 2008; Silenas et al., 2008).

The vast expansion of mission profile from purely kinetic operations to peace keeping, nation stabilization and nation building, combined with a wide range of humanitarian and disaster relief operations, exposed the armed forces to the unprecedented change in the "operational climate." Consequently, both the US and NATO military establishments were forced to cooperate at a hitherto unprecedented scale not only within their own already very complex structures, but also across the broad spectrum of civilian governmental agencies, private organizations, and, frequently, inhabitants of small communities involved in a desperate struggle to survive. It is thus not very surprising the concept of ToL emerged from within the US Army bearing the brunt of these efforts.

It is unquestionably a paradox when military medical units deliver healthcare in the jungles of Borneo, while the enthusiastic acceptance of IT, IM, and KM by Western healthcare professions creates the definition of "continuum of care" by the National Cancer Institute (http://ncim.nci.nih.gov see also http://www.cancer.gov/dictionary/?CdrID=561395) that sounds painfully similar to the definition of supply chain management (e.g., http://jpfarrell.blogspot.com/2008/08/glossary-of-terms-used-on-site.html). The Western quest to incorporate almost every aspect of business practice (and verbosity) into healthcare (e.g., Wickramasinghe and Schaffer, 2006) converted the latter into the increasingly mechanized and bureaucratically distant activity in which its ultimate target – people – have been swept aside by "technology and processes" (Wickramasinghe and Schaffer, 2006).

ToL changes all that. It brings to the forefront the fact that technology (such as grid computing), no matter how powerful, provides but the tool to be used in solving tasks whether simple or unimaginably complex. Processes (such as IM and KM) or their combination (network-centric operations) lead to the formulation and operational implementation of actionable knowledge, typically in a very task specific (i.e., narrow) context. Technology alone will not bring the required change and therein lies the strength of ToL. By bringing together those who implement technology and processes, by allowing maximum exploitation of their intellectual capabilities, and by rooting all activities in the *maximum, platform-independent use of all relevant technologies and processes*, ToL permits to develop the *strategy* necessary for the successful execution of the mission (Figures 4,5,6). The latter cannot be devised by even the most intense application of either technology or processes alone. ToL serves therefore as the *force multiplier*. It is the latter attribute of ToL that, contrary to the "within the profession" approach, supports development of evidence-based methods and of best practices among a much wider range of professionals, disciplines and agencies than it was ever possible.

On a less "luminous" but just as critical level, ToL demonstrates its value not only in the operational context (Table 6), but also as a significant tool in the development of foundations for a highly efficient training with the quality of outcomes that can be determined *prior* to real life practice (von Lubitz, 2008). "Just-in-time" training and adequate preparation of responders for the conditions likely to be encountered during forthcoming activities is a highly intricate and often multidisciplinary task (e.g., Williams, 2008, Kyle and Bosseau, 2008; von Lubitz, 2008**c).** Its inadequacies emerge, often with catastrophic results (e.g., Cooper and Block, 2006; Ricks, 2007), during complex operations where personnel of several, often multinational agencies, all of whom are endowed with more than adequate and shared knowledge and skills, miss the critical ingredient of shared attitudes (Brown and Bradford, 2008). By promoting mutual trust, ToL furthers rapid development and coalescence of such attitudes among all actors. In the end, the exponential growth of mission-oriented cohesion and coordination of effort that ToL fosters provides the cornerstone for mission success (Bradford and Brown, 2008)

The latter attribute of ToL attains the level of absolutely critical significance in international and multinational healthcare operations. It has

Table 6. Operational consequences of ToL implementation in large scale (national/international/multinational) healthcare activities

TARGET	ACTION
Mission Definition (criticality)	Prevention - Determination of what must be protected, to what extent, and what assets are critical to mission execution Correction - Determination of mission criticality level: a. critical b. essential c. required d. non-essential
Threat reduction	Prevention - Through the building of trust in the quality and reliability of people, processes, practices, platforms and systems of platforms and in the information quality/reliability handled by involved actors Detection - Cross-domain extraction of data, establishment of links, correlations, and dependencies leading to detection of unanticipated threats at pre-critical level Correction - Early mitigation and elimination of unanticipated and anticipated threats through timely development of corrective procedures and processes
Personnel	Prevention - Development of intellectually agile, alert, and decisive, mission oriented personnel Detection - Detection of weak links in personnel and command structure, detection of security threats Correction - Development of training, facilitation of simulation exercises
Problem Detection	Detection - Active search for anomalies, exacerbation of known or potential problems/threats in all responsible areas using all available KM systems within related/non-related domains*)
Response	Prevention - Timely detection of asset inadequacies, preemptive, strategic asset deployment Detection - Early detection of failures in operational deployment of assets, early detection of logistic difficulties and breakdowns Correction - "Preventive maintenance" through detection/correction of non-critical events with potential future criticality, selection of appropriate assets-personnel, technology and their deployment, founding of collaborative task forces and command entities; rapid involvement of commercial entities in response/recovery processes

been said that, in the context of issues facing healthcare at the global scale, the strategies of the developed nations are rooted within their mono-cultural, ethno-centric concepts and the remedies proposed by the rich may therefore be both beyond the reach and without any relevance to the present and future problems of the poor (Fernandez, 2002). ToL not only allows for fully empowered inclusion of the representatives of all affected groups – in order to be effective, the concept of ToL *demands* such inclusion. Only then can problems be addressed effectively and efficiently.

Harsh criticism leveled at the Western nations for their proclaimed indifference to the healthcare plight of the Third World notwithstanding, there is no doubt that healthcare issues facing the Western countries are just as equally daunting and demand increasingly larger fiscal outlays merely (and barely) to be contained at the level of their current intensity (e.g., OECD, 2004; National center for Health Statistics, 2002). With the existing atmosphere of conflicting agendas and failing mutual trust (Taylor-Gooby, 2006; European Policy

Centre, 2008; Taylor, 2007), ToL may provide a foundation for effective solutions also here.

To reduce the burden, Western healthcare managers place increasing emphasis on information, computer, and communication technologies (IC^2T) as the most effective means to reduce costs and increase operational efficiency (e.g., European Institute of Medicine, 2003; National Coalition on Healthcare, 2004). However, with the effort aimed primarily at the Western healthcare markets, the divergence between the wealthy and those belonging to the "non-integrating gap' (Barnett, 2004) increases steadily. Paradoxically, despite technological and economical ability to reduce much of the healthcare-related difficulties of the developing world, the absence of adequate profit incentives limits the eagerness of the corporate world to participate with equal vigour in global programs as in those of solely Western national/ regional significance (Fernandez, 2002).

There is thus absolutely no doubt that, despite increasing determination to implement technology and to increase funding as a dam stemming its eventual collapse, the state of disarray pervading both national and global healthcare increases almost uncontrollably. Disagreements and growing polarization (clearly indicated by the healthcare debates preceding the US presidential election of 2008 and the current attempts at modifying the US healthcare by the Obama administration) indicate the very clear need for the development of an approach based on a new philosophy, and centered on solutions that clearly break with what has been hitherto proposed or practiced. No matter how advanced or powerful they may ultimately become, neither technologies nor processes (including the two presently in the forefront, i.e., grid computing and network-centric) can provide a unifying setting to assure inter-domain cooperation and collaboration critical for "healing the healthcare."

It would be exceedingly naïve to expect ToL to offer a dilemma-solving panacea. Nonetheless, its rapid and consequent implementation within the broadest realm of healthcare may provide the starting point for generation of effective remedies. ToL, despite its reliance on advanced technology employs that technology as tools not solutions. ToL is people- rather than technology driven. Hence, it is endowed with a number of distinct and unique advantages. First of all, the essential physical constituents already exist, several of which have been discussed in this chapter. Furthermore, the ToL concept has been very successfully implemented by the US European Command (EUCOM) as part of its extensive interactions with the civilian authorities of several European countries (which also include healthcare issues, e.g., Bradford and Brown, 2008). It is not a "new-fangled idea" but a well proven approach whose "lessons learned" can be readily adopted and implemented in the environment of healthcare operations. Most importantly, however, implementation of ToL will unify the currently disconnected entities and fields of healthcare and foster rapid development of actionable understanding rather than actionable knowledge.

As argued in the preceding sections, it is actionable understanding rather than actionable knowledge that serves both as the prerequisite and the *essential* prelude to creating a solid foundation for the development of the very badly needed collaboration and cooperation among all involved healthcare actors. Without such understanding, all efforts to relieve the mounting pressures of conflicting demands, inequities, and deficiencies will ultimately fail. The signs of the approaching collapse are clearly visible already, and the currently favoured erratic application of ever larger amounts of money to avert the inevitable is, equally clearly, utterly inadequate.

REFERENCES

Abel-Smith, B. (1989). Health economies in developing countries. *The Journal of Tropical Medicine and Hygiene*, *92*, 229–241.

Afford, W. (2003). *Corrosive reform: failing health systems in Eastern Europe, ILO Socio-Economic Security Programme, Geneva 2003*. Accessible at http://www.ilo.org/public/english/bureau/inf/features/03/health.htm

After the outbreak. (2003, April 3rd). *Economist*.

Akhtar, R. (Ed.). (1991). *Health Care Patterns and Planning in Developing Countries* (pp. 1–336). New York: Greenwood Press.

Alberts, D. S., Garstka, J. J., Hayes, R. E., & Signori, D. A. (2001). *Understanding Information Age Warfare*. Washington, DC: CCRP Press. Retrieved from http://%20www.dodccrp.org/publications/ pdf/ Alberts_UIAW.pdf

Alberts, D. S., Garstka, J. J., & Stein, F. P. (2000). *Network Centric Wardare: Developing and Leveraging Information Superiority*, (pp 1-284). Washington, DC: CCRP Publication Series. Retrieved from http://www.dodccrp.org/publications/pdf/Alberts_NCW.pdf

Aloisio, G., Barba, M. C., Biasi, E., Cafaro, M., Fiore, S., & Mirto, M. (2005). A web service-based Grid portal for Edgebreaker compression. *Methods of Information in Medicine*, *44*(2), 233–238.

Alonso, J. M., Ferroero, J. M. Jr, Hernánde, Z. V., Moltò, G., Saiz, J., & Trénor, B. (2008). A grid-based approach for the acce;eration of simulation in cardiology. *IEEE Transactions on Information Technology in Biomedicine*, *12*(2), 138–144.

Andalusi, I., Blanquer, I., Breton, V., Dobrev, A., van Dooselaere, C., & Hernandez, V. (2008). The SHARE road map: healthgrids for biomedical research and healthcare. *Studies in Health Technology and Informatics*, *138*, 238–278.

Anderson, P. (2007). What is Web 2.0? Ideas, technologies and implications for education. *JISC Technology and Standards Watch,* (Feb. 2007). Retrieved from http://www.jisc.org.uk/media/documents/techwatch/tsw0701b.pdf

Andronico, G. Barbera, R. Falzone, A. Lo Re, G., Pulvirenti, A., Rodolico, A. (2005). The GENIUS web portal – an easy way yo access the Grid. *Methods Inf. Med.*

Anirban, G., Anirban, C., Dheepak, R. A., & Shaken, A. (2007). Streamlining drug discovery research by leveraging grid workflow manager. *Infosys Nov. 2007*. Retrieved from http://www.infosys.com/industries/life-sciences/white-papers/streamlining-drug-discovery.pdf

Arbona, A., Benkner, S., Engelbrecht, G., Fingberg, J., Hofmann, M., & Kumpf, K. (2007)... *IEEE Transactions on Nanobioscience*, *6*(2), 136–141.

ASME. *(Assoc. for the Study of Med. Educ.)*. (2008). Understanding Medical Education Series, description available at http://www.asme.org.uk/pub_ume.htm

Associated Press. (2007). FDA is rejecting more drugs than in the past. Retrieved from http://www.msnbc.msn.com/id/20321830/

Attaran, A. (2004). Where did it go wrong. *Nature*, *430*, 2–3.

Auf der Heide, E. (2006). The importance of evidence-based disaster planning. *Annals of Emergency Medicine*, *1*, 34–49.

Ballester, F., Michelozzi, P., & Iñiguez, C. (2003). Weather, climate, and public health. *Journal of Epidemiology and Community Health*, *57*, 759–760.

Barnett, T.P.M., (20040. *The Pentagon's New Map*, (pp. 1-435). New York: G.P. Putnam & Sons.

Bartocci, E., Cacciagrano, D., Cannata, N., Corradini, F., Merelli, E., Milanesi, L., & Romano, P. (2007)... *IEEE Nanobioscience*, *6*(2), 142–148.

Beier, K. P., Freer, J., Griffiths, J. M., Levine, H., Sauter, J., & Treloar, D. (2001). The VIBE of the burning agent: simulation and modeling of burns and their treatment using agent-based programming, virtual reality, and human patient simulation. In Westwood, J. D. (Eds.), *Medicine Meets Virtual Reality 2001* (pp. 551–560). Amsterdam: IOS Press.

Bello, I. S., Arogundade, F. A., Sanusi, A. A., Ezeoma, I. T., Abioye-Kuteyi, E. A., & Akinsola, A. (2004). Knowledge and utilization of Information Technology among health care professionals and students in Ile-Ife, Nigeria: a case study of a university teaching hospital. *I. Med. Internet Res.*, *6*(4), e45.

Bescos, C., Schmitt, D., Kaas, J., Garcia-Barbero, M., & Kentchev, P. (2005). Interoperability and HealthGrid. *Methods of Information in Medicine*, *44*(2), 190–192.

Biomoby Consortium. (2008). Interoperability with Moby 1.0 – it's better than sharing your toothbrush. *Briefings in Bioinformatics*, *9*(3), 220–231.

Blignaut, P. J. (1999). Software for primary healthcare in a developing country. Background and problem statement. *Computers in Nursing*, *17*(6), 291–296.

Bologna Declaration. (1999). Retrieved from http://www.bologna-bergen2005.no/Docs/00-Main_doc/990719BOLOGNA_DECLARATION.PDF

Bouchama, A. (2005). The 2003 European heat wave. *Int. Care Med.*, *30*(1), 1–3.

Boyd, C., Williams, W., Skinner, D., & Wilson, S. (2005). *A comparison of approaches to assessing network-centric warfare (NCW) concept implementation, Systems Engineering/Test and Evaluation Conference (SETE) 2005*. Retrieved from http://www.concepts.aero/ documents/ SETE-2005- NPI.pdf#search=%22Boyd%20 C%20Williams%20 W%20 Skinner%20D%20 Wilson%20S%20a%20comparison%20of%20 approaches%22

Boyd, J. R. COL. USAF. (1987). *Patterns of Conflict*. unpubl Briefing (accessible as "Essence of Winning and Losing", http://www.d-n-i.net).

Bradford, Z. B., & Brown, F. J. (2008). *America's Army: A Model for Interagency Effectiveness,* (pp. XIV + 1-250). Westport, CN: Praeger Security International.

Braverman, A. M. (2004). Father of the Grid. *University of Chicago Magazine 96*(4). Retrieved from http://magazine.uchicago.edu/0404/features/index.shtml

Brennan, R. J., & Nandy, R. (2001). Complex humanitarian emergencies: a major global challenge. *Emerg. Med.*, *13*(2), 147–156.

Brown, F. J. (2002). Imperatives for tomorrow. *Military Review*, (September-October): 81–91.

Byrne, J. P. (2006). *Daily Life During the Black Death* (pp. 1–344). Westport, CT: Greenwood Press.

Callen, J. L., Buyankhishig, B., & McIntosdh, J. H. (2007). Clinical information sources used by hospital doctors in Mongolia. *International Journal of Medical Informatics*, (Jul): 21.

Cavalier, J. C., & Klein, J. D. (1998). Effects of cooperative versus individual learning and orienting activities during computer-based instruction. *ETR&D*, *46*(1), 5–17.

Cebrowski, A. K., & Garstka, J. J. (1998). Network-centric warfare: its origin and future. *US Nav. Inst. Proc. 1*, (pp. 28-35). Retrieved from http://www.usni.org/magazines/proceedings/ archive/month.asp?ID=205

Chang, W. (2008). *Network-centric Service Oriented Enterprise* (pp. 1–540). Dordrecht, The Netherlands: Springer.

Chen, L., Evans, T., Anand, S., Boufford, J.I., & Brown, H., Chowdhury, et al. (2004). Human resources for health: overcoming the crisis. *Lancet*, *364*, 1984–1990.

Claus, B. L., & Johnson, S. R. (2008). Grid computing in large pharmaceutical molecule modeling. *Drug Discov. Today 13*(13-14), S 78-83, Collins, F.S. & McKusick, V.A. (2001). Implications of the Human Genome Project for Medical Science. *Journal of the American Medical Association*, *285*, 540–544.

Cooper, C., & Block, R. (2006). *Disaster: Hurricane Katrina and the Failure of Homeland Security* (pp. 3–333). New York: Times Books/ Henry Holt and Company.

Coulter, A., & Ham, C. (2002). *The global challenge of health care rationing* (pp. 1–267). Buckingham, UK: Open University Press.

Coveney, P. V., & Fowler, P. W. (2005). Modelling biological complexity: a physical scientist's perspective. *J.R. Soc. Interface*, *2*(4), 267–280.

Curran, V. R., Sharpe, D., Forristall, J., & Flynn, K. (2008). Student satisfaction and perceptions of small group process in case-based interprofessional learning. *Medizinische Technik*, *30*(4), 431–433.

Davis, D. (1998). Continuing medical education: Global health, global learning. *BMJ (Clinical Research Ed.)*, *316*(7128), 385–389.

Day, B., Mckay, R. B., Ishman, M., & Chung, E. (2004). The new normal: lessons learned from SARS for corporations operating in emerging markets. *Management Decision*, *42*(6), 794–806.

Devitt, N., & Murphy, J. (2004). A survey of the information management and technology training needs of doctors in an acute NHS trust in the United Kingdom. *Health Information and Libraries Journal*, *21*(3), 164–172.

Dianic, A. (2006). The need for scalability in network-centric warfare – it's all in the semanitcs. *SEC BSSD Bulletin January*, 1-11. Retrieved from http://www.pdf-search-online.com/dianic-pdf-40.html

Dixon, N. M., Allen, N., Burgess, T., Kilner, P., & Dchweitzer, S. (2005). *Company Command: Unleashing the Power of the Army Profession* (pp. 1–198). NY: West Point.

Drews, J. (2000). Drug discovery: a historical perspective. *Science*, *287*(5460), 1960–1964.

Eddrippulige, S., Marasinghe, R. B., Smith, A. C., Fujisawa, Y., Herath, W. B., & Jiffry, M. T. (2007). Medical students' knowledge and perception of e-health: results of a study in Sri Lanka. *Medinfo*, *12*(Pt.2), 1406–1409.

ESRI. (n.d.). Retrieved from http://www.esri.com/library/brochures/pdfs/gis-for-defense

EUCOM. (2009). *Teams of Leaders Coaching Guide 1.0*. Stuttgart, Germany: US Army European Command.

European Commission. (2007). *From Bergen to London*. Retrieved from http://ec.europa.eu/education/policies/educ/bologna/report06.pdf

European Institute of Medicine. (2003). *Health is Wealth: Strategic Vision for European Healthcare at the Beginning of the 21st Century*. Salzburg, Austria: European Academy of Arts and Sciences.

European Policy Center. (2008, 1st November). *European Health Policy in an International Perspective Report*. Retrieved from http://www.epc.eu/en/er.asp?AI=439&LV=293&PG=ER/EN/detail&TYP=ER&see=y&t=2

Evans, G. (1993). Health and security in the global village. *World Health Forum*, *14*, 133–135.

Evans, W. E., & McLeod, H. L. (2003). Pharmacogenomics – drug disposition, drug targets, and side effects. *The New England Journal of Medicine*, *348*(6), 538–549. Retrieved from http://content.nejm.org/cgi/content/full/348/6/538.

FDA (US Food and Drug Administration). (2004). *Innovation or Stagnation. White Paper.* Washington, DC: Author.

Fernandez, I. (2002). Barcelona 2002: law, ethics, and human rights. Global battle cry: health is a right, not a commodity. *Canadian HIV/AIDS Policy & Law Review*, *7*, 80–84.

Fogg, B. J. (2003). *Persuasive Technology: Using Computers to Change What We Think and Do* (pp. 1–282). San Francisco: Morgan Kaufman.

Foster, I., & Kesselman, C. (2003). *The Grid 2: Blueprint for a new Computing Infrastructure,* (The Elsevier Series in Grid Computing, pp. 1-748). San Francisco, CA: Morgan Kaufman.

Frenk, J., Sepulveda, J., Gomez-Dantes, O., McGuinness, M. J., & Knaul, F. (1997). The future of world health: the new world order and international health. *BMJ (Clinical Research Ed.)*, *314*, 1404–1407. Retrieved from http://www.ncbi.nlm.nih.gov/pmc/articles/PMC2126640/pdf/9161318.pdf.

Frost & Sullivan Country Industry Forecast – European Union Healthcare Industry. (2004, May 11). Retrieved from http://www.news-medical.net/print_article.asp?id=1405

Galperin, M. Y. (2005). The molecular biology database collection: 2005 update. *Nucleic Acids Research*, *33*, D5–D24.

Galperin, M. Y. (2008). Genomes of model organisms: know thy tools. *Environ. Biol.*, *10*(6), 1383–1391.

GAO. (2004). *Emerging Infectious Diseases: Review of State and Federal Disease Surveillance Efforts* (GAO 04-877, I-IV, pp. 1-64). Washington, DC: Government Accounting Office.

Garrett, L. (1994). *The Coming Plague: Newly Emerging Diseases in the World out Of Balance* (pp. 3–750). New York: Penguin.

Garstka, J. J. (2000). Network Centric Warfare: an overview of emerging theory. *Phalanx*, *4*, 28–33.

Garstka, J. J. (2004, 28th January). Implementation of network centric warfare. *Force Transformation Trends*. Retrieved from http://www.oft.osd.mil

Gilelet, F., Fichera, R., Schreck, G., Yates, S., & Wenninger, S. (2004). *Grid gets big, but the term is confusing*. Retrieved from http://www.egenera.com/reg/pdf/forrester_grid.pdf

Gokhale, A. A. (1995). Collaborative learning enhances critical thinking. *J. Technological Education*, *7*(1), 22–30.

Gray, C. S. (2006). Clausewitz, history, and the future strategic world. In Murray, W., & Sinnreich, R. H. (Eds.), *The Past as Prologue: the Importance of History to the Military Profession* (pp. 111–132). Cambridge, UK: Cambridge University Press.

Grifftihs, J.-M., Sauter, J., Parunak, H. V. D., Wolf, E., & von Lubitz, D. K. J. E. (2000). Models, models everywhere: brain injury, datapocalypse, and the art of computing. In C. Webb (Ed.), *Proc. NIH Pulse Workshop*, NIH, Leesburg, VA, June 29-30.

Haine, J.-Y. (2005). Military matters: ESDP transformed? *NATO Review,* Summer. Retrieved from http://www.nato.int/docu/review/2005/issue2/english/military.html

Hernandez, V., & Blanquer, I. (2005). The grid as a healthcare provision tool. *Methods of Information in Medicine*, *44*(2), 144–148.

Hubbard, T. (2002). Biological information: making it accessible and integrated (and trying to make sense of it). *Bioinform.*, *18*(Suppl. 2), S140.

Ichikawa, K. date, S., Kaishima, T., & Shimojo, S. (2005). A framework supporting the development of a Grid portal for analysis based on ROI. *Methods of Information in Medicine*, *44*(2), 265–269.

Johansson, F. (2006). *The Medici Effect* (pp. 1–206). Boston: Harvard Business School Press.

Jonas, K. W. (2005). *Network-centric operations: European capabilities*, Report A1899. Assembly of WEU, Interparliamentary European Security and Defense Assembly

Kalawsky, R.S., Nee, S.P., Homes, I. & Coveney, P.V. (2005). A grid-enabled lightwiright computational steering client: a .NET PDA implementation. *Philos. Trans. A. math. Phys. Eng. Sci.*, *363*(1833), 1885-94.

Kalawsky, R.S., O'Brien, J., & Coveney, P.V. (2005). Improving scientists' interaction with complex computational-visualization environments based on a distributed grid infrastructure. *Philos. Trans. A. Math. Phys. Eng. Sci*, *363*(1833), 1867-84.

Kamel Boulos, M. N., Hetherington, L., & Wheeler, S. (2007). Second Life: an overview of the potential of 3-D virtual worlds in medical and health education. *Health Information and Libraries Journal*, *24*(4), 233–245.

Kamel Boulos, M. N., & Wheeler, S. (2007). The emerging Web 2.0 social software: an enabling suite of sociable technologies in health and health care education. *Health Information and Libraries Journal*, *24*(1), 2–23.

Karasavvas, K. A., Baldock, R., & Bureger, A. (2004). Bioinformatics integration and agent technology. *Biomed. Inform.*, *37*(3), 205–219.

Kersten, H. B., Thompson, E. D., & Frohna, J. G. (2008). The use of evidence-based medicine in pediatrics: past, present, and future. *Current Opinion in Pediatrics*, *20*(3), 326–331.

Kola, I., & Landis, J. (2004). Can the pharmaceutical industry reduce attrition rates? *Nature Reviews. Drug Discovery*, *3*(8), 711–715.

Kulkarni, R., & Nathanson, L. A. (2005). Medical Informatics in medicine. *E-Medicine.* Retrieved from http://www.emedicine.com/emerg/topic879.htm

Kun, L. (2001)... *Computer Methods and Programs in Biomedicine*, *64*(3), 155–167.

Kyle, R., & Murray, B. (Eds.). (2008). *Clinical Simulation: Operations, Engineering, and Management* (pp. 1–821). Amsterdam: Elsevier Press.

Kyprianou, M. (2005). Healthcare: Is Europe getting better? *The new European Healthcare Agenda – The European Voice conference.* Retrieved from http://www.noticias.info/asp/aspcommunicados.asp?nid=45584

Lacher, D., Nelson, E., Bylsma, W., & Spena, R. (2000). Computer use needs of internists: a survey of members of the American College of Physicians-American Society of Internal medicine. *In Proc. AMIA Symp.*, *2000*, 453–456.

Lagadec, E. (2007). *Unconventional Crises, Unconventional Responses: Reforming Leadership in the Age of Catastrophic Crises and Hypercomplexity* (pp. 1–68). Baltimore, MD: Johns Hopkins University Press.

Lee, J. W., & McKibbin, W. J. (2003). Globalization and disease: the case of SARS. *Asian Economic Papers*, *3*(1), 113–131. doi:. doi:10.1162/1535351041747932

Lee, M. Y., Albright, S. A., Alkasab, T., Damassa, D. A., Wang, P. J., & Eaton, E. K. (2003). Tufts Health Sciences Database: lessons, issues, and opportunities. *Academic Medicine*, *78*, 254–264.

Leeder, S., Raymond, S., & Greenberg, H. (2007). The need for leadership in global health. *The Medical Journal of Australia*, *187*(9), 532–535.

Lewis, W. W. (2006). *The Power of Productivity: Wealth, Poverty, and the Threat to Global Stability* (pp. 1–339). Chicago: Chicago University Press.

Li, M., & Easrman, C. J. (2003). Working with funding agencies in the delivery of healthcare in the Asia Pacific region. *MJA*, *178*, 13–16.

Lindsay, M. A. (2005). Finding new drug targets in the 21st century. *Drug Discovery Today*, *10*(23-24), 1683–1687.

Lipnack, J., Stamps, J., Prevou, M., Hannah, M., (in press). *Teams of Leaders Handbook,* (pp. 1-175). Fort Leavenworth, KS: Battle Command Knowledge System Combined Arms Center – Knowledge.

Littler, D., Leverick, F., & Wilson, D. (1998). Collaboration in new technology based product markets. *International Journal of Technology Management*, *15*(1-2), 139–159.

Lou, Y. (2001). Small group and individual learning with technology. *Review of Educational Research*, *71*(3), 449–521.

Lure Wasko, M., & Sara, F. (2000). "it's what one does": why people help others in electronic communities of practice. *The Journal of Strategic Information Systems*, *9*(1-3), 155–173.

Maresko, D. (n.d.). Development, relief aid, and creating peace: humanitarian aid in Liberia's war of the 1990s. *OJPCR (The Online Journal of Peace and Conflict Resolution* *6*(1), 94-120.

Martin, R., & Hoover, J. N. (2008). Guide to cloud computing. *Information Week, June 21*. Retrieved from http://www.informationweek.com/news/services/hosted_apps/show Article.jhtml?articleID=208700713

McEntire, D. A. (1999). Issues in disaster relief: progress, perpetual problems and prospective solutions. *Intl. J. Disaster Prevention and Management*, *8*(5), 351–361.

Michelon, T., Magne, P., & Simon-Delavell, F. (2005). Lessons of the 2003 Heat-Wave in France and action taken to limit the effects of future heat waves. In Kirch, W., Bertollini, R., & Menne, B. (Eds.), *Extreme Weather Events and Public Health Responses* (pp. 131–140). Berlin: Springer.

Nash, D. B., & Quigley, G. D. (2008). Looking forward to the end of autonomy. *Headache*, *48*(5), 719–726.

National Center for Health Statistics. *Health Expenditures*. (2002). Hyatsville, MD: CDC/NCHS. Retrieved from http://www.cdc.gov/nchs/fastats/hexpense.htm

National Coalition on Healthcare. (2004). *Building a Better Health: Specifications for Reform*. Washington, DC: Author.

NATO. (2005). *NATO Network Enabled Capability; Feasibility Study*. Brussels: NATO Consultation, Command and Control Agency.

Neerincx, P. B. T., & Leunissen, J. A. M. (2005). Evolution of web services in bioinformatics. *Briefings in Bioinf.*, *6*(2), 178–188.

Noji, E. K. (2005). Disasters: introduction and state of the art. *Epidemiologic Reviews*, *27*(1), 3–8.

OECD (Organization for Economic Co-operation and Development). (2004). *OECD Health Data 2004,* CD-ROM, (also downloadable at www.oecd.org/health/healthdata).

Olive, M., Rahmouni, H., & Solomonides, T. (2008). *SHARE the journey: a European Healthgrid Roadmap, EU Commission: Information Society and Media*. Retrieved from http://ec.europa.eu/information_society/activities/health/docs/publications/200810share-roadmap.pdf

Olive, M., Rahmouni, H., Solomonides, T., Solomonides, T., Breton, V., & Legré, Y. (2008). SHARE, from vision to road map: technical steps. *Studies in Health Technology and Informatics, 129*(Pt.2), 1149–1153.

Oliveira, I. C., Oliveiura, J. L., Lopéz-Alonso, V., Martin-Sanchez, F., Maojo, V., & Sousa Pereira, A. (2005). Grid requirements for the integration of biomedical information resources for health applications. *Methods of Information in Medicine, 44*(2), 161–167.

Onen, C. L. (2004). Medicine in resource-poor settings: time for a paradigm shift? *Clinical Medicine (London, England), 4*, 355–360.

Oster, S., Langella, S., Hastings, S., Ervin, D., Madduri, R., & Phillips, J. (2008). caHrid 1.0: an enterprise grid infrastructure for biomedical research. *Journal of the American Medical Informatics Association, 15*(2), 138–149.

Osterholm, M., & Branswell, H. (2005). *Emerging pandemic: costs and consequences of an avian influenza outbreak, Global health Initiative/Woodrow Wilson International Center for Scholars*. Retrieved from http://www.wilsoncenter.org/index.cfm?event_id=142787&fuseaction=topics.event_summary&topic_id=116811

Pal, S. K., & Mittal, B. (2004). Fight against cancer in countries with limited resources: the post genomic era scenario. *Asian Pacific Journal of Cancer Prevention, 5*, 328–333.

PandemicFlu.gov. (n.d.). Retrieved from http://www.pandemicflu.gov/global/index.html

Perry, M. (2006). *Humanitarian relief challenges in the wake of South East Asian tsunami disaster*. Department of Management Working Paper Series, Monash University, Austalia. Retrieved from http://www.buseco.monash.edu.au/mgt/research/working-papers/2006/wp16-06.pdf

(2005). *Plunkett's Health Care Industry Almanac*. Houston, TX: Plunkett Research, Ltd.

Porter, R. (1997). *The Greatest Benefit to Mankind: A Medical History of Humanity* (pp. 3–831). New York: Norton.

Porter, R. (2006). *The Cambridge History of Medicine* (pp. 1–408). New York: Cambridge University Press.

Radetzky, U., Leser, U., Schultze-Rauschenbach, S. C., Zimmermann, J., Lüssem, J., Bode, T., & Cremers, A. B. (2006). Adapters, shims, and glue – services interoperability for in silico experiments. *Bioinform., 22*(9), 1137–1143.

Redfern, S., & Naughton, N. (2002). Collaborative virtual virtual environments to support communication and community in internet-based distance education. *Journal of Information Technology Education, 1*(3), 202–211.

Richards, C. (2004). *Certain to Win: the Strategy of John Boyd Applied to Business* (pp. 1–187). St. Paul, MN: Xlibris.

Richards, C. (2008). Operations other than war: what they are, and why. *Intl. J. Risk Assessment and Management, 9*(4), 376–393.

Ricks, T. E. (2007). *Fiasco: the American Military Adventure in Iraq* (pp. 3–492). New York: Penguin.

Rifkin, J. (1998). *The Biotech Century: Harnessing the Gene and Remaking the World* (pp. 1–271). New York: Tarcher.

Rifkin, J. (2001). *The Age of Access* (pp. 3–312). New York: Tarcher/Putnam.

Rifkin, J. (2005). *The European Dream: How Europe's Vision of the Future Is Quietly Eclipsing the American Dream,* (pp. 1-434). New York: Tarcher (Penguin).

Rosenthal, U., Boin, A. R., & Comfort, L. K. (1993). *Managing Crises: Threats, Dilemmas, Opportunities* (pp. 5–354). Springfield, IL: Charles C. Thomas.

Rubin, C. (Ed.). (2007). *Emergency Management: The American Experience 1900-2005* (pp. 1–274). Fairfax, VA: PERI.

Ruiz, J. G., Mintzer, M. J., & Leipzig, R. M. (2006). The Impact of E-Learning in Medical Education. *Academic Medicine, 81*(3), 207–212.

Sadiq, S.K., Mezzeo, M.D., Zasada, S.J., Manos, S., Stoica, I., Gale, C.V. et al. (2008). Patient-specific simulation as a basis for clinical decision-making. *Philos. Transact. A. Med. Phys. Eng. Sci. 366*(1878), 3199-219.

Salmoni, A. J., & Gonzales, M. L. (2008). Online collaborative learning: quantifying how people learn together online. *Medizinische Technik, 30*(7), 710–716.

Saltz, J., hastings, S., Langella, S., Oster, S., Kurc, T., & payne, P. et al. (2008). The roadmap for caGrid, an enterprise Grid architecture for biomedical research. *Studies in Health Technology and Informatics, 138*, 224–237.

Sams-Dodd, F. (2005). Target-based drug discovery: is something wrong? *Drug Discovery Today, 10*(2), 139–147.

Scheffler, R. M., Liu, J. X., Kinfu, J., & Dal Poz, M. L. (2008). Forecasting the global shortage of physicians: an economic- and needs-based approach. *Bull. World health Organ,* Geneva. Retrieved from http://www.scielosp.org/pdf/bwho/v86n7/a11v86n7.pdf

Seely Brown, J. & Duguid, P. (1991). Organizational learning and communities of practice: toward a unified view of working, learning, and innovation. *Organization Science 2*(1 -Special Issue: Papers in honor of (and by) James G. March), 40-57.

Seers, K. (2007). Evaluating complex interventions. *Worldwide Evid. Based Nurs., 4*(2), 67–68.

Shefter, S. M. (2006). Workflow technology: the new frontier. How to overcome the barriers and join the future. *Lippincott's Case Management, 11*(1), 25–34.

Shostak, S. (1999). *Evolution of Sameness and Difference: Perspectives on the Human Genome Project* (pp. 3–342). Boca Raton, FL: CRC Press.

Silenas, R., Waller, S. G., D'Amore, A. R., & Carlton, P. K. (2008). US Armed Forces medical operations other than war. *Int. J. Risk Assessment and Management, 9*(4), 367–375.

Sloot, P., Coveney, P., Bubak, M.T., Vandamme, A.M., & Nuallain, O, B., van de Vijver, D. & Boucher, C. (2008). Multi-science decision support for HIV drug resistance treatment. *Stud. Health Inform., 138*, 188–198.

Taylor, H. (2007). Lack of trust in both FDA and pharmaceutical companies makes drug safety a concern. *Healthcare News 7*(6), April 25. Retrieved from http://www.harrisinteractive.com/news/newsletters/healthnews/HI_HealthCare-News_2007_v07_i06.pdf

Taylor-Gooby, P. (2006). Trust, risk, and healthcare reform. *Health Risk & Society, 8*(2), 97–103.

The Economist. (2003, April 10). Epidemics and economies.

The Healthgrid White Paper. (2005)... *Stud. Technol. Inform., 112*, 249–321.

Tierney, K. J. (2006). Testimony on needed emergency management reforms. *J. Homeland Security and Disaster Management 4*(3), Article 15.

US Mission to the UN Release 65. (2002). USAI leads public and private partners to improve health and save lives through food fortification, USUN, New York, May 8, 2002.

Vallat, B. (2007). Avian influenza epizootie: where do we stand in 2007. *CSIRO Snowdon Lecture*, 11 July 2007 (chapter 2). Retrieved from http://www.csiro.au/files/files/pqlo.pdf

Van Rooyen, M. J., Hansch, S., Curtis, D., & Burnham, G. (2001). Emerging issues and future needs in humanitarian assistance. *Prehospital and Disaster Medicine*, *16*(4), 216–222.

von Lubitz, D. K. J. E. (2008). Medical readiness for operations other than war: Boyd's OODA Loop and training using advanced distributed simulation technology. *Intl J. Risk Assessment and Management*, *9*(4), 409–432.

von Lubitz, D. K. J. E., & Beakley, J. (in press). "Teams of Leaders" concept in homleland security and disaster management operations. *Int l.J. Homeland Security and Disaster Management.*

von Lubitz, D. K. J. E., Beakley, J., & Patricelli, F. (2008a). "All hazards approach" to network-centric disaster management: the role of information and knowledge management, and Boyd's OODA Loop in disaster leadership. *The Journal of Disaster Study, Policy and Management,* May 13. doi:10.1111/j.0361-3666.2008.01060.x, available at http://www.blackwell-synergy.com/toc/disa/0/0

von Lubitz, D. K. J. E., Beakley, J., & Patricelli, F. (2008b). Disaster Management: The Structure, Function, and Significance of Network-Centric Operations. *Journal of Homeland Security and Emergency Management, 1/1*(5). Available at: http://www.bepress.com/jhsem/vol5/iss1/1

von Lubitz, D. K. J. E., Beier, K. P., & Freer, J. Griffiths, J.M., Levine, H., Sauter, J., et al. (2001). *IMERSEME in VIBEs: Interactive/Immersive Medical Education/Research Simulation and Modeling Environment (IIMERSME) and Virtual Interactive Burn Environment (VIBE) as a "New Generation" approach to global biomedical education, training, and research.* Proc ITEC 2001, Lille (France), April 24-26, 2001.

von Lubitz, D. K. J. E., Carrasco, B., Fausone, C. A., Gabbrielli, F., Kirk, J., Lary, M. J., et al. (2005). Bioterrorism, medical readiness, and distributed simulation training of first responders. In J. Johnson, M. Cwiek, G. Ludlow, (eds.), *Community and Response to Terrorism (Vol. II): A Community of Organizations: Responsibilities and Collaboration Among All Sectors of Society,* (pp. 267-312). Westport, CT: Praeger/Greenwood Publ. Group.

von Lubitz, D. K. J. E., Levine, H., & Wolf, E. (2002). The Goose, the Gander, or the Strasbourg Paté for All: Medical Education, World, and the Internet. In Chin, W., Patricelli, F., & Milutinovic, V. (Eds.), *Electronic Business and Education: Recent Advances in Internet Infrastructures* (pp. 189–210). Boston: Academic Publishers.

von Lubitz, D. K. J. E., & Patricelli, F. (2006). Networkcentric Healthcare Operations; Data Warehousing and the Associated Telecommunication Platforms. *Intl. J.Services and Standards*, *3*(1), 97–119.

von Lubitz, D. K. J. E., & Patricelli, F. (2008). Telecommunications infrastructure for worldwide network-centric healthcare operations and the associated information system. *Intl. J. Business and Systems Research*, *2*(1), 34–51.

von Lubitz, D. K. J. E., & Wickramasinghe, N. (2006a). Healthcare and technology: the doctrine of network-centric healthcare. *International Journal of Electronic Healthcare*, *4*, 322–344.

von Lubitz, D. K. J. E., & Wickramasinghe, N. (2006b). Networkcentric healthcare and bioinformatics: unified operations within three domains of knowledge. *Expert Systems with Applications*, *30*, 11–23.

von Lubitz, D. K. J. E., & Wickramasinghe, N. (2006c). Dynamic Leadership In Unstable And Unpredictable Environments. *Intl. J. Innovation Learning*, *4*, 339–350.

von Lubitz, D. K. J. E., & Wickramasinghe, N. (2006d). Networkcentric healthcare: outline of entry portal concept. *Intl. J. Electronic Business Management*, *4*(1), 16–28.

von Lubitz, D. K. J. E., & Wickramasinghe, N. (2006e). Creating germane knowledge in dynamic environments. *Int. J. Innovation and Learning*, *3*(3), 326–347.

von Lubitz, D. K. J. E., Wickramasinghe, N., & Yanovsky, G. (2006). Networkcentric healthcare operations: the telecommunications structure. *Int. J. Networking and Virtual Org.*, *3*(1), 60–85.

Ward, R., Stevens, C., Brentnall, P., & Briddon, J. (2008). The attitudes of healthc care staff to information technology: a comprehensive review of the research literature. *Health Info Libr.*, *25*(2), 81–97.

Ward, R., & Wamsley, G. (2007). From a painful past to an uncertain future. In Rubin, C. (Ed.), *Emergency Management: The American Experience 1900-2005* (pp. 207–242). Fairfax, VA: PERI.

WHO. (1946). *Constitution of the World Health Organization*. Retrieved from http://www.who.int/gb/bd/PDF/bd46/e-46_p2.pdfhttp://www.who.int/gb/bd/PDF/bd46/e-bd46_p2.pdf

Wickramasinghe, N., & Schaffer, J. L. (2006). Creating knowledge-driven healthcare processes with the Intelligence Continuum. *International Journal of Electronic Healthcare*, *2*(2), 164–174.

Wickramasinghe, N., & von Lubitz, D. K. J. E. (2007). *Knowledge-Based Enterprise: Theories and Fundamentals* (pp. 1–380). Hershey, PA: IDEA Group Publishing.

Wiecha, J., & Barrie, N. (2002). Collaborative online learning: a new approach to distance CME. *Academic Medicine*, *77*(9), 928–929.

Wiese, C.R. (2006). Organizing Homeland Security after Katrina: is adaptive management what's missing. *Publ. Adm. Rev. May-June 2006*, 302-318.

Williams, K. A., Sullivan, F., Suner, S., Shapiro, M., Kobayashi, L., Woolard, B., & Hill, W. (2008). Rhode Island disaster initiative. *Intl. J. Risk Assessment and Management*, *9*(4), 394–408.

Wilson, C. (2004). *CRS Report for Congress, 2004, Network Centric Warfare: Background and Oversight Issues for Congress* (pp. 1–35). Washington, DC: Congressional Research Service and The Library of Congress.

Wong, J. G. (1996). Efficiency and effectiveness in the urgent care clinic. *Postgraduate Medicine*, *99*(4), 161–166.

Workman, P. (2001). New drug targets for genomic cancer: therapy successes, limitations, opportunities, and future challenges. *Current Cancer Drug Targets*, *1*(1), 33–47.

World Economic Forum, Eurasia Economic Summit 2002: Health and the Future of Business, the Global Health Initiative of the World Economic Forum. (2002, August 8th).

World Federation on Medical Education. (1998). International standards in medical education: assessment and accreditation of medical schools'--educational programmes. A WFME position paper. The Executive Council, The World Federation for Medical Education. *Medical Education*, *32*(5), 549–558.

World Federation on Medical Education. (2000). WFME task force on defining international standards in basic medical education. Report of the working party, Copenhagen, 14-16 October 1999. *Medical Education*, *34*(8), 665–675.

World Health Organization Report. (2004). *Changing History,* (pp. 1-167). Geneva: Author.

Wyle, M. D., Lind, W. S., & Trainor, B. E. (1981). Maneuver/Fluid Warfare. *The Marine Corps Gazette*, *65*(April), 49–54.

Zara, C., Torralba, M., Sotoca, J. M., Prat, A., Faixedas, M. T., & Gilalbert, A. (2004). The impact of new drug introduction on drug expenditure in primary health care in Catalunya, Spain. *The Annals of Pharmacotherapy*, *39*(1), 177–182.

Zupan, J. (2003). Perinatal mortality and morbidity in developing countries: a global view. *Med Trop*, *63*(Mars), 366–368.

Chapter 5
Grid Architecture and Components in Diagnostic Pathology

Gloria Bueno García
Universidad de Castilla-La Mancha, Spain

Marcial García Rojo
Hospital General de Ciudad Real, Spain

Roberto González Morales
Universidad de Castilla-La Mancha, Spain

Oscar Déniz Suárez
Universidad de Castilla-La Mancha, Spain

Jesús García González
Hospital General de Ciudad Real, Spain

ABSTRACT

The Grid vision has been described as a world in which computational power (resources, services, data) is as readily available as different utilities. They are available to users by means of computational, data, application, information and knowledge services at different levels and areas. These services can interact to perform specified tasks in an efficient and secure way. Their main applications include large-scale computational and data intensive problems in science and engineering. Therefore, Grids are likely to have a deep impact on health related applications. Moreover, they seem to be suitable for tissue-based diagnosis. This chapter analyzes the general structures and functions of a Grid environment implemented for tissue-based diagnosis on digital images. Moreover, it describes the web-based automated image analysis system developed by the authors for diagnostic pathology.

DOI: 10.4018/978-1-61692-010-4.ch005

INTRODUCTION

Grid technology has enabled the clustering and access to and interaction among a wide variety of geographically distributed resources such as: supercomputers, storage systems, data sources, instruments and special devices and services (Roure, 2005), that is network-centric operations (Alberts, 1999), (von Lubitz, 2006). Therefore Grid infrastructures and services have presented significant challenges at different levels, including: a) Models, from conceptual to implementation, b) Application: formulation and development, c) Programming systems, d) Infrastructures and services, e) Resources management, f) Networking and g) Security (Parashar, 2005).

Grid technologies have been developed for applications with large storage and computation requirements (Montagnat, 2003). They offer a powerful tool to deal with current challenges in many biomedical domains involving complex anatomical and physiological modelling of structures from images or large image database assembling and analysis. Indeed, grids are suitable for:

- allowing distribution of large datasets over different sites
- enforcing the use of common standards for data exchanges
- enlarging the datasets available for large scale studies in many sites
- opening new studies, perspectives and application fields

On the other hand, institutions involved in tissue-based diagnosis, including conventional, prospective, indicative and risk-assigned diagnosis, should have access to a variety of sources for data, information, and knowledge, to enable working in an efficient manner (Görtler, 2006). That is why Grids are a promising technology for Diagnostic Pathology. Particularly, medical image processing and the introduction of virtual slides will promote Grid applications in tissue-based diagnosis to fulfil the requirements of Anatomic Pathology applications.

BACKGROUND

Grid computing has been applied in several large-scale projects in biomedicine, such as: BIRN, MammoGrid, Health-e-Child, eDiamond, MEDIGRID, caBIG™ and EAMUS™. The Biomedical Informatics Research Network (BIRN) (Peltier, 2003) initiative focuses on support for collaborative access to and analysis of datasets generated by neuroimaging studies. Both MammoGrid (Amendolia, 2004) and eDiamond (Solomonides, 2003) projects are funded by the European Union (EU) to apply Grid user level middleware and network resources to build and research on a distributed database of mammograms. These projects develop and promote standardization in medical image databases for mammography and other cancer diseases. MEDIGRID (Tweed, 2003) is another multi-institutional project investigating the application of Grid technologies for manipulating large medical image databases. The European project Health-e-Child (2006-2009) aims at developing a biomedical information platform, including image analysis and computational models, to share paediatric knowledge and clinical data based on grid technologies (Health-e-Child, 2008).

Another example of a grid information service is the EU project Virolab Grid. This project deals with viral infection (HIV/AIDS) analysis. Its service offers the integration of biomedical information, advanced applications and data services under secure distributed resources (Virolab, 2006), (Görtler, 2006).

In Anatomic Pathology, the caBIG™ (cancer Biomedical Informatics Grid) project (caBIG, 2006) released in 2006 tries to develop applications and the underlying systems architecture that connects together data, tools, scientists and organizations in an open federated environment. caBIG™ used caGrid as the underlying SOA (service oriented network architecture) that provides the basis for connectivity between all of the cancer community institutions. caTissue is a project developed in 2007 and integrated within caBIG™ to develop software repository tools for bio-specimen inventory, tracking and basic Pathology Annotation (CAP protocol pathology annotation), caTIES-like Pathology Report Annotation, Custom Annotation (Dynamic Extensions) and Advanced Query "Wizard". caTissue allows users to track the collection, storage, quality assurance and analyzes them. It also allows users to find and request specimens that may then be used in molecular, correlative studies. The objectives of caTissue encompass establishing: a) Common Data Elements, b) protocols for the new tracking system and data fields and c) adoption of caBIG™ compatible caTissue systems. The tool will enhance the ability of pathologists, bio-specimen bankers and other researchers to share databases and locate and acquire specimens with the long term goal of catalyzing translational research and optimizing bio-specimen banking efforts (caTissue, 2007).

In tissue-based diagnosis, the EAMUS™ project (Kayser, 2006-b) can be considered as a simple, one-node implementation of the application service. The *application services* manage Grid application and give access to remote software, libraries and Web services (Görtler, 2006). Moreover, the EAMUS™ project may be used for a grid information service by combining it with an existing telepathology information system such as UICC-TPCC, or iPATH (Oberholzer, 2003). *Information services* try to extract and present information provided by data and/or other grid services, and to put these into relationship.

Other grid solutions in diagnostic pathology for *data* and *computational services* have been developed. That is: a) to offer secure access to distributed datasets, managing access, retrieval, storage, replication, or catalogues of individual or distributed libraries, in the case of data services, and b) to deal with secure distributed computational resources for executing application jobs in the case of computational services. These solutions are based on PACS (Picture Archive and Communication System) applications developed for live imaging, neurosurgery, or dermatology. (Germain, 2005), (Liu, 2005), (Balogh, 2006), and systems that automatically evaluate cytology smears (Husain, 1987), or measure DNA content or expression of antigens (Haroske, 1998), (Haroske, 2000). Also the application of the workflow system DataCutter (Beynon, 2001) for efficient image processing workflows on very large microscopy image datasets across Grid-nodes have been used for mouse brain analysis (Kumar, 2008) and prognosis of neuroblastoma (Cambazoglu, 2007).

These examples show how Grids have emerged as a promising technology to handle large amounts of data and compute the specific biomedical and bioinformatics requirements for several applications in radiology, laboratory, neurosurgery, etc. Moreover, grid technology is part of the solution of the operative system underlying that is of network-centric operations (NCO). NCO is an emerging but rapidly dominating concept created by Albert and Garstka in the early 90's at the Pentagon (Alberts, 1999), originally aimed at extreme complexities of modern battle field, is now implemented in healthcare (von Lubitz, 2006), business, transport, etc. The concept of NCO is about the relationships among things and people, as well as achieving and maintaining information superiority; that is, getting the right information to the right place in the right format at the right level of precision and accuracy at the right time (Alberts, 1999).

However, grid technologies are still in their infancy and they often propose only very generic services for secure access. Higher level services, in terms of user and core level middleware as well as network resources, should be developed to take into account the specific requirements in biomedical applications and particularly in diagnostic pathology. The above mentioned tools can only be considered as precursors and do not meet the performance of a Grid in general, as they are designed for one analysis system with open access. Implementations of Grids to be applied in tissue-based diagnosis have not been published yet (Görtler, 2006).

The following sections contain a brief introduction to a general workflow scheme in Diagnostic Pathology connecting this to grid architecture and individual components. Then the features of the Grid Distributed Architecture will be described. The chapter ends with the explanation of the grid middleware application implemented by the authors for Diagnostic Pathology applications.

DIAGNOSTIC PATHOLOGY AS A GRID APPLICATION

Workflow in Diagnostic Pathology

The workflow in a department of pathology usually follows this sequence: tissue identification, slide production, processing, diagnostics, clerical work and final diagnosis submission. The described workflow is not a simple straightforward procedure but there might be several feedback mechanisms due for example to slide quality and additional clinical information.

Moreover, emerging technologies in anatomic pathology imaging, that is the introduction of virtual microscopy, will cause several changes on the workflow of the pathology department. At a low level it will offer the chance to interact with all feedback mechanisms directly. At a higher level, introducing user and core level middleware as well as hardware will offer the possibility to provide tools that help pathologist carry out more accurate and objective diagnostics. For example, additional data, clinical information and second opinions can be requested prior to diagnosis and report. The current pathology information system will also change to allow storage and retrieval of the digital slides, as well as to include diagnosis databases linked to the images (Schrader, 2006), (Kayser, 2008). Figure 1 shows the workflow in diagnosis pathology in institutes with digitalised pathology for two use cases, that is a) referring center owner of digitization system and b) Expert's role (consultant).

According to the workflow, several grid functions may be distinguished in at least five different grid levels (Kayser, 2006). These levels are:

- **Application Level**: Laboratory and diagnostic quality assurance, slide screening, measurements, digital diagnosis reports, expert consultation, clinical history archive.
- **User Level MiddleWare:** Software environment and tools (programming languages, libraries, etc…), diagnosis management, data selection.
- **Core Level MiddleWare:** Pathology – hospital, institutions coupling services. Private security, images and clinical data, diagnosis status.
- **Local resources management:** Laboratory, pathology operating and queuing systems, libraries, hospital archive, internet protocol.
- **Network resources (hard ware):** Computers, line connections, storage systems, scanners, monitors, tissue embedding and slide preparation instruments.

This again is in accordance with the concept of NCO (Alberts, 1999), previously mentioned.

This concept has been used also in healthcare by von Lubitz, Wickramasinge and Patricelli, (von Lubitz, 2006). (von Lubitz, 2007). According to von Lubitz et al. healthcare globally is failing to meet its objectives of delivering appropriate medical attention to patients. They suggest that by adopting a NCO approach healthcare operations and delivery will be dramatically enhanced with the ultimate beneficiary being the patient. Underlying the NCO in healthcare is the use of information, computer and communication technologies,

Figure 1. Workflow in Diagnostic Pathology

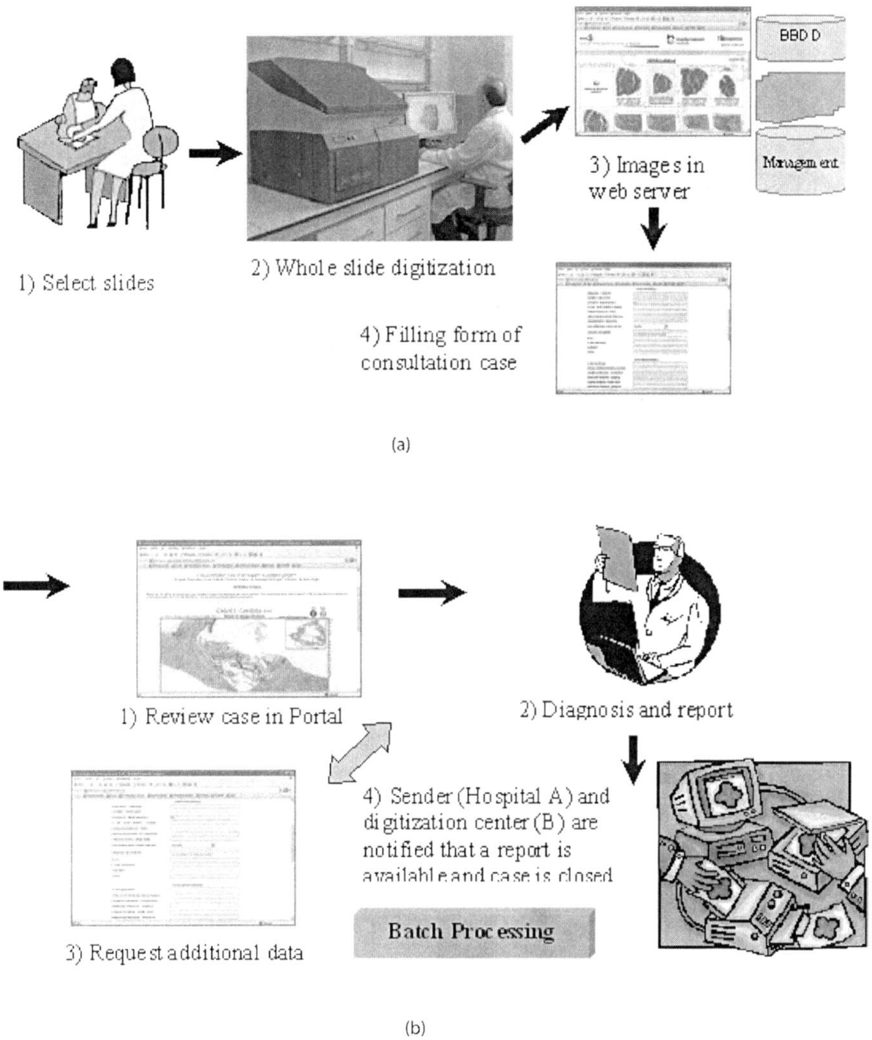

already existing, focus on how to combine them and facilitates transition from non-collaborative, platform-centric activities to fully federated, network-centric operations so that network centric healthcare can in fact become a reality.

a) Use Case: referring center owns digitization system
b) Use Case: Expert's role (consultant)

In this chapter we will deal with an application for the User Level Middleware. The objective of the application is the implementation of a Web based application which is accessible, efficient and useful in diagnostic pathology to visualize and analyze different types of image formats (JPEG, JPG, TIF, GIF, BMP, PPM) at different zoom levels. The application, obviously, must also take into account that the size of a pathology image is typically in the order of several gigabytes. This is also one of the aspects that call for the use of Grid technologies and therefore distributed architectures for diagnosis pathology. At the same time the application should give support to medical requirements, that is to integrate collaborative tools, editing and navigation tools as well as

Figure 2. Middleware Scheme. Distributed Parallel Processing for Diagnostic Pathology.

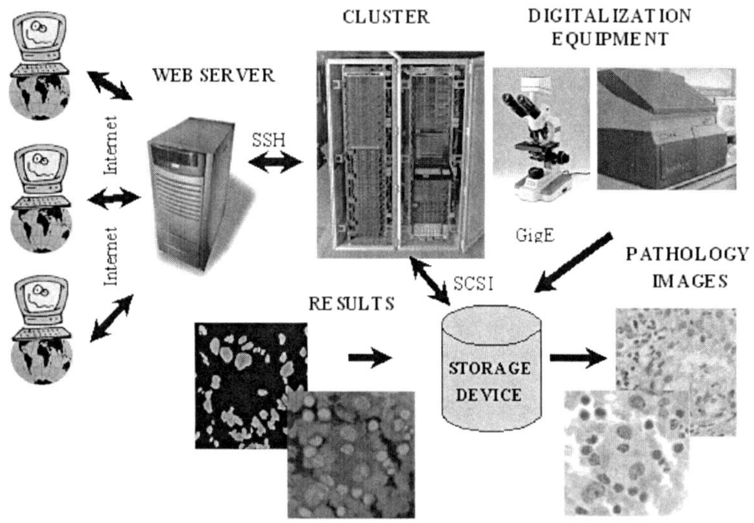

image pre-processing and processing methods. Figure 2 shows a scheme of the middleware grid application.

MIDDLEWARE IN DIAGNOSTIC PATHOLOGY

Distributed Architecture

Distributed programming models and systems are the basis of most existing Grid programming and applications. They allow a very efficient environment to integrate different type of data and algorithms (Parashar, 2005). Their characterization, requirements and classifications are as follows.

Characteristics of Grid Execution Systems and Applications

There are four main characteristics of Grid execution systems and applications:

- **Heterogeneity:** Grid environments aggregate large numbers of independent and geographically distributed computational and information resources.
- **Dynamism:** The grid computation, communications and information environment is continuously changing during the lifetime of an application. Moreover, the organization and interactions of the component/services can also change.
- **Uncertainty:** caused by multiple factors, including: a) Dynamism, which introduces unpredictable and changing behaviours, b) Failures, which have an increasing probability of occurrence as systems/application scales increase, c) Incomplete knowledge of global system state, which is intrinsic to large distributed environments.
- **Security:** Grid has secure hardware/software resources for authentication, authorization and access control.

Requirements for Grid Systems

The above mentioned characteristics make necessary for grid systems to be able to specify applications which can detect and respond to changes in both the execution and application states. That is:

- Grid applications should be composed of discrete, self-managing components which incorporate separate specifications for all states:
  a) functional: computational,
  b) non-functional: performance, fault detection and recovery,
  c) interaction and coordination.
- The specifications of the different states or behaviours should be separated and their combinations should be re-composed.
- The interface definitions of these components should be separated from their implementation to enable heterogeneous components to interact and to enable dynamic selection of components.

Classification for Grid Systems

The programming models for grid systems may be classified as:

1) Models based on the addition of communication/interaction models and mechanism to sequential programming models, that is: Message Passing Interface (MPI), Parallel Virtual Machine (PVM), shared-space models and RPC (remote procedure calls).
2) Distributed object models, for example Common Object Request Broker Architecture (CORBA).
3) Component based models such as: JavaBean, CORBA Component Model (CCM), and Common Component Architecture (CCA).
4) Services models, for example: Web Service, Open Grid Services Architecture (OGSA) and Web Service Resource Framework (WSRF)

Distributed Architecture for Diagnosis Pathology

The distributed programming application implemented by the authors is a joint application that mixes both Web and Grid Service Architecture around a distributed architecture for image processing. It makes use of servlets-Java and Java Server Pages, as well as models based on MPI and MPI2. The application gives support to multiple users by means of a server (Apache Tomcat) and it may be integrated within a netplatform. Figure 3 shows the scheme to integrate the web services within a network platform.

The service based models (Web Service) exist across applications against component-based models that has meaning during the life time and in the context of an application. Web services are easy to create, to access and to integrate different data and programming models. Message Passing models /Interface (MPI) provide messaging abstraction that enable entities defined by sequential programming models to communicate; that is message passing operators to sequential languages such as C and Fortran. MPICH-G2 and MPI-2, a grid enabled implementation of MPI, support heterogeneity using services provided by Globus toolkit, dynamism and uncertainty.

For the system design, unified process and conceptual design (UML) was used for case diagrams. Also a logical design for services and client objects by means of UML diagrams was done and divided into 3 layers:

- Functional: computational domain.
- Non-functional: performance, output processing, etc.
- Interaction-coordination: presentation for the Graphical User Interface (GUI).

Architecturally, the application may be divided into three main parts:

- Visualization: virtual microscopy viewer, using: a) Applet (Java): Hypertext Transfer Protocol (HTTP) over TCP at port 80, security for external institutions, b) HTTP Tunnelling: applet communication with remote servers, c) HTTP Basic

Figure 3. Web-Grid Service Architecture Integrated within a Network for Platform

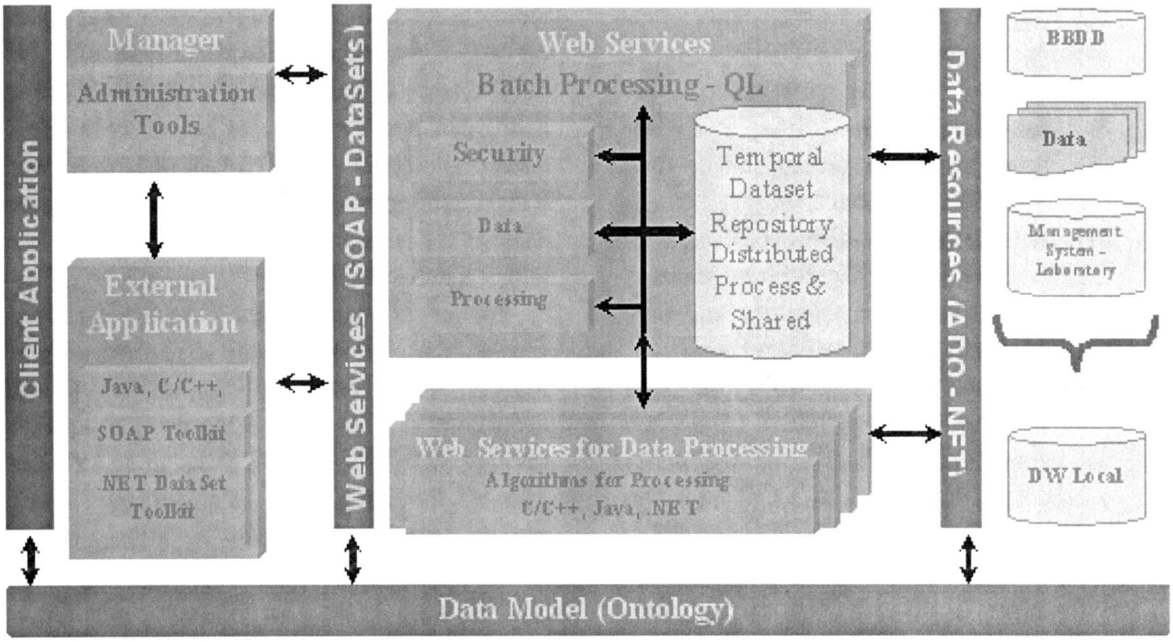

Authentication of client (login and password), d) Java library for GUI, data-file interchange and pre-processing.

- Processing: web servlets processing, using: a) C, C++ for an efficient parallel image processing, b) .NET: Platform integration for the web application, c) General platform IQL, for example INBIOMED/ COMBIOMED (Pérez del Rey, 2005).
- Storage: data storage, using: Servlets technology, Java 2 Enterprise Edition (J2EE) and Java Server Pages (JSP), and looking for efficiency when manipulating the gigabyte size images.

An MPP architecture with a cluster of 17 nodes interconnected using INFINIBAND, each node having one processor Intel XEON of 3.2GHz and 2GB of RAM memory was the hardware configuration used.

Figure 4 shows working sessions of the implemented system for diagnostic pathology. The systems support visualization and editing tools for all pathologic images and processing for just biopsy, cytology and autopsy histological images. Figure 4.a) shows a zoom of biopsy images at 40x for visualization and pre-processing regions of interest (ROI). Figure 4. b) shows the ROI detection and diagnosis carried out by the system after the application of artificial intelligence techniques.

a) Tools for image pre-processing
b) ROI detection and diagnosis

FUTURE RESEARCH DIRECTIONS

Grids have emerged as a promising technology to handle large amounts of data and compute the specific biomedical requirements in different areas such as radiology, bioinformatics and neurosurgery. However, further efforts should be made to implement Grids for tissue-based diagnosis. These efforts will be fuelled with the use of virtual microscopes.

However, only secured and specialized infrastructures with high level services including

Figure 4. Working sessions of the implemented Web-Grid system for diagnostic pathology

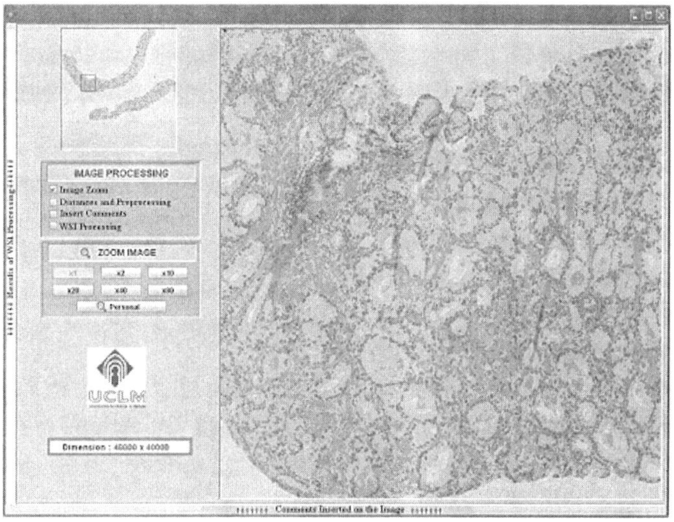

(a)

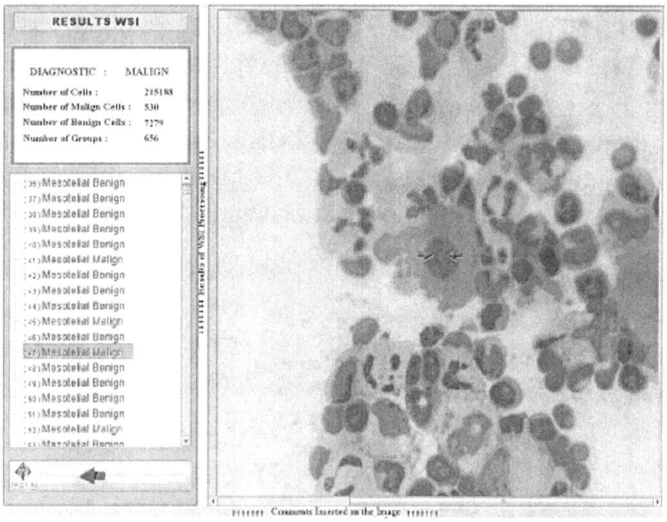

(b)

automated diagnostic procedures and appropriate standards will really allow a large scale acceptance and deployment of grid environments for diagnostic pathology applications.

CONCLUSION

This chapter has given a general view of Grid distributed programming models, their features and requirements applied to diagnostic pathology. It has been shown how grids have been used for biomedical applications. Moreover, basic middleware are today available and there is a big potential in grid technologies to tailor specific applications. Therefore, grid technology is also being taken into consideration in diagnostic pathology. The use of digital imaging requires the use of grid technology in order to combine all available information resources and establish tissue-based diagnosis in the medical environment.

A Grid middleware application for diagnostic pathology, implemented by the authors, has been described. The system supports different image analysis operations commonly applied in anatomic pathology. The system takes into account secured aspects and specialized infrastructures with high level services designed to meet application requirements. However, there is still room for further improvements within the system. Further tools for pathology image processing including artificial intelligence methods for pattern recognition and automated diagnostic procedures are under development.

REFERENCES

Alberts, D. S., Garstka, J. J., & Stein, F. P. (1999). Network Centric Warfare: Developing and Leveraging Information Superiority. *CCRP Publ.* From: http://www.dodccrp.org/files/Alberts_NCW.pdf

Amendolia, R., Estrella, F., Hauer, T., Manset, D., McCabe, D., McClatchey, R., et al. Grid databases for shared image analysis in the mammogrid project. In *Proc. 8th Int. Database Eng. Appl. Symp. (Ideas2004)*, pp. 302–311.

Balogh A.A., Preul M.C., Laszlo K., Schornak M., Hickman M., Deshmukh P., & Spetzler R.F. (2006). Multilayer image grid reconstruction technology: four-dimensional interactive image reconstruction of microsurgical neuroanatomic dissections. *Neurosurgery, 58*(1 Suppl):ONS157-65. Discussion ONS157–65.

Beynon, M. D., Kurc, T., Catalyurek, U., Chang, C., Sussman, A., & Saltz, J. (2001). Distributed processing of very large datasets with DataCutter. *Parallel Computing, 27*(11), 1457–1478. doi:10.1016/S0167-8191(01)00099-0

caBIG, caTissue. (2006). Retrieved from https://cabig.nci.nih.gov/tools/catissuecore; https://cabig.nci.nih.gov/workspaces/Architecture/caGrid; http://gforge.nci.nih.gov/projects/cacorecvs/

Cambazoglu, B., Sertel, O., & Kong, J. (2007). Efficient processing of pathological images using the grid: Computer-aided prognosis of neuroblastoma. In *Proc. Challenges of Large Applications in Distributed Environments,* CLADE'07, June 25, 2007, (pp. 35-41), Monterey, California.

Germain, C., Breton, V., Clarysse, P., Gaudeau, Y., & Glatard, T., Jeannot, et al. (2005). Grid-enabling medical image analysis. *Journal of Clinical Monitoring and Computing, 19*(4–5), 339–349. doi:10.1007/s10877-005-0679-9

Görtler, J., Berghoff, M., Kayser, G., & Kayser, K. (2006). Grid technology in tissue-based diagnosis: fundamentals and potential developments. *Diagnostic Pathology, 1*, 23. August 24, 2006, from: http://www.diagnosticpathology.org/content/1/1/23

Haroske, G., Meyer, W., Kunze, D., & Boeking, A. (1998). Quality control measures for dna image cytometry in a telepathology network. *Advances in Clinical Pathology, 2*(2), 143–145.

Haroske, G., Meyer, W., Oberholzer, M., Bocking, A., & Kunze, K. D. (2000). Competence on demand in DNA image cytometry. *Pathology, Research and Practice, 196*(5), 285–291.

Health-e-Child. (2008). Retrieved from http://www.health-e-child.org/

http://www.gridwisetech.com/virolab

Husain, O. A., & Watts, K. C. (1987). Preparatory methods for DNA hydrolysis, cytochemistry, immunocytochemistry and ploidy analysis. Their application to automated and routine diagnostic cytopathology. *Analytical and Quantitative Cytology and Histology, 9*(3), 218–224.

Kayser, G., Radziszowski, D., Bzdyl, P., Sommer, R., & Kayser, K. (2006). Theory and implementation of an electronic, automated measurement system for images obtained from immunohistochemically stained slides. *Analytical and Quantitative Cytology and Histology*, *28*(1), 27–38.

Kayser, K., Görtler, J., Goldmann, T., Vollmer, E., & Hufnagl, P. & Kayser G. (2008). Image standards in tissue-based diagnosis (diagnostic surgical pathology). *Diagnostic Pathology, 3*, 17. Retrieved from http://www.diagnosticpathology.org/content/3/1/17

Kayser, K., Molnar, B., & Weinstein, R. S. (2006). *Virtual Microscopy*. Berlin: VSV Interdisciplinary Medical Publishing.

Kumar, V. S., Rutt, B., Kurc, T., Catalyurek, U. V., Pan, T. C., & Chow, S. (2008). Large-Scale Biomedical Image Analysis in Grid Environments. *IEEE Transactions on Information Technology in Biomedicine*, *12*(2), 154–161. doi:10.1109/TITB.2007.908466

Liu, B. J., Zhou, M. Z., & Documet, J. (2005). Utilizing data grid architecture for the backup and recovery of clinical image data. *Computerized Medical Imaging and Graphics*, *29*(2–3), 95–102.

Montagnat, J., Breton, V., & Magnin, I. E. (2003). Using grid technologies to face medical image analysis challenges. In *Proceedings of BioGrid 2003: 3rd Int. Symp. Cluster Comput. Grid (CC-Grid 2003)*, (pp. 588–593).

Oberholzer, M., Christen, H., Haroske, G., Helfrich, M., Oberli, H., & Jundt, G. (2003). Modern telepathology: a distributed system with open standards. *Current Problems in Dermatology*, *32*, 102–114. doi:10.1159/000067381

Parashar, M., & Browne, J. C. (2005). Conceptual and implementation models for the grid. *Proceedings of the IEEE*, *93*(3), 653–668. doi:10.1109/JPROC.2004.842780

Peltier, S., & Ellisman, M. (2003). The Grid, blueprint for a new computing infrastructure. in *The Biomedical Informatics Research Network*, (2nd ed.). Amsterdam, The Netherlands: Elsevier. Retrieved from http://www.nbirn.net

Pérez del Rey, D., Crespo, J., Pérez, L. J., Dorado, J., Bueno, G., & Feliu, V. (2005). Biomedical Image Processing Integration through INBIOMED: A Web Services-Based Platform. *Lecture Notes in Computer Science, (. LNBI*, *3745*, 34–43.

Roure, D., Jennings, N. R., & Shadbolt, N. R. (2005). The semantic grid: past, present and future. *Proceedings of the IEEE*, *93*(3), 669–681. doi:10.1109/JPROC.2004.842781

Schrader, T., Niepage, S., Leuthold, T., Saeger, K., Schluns, K., Hufnagl, P., et al. (2006). The diagnostic path, a useful visualisation tool in virtual microscopy. *Diagnostic Pathology*. doi:10.1186/1746-1596-1-40, 08 November 2006, 1:40, from: http://www.diagnosticpathology.org/content/1/1/40

Solomonides, A., McClatchey, R., Odeh, M., Brady, M., Mulet-Parada, M., Schottlander, D., & Amendolia, S. (2003). Mammogrid and ediamond: Grids applications in mammogram analysis. In *Proc. International Association for Development of the Information Society International Conference, IADIS Int. Conf.: e-Soc.*, (pp. 1032–1033).

Tweed, T., & Miguet, S. (2003). Medical image database on the grid: Strategies for data distribution. In *Proc. HealthGrid 2003 Workshop*, (pp. 152–162).

Virolab. (2006). Retrieved from http://www.virolab.org:8080/virolab/ and

von Lubitz, D., & Patricelli, F. (2007). Network-centric healthcare operations: data warehousing and the associated telecommunications platforms. *International Journal of Services and Standards*, *3*(1), 97–119. doi:10.1504/IJSS.2007.011830 von Lubitz D. & Wickramasinghe N. (2006). Networkcentric healthcare: applying the tools, techniques and strategies of knowledge management to healthcare. *International Journal of Management*, 60-85.

KEY TERMS AND DEFINITIONS

Histology: Histology is the study of the microscopic morphology of cells and tissues. It is performed by examining a thin slice (section) of tissue under a light microscope or electron microscope. The ability to visualize or differentially identify microscopic structures is frequently enhanced through the use of histological stains. Accurate diagnosis of cancer and other diseases usually requires **histopathological** examination of samples. That is the microscopic study of diseased tissue. Histopathology is an important tool in anatomic pathology or diagnosis of disease based on the gross, microscopic and examination of organs, tissues and autopsy.

Virtual Slide: A virtual slide is a high resolution digital image obtained when glass slides are digitally scanned in their entirety using a digital scanning system for the purpose of medical digital image analysis. Digital slides can be retrieved from a storage system, and analyzed in a similar way as on a microscope.

Virtual Microscope: It is the practice of create a virtual slide. That is, converting histological sections mounted glass slides into high-resolution digital images. Virtual microscopy offers several advantages over traditional microscopy, including remote viewing and data sharing, annotation, and various forms of data mining.

Tissue-based Diagnosis: It is the process of identifying a medical condition or disease by its signs and from the results of various diagnostic procedures, including conventional, prospective, indicative and risk-assigned diagnosis, to analyze spatial configurations of biological functional units. Most frequently cells, cellular agglutinations such as vessels, nerves, glands, etc. are being investigated

Globus Toolkit: is an open source toolkit for building computing grids developed and provided by the **Globus Alliance**. The Globus Alliance is an international association dedicated to developing fundamental technologies needed to build grid computing infrastructures. The Globus Alliance was officially established in September 2003, however it was created out of the previous Globus Project in 1995 (http://www.globus.org/alliance/news/prGAannounce.html).

InfiniBand: is a network topology communications link where network nodes connect with each other via one or more network switches, and primarily used in high-performance computing. Its features include quality service and the capability to switch over automatically to a redundant or standby computer server, system, or network upon the failure computer server, system, or network upon the failure or abnormal termination of the previously active server, system, or network, and it is designed to be scalable. The InfiniBand architecture specification defines a connection between processor nodes and high performance Input/Output nodes such as storage devices. It is a superset of the Virtual Interface Architecture.

MPI: is a language-independent communications protocol used to program parallel computers. Both point-to-point and collective communication are supported. MPI is a message-passing application programmer interface, together with protocol and semantic specifications for how its features must behave in any implementation, where communication is made by the sending of messages to recipients. MPI's goals are high performance, scalability, and portability. MPI remains the dominant model used in high-performance computing today.

Chapter 6
Grid Technology in Telepatology and Personalised Treatment

O. Ferrer-Roca
University of La Laguna, Spain

F. Marcan
University of La Laguna, Spain

ME. Vidal
University Simon Bolivar, Venezuela

E. Ruckhaus
University Simon Bolivar, Venezuela

X. Santos
University of La Laguna, Spain

E. Iglesias
University Simon Bolivar, Venezuela

ABSTRACT

Histopathology requires automation, quality control and global collaborative tools. Usually the PIMS (Pathology information management system) automates samples, images and reports and progressively incorporates the PI (Pathology informatics), the D-PATH (digital pathology), e-PATH (electronic pathology), the PPH (Patho-pharmacology), virtual autopsy (VA) and all type of translational research in the PMIS. Not being subject to a specific standard, quality control follows ISO-13485:2003 on services and medical devices, ISO 17025:2005 on technical aspects; and ISO-15198:2003 for automate and quantifiable procedures that will be affected by the new European Directive on medical devices. For the non-standardized pathology procedures, consumer's requirements are what define test and calibration procedures. The paper analysed the non-standardized procedures: VS (Virtual Slides), GRID networking and Literature Based Discovery as tools for knowledge discovery of relevant relationships on image-diagnosis and personalized treatments. Standardized procedures available for search and annotation are the ISO/IEC 11179 Information Technology Metadata Registries specification, the ISO/IEC 13250:2003 for topics maps or MPEG-7 & 21 for images and the ISO/IEC 24800-3 for JPEG query search. The

DOI: 10.4018/978-1-61692-010-4.ch006

forthcoming innovations prepare to quality certify the so called "solo-pathology" robotic labs, supported by telepathology to reduce diagnostic errors and carrying out a relevant task on personalized treatment through GRID technology. In this environment the JPEG query search play a relevant role on images which metadata can be annotated on natural language.

INTRODUCTION

Quality control of the health-care laboratories include: (1) Management requirements according to ISO 9001:20001 norm or its equivalent ISO-13485:2003 (ISO 13250, 2003) for medical devices and services. (2) Technical requirements inside of the ISO 17025:2005 (ISO17025, 2005) norm for testing and calibration, the (3) ISO 15189:2007 or quality and competence of microbiological and clinical laboratories and (4) finally the norm ISO/TS 22367:2008, which are the technical specifications of risk reduction and risk management in laboratories.

The ISO 15189 norm was intended for microbiology and clinical laboratories, peculiar because their reports only have objective results without diagnostic interpretation.

The ISO 15189 includes management issues following ISO 9001 norm and technical issues following ISO 17025 norm. The technical direction responsible of quality-DTC is in charge to define **politics** and **objectives** (Service goal, level of services, Quality objectives) (Gimenez, 2007; SEAP, 2003) including **internal** and **external controls** (instrument calibration, reactive and systems). Everything should be documented in a **quality manual.**

Nowadays differences between clinical laboratories and pathology departments have shorted due to automation (VLA, 2006; Garcia-Rojo, 1998), quantitative pathology (FISH-HISH-cytogenetic and tumour markers, IHQ etc.) and pharmaco-pathology for therapeutic targets involving or not GRID diagnostic support of distributed computation (Schmitt, 2007).

A pathology department should consider the quality standards and risk management of the new EU directive of medical devices (ISO11073, 2008; IEC60601, 2006; ISO14971, 2007; DIR2007, 2007) together with technical advances of informatics (PI, 2008; Becich, 2008)

Table 1. ISO 15189:2007 Critical points in laboratories

Personnel competency
Laboratory installations and devices
Validation of the analytical process
Validation of the ICT
Ethic code, confidentiality and data security
Post-analytic processes. Laboratory reports.
Implementation, follow up and improvement.
Risk management / priorities
Quality assurance of analytical processes
Auditing, Review of system quality management by the direction

digital pathology (D-AP) electronic pathology (e-AP), la tele-pathology (TP), virtual autopsy, pharmaco-pathology and translational research on aetiology and physiopathology of the illnesses. On this regard its patho-informatics service will be in charge of the LIS2 (Pearson, 2006)- PIS3 data and specimen flow, of reproducibility and traceability of digital images, of HIS4 and PACS5 integration and of data/image availability for cooperative work (autopsy room, operating theatre of the future etc.), automatic classification and annotation; together with anonymization, biobanking, mining etc. Aspects not yet considered in the pathology competency in some countries (SNCFP, 2005).

To be specific, the patho-informatics started with Tom Lincoln and Don Connelly in the 80s defining theoretical bases. In 1987 Ralph Korpman stressed the role of pathologist in medical informatics systems and in 1990 Bruce Friedman established the term "*pathology informatics*" (PI). At that time 1993 Greg Buffone and Bob Beck propose its sub-speciality in the field of pathology. Finally in 2002, Friedman carried out the first meeting in which the discipline of "*pathology bioinformatics*" was defined inside of the Bioinformatics. Since then, informatics in pathology is taking care of

1. Basis of the illnesses (aetiology-physiopathology) merging pathology, biochemistry and pharmacology (translational research).
2. Patient data security and confidentiality as well as access and responsibility in the clinical environment.
3. Tissue Banks, Management and mission (diagnostic and specimen provision).
4. Data exchange and its standards. Since the main mission of the patho-informatics is translational and interdisciplinary.
5. Web distance access and Management of big longitudinal and relational data bases from standardized clinical and research data.

Figure 1. Role of the patho-informatics. GLP = good laboratory practice: The LIMS have to be substituted by PIMS = pathology informatics management system.

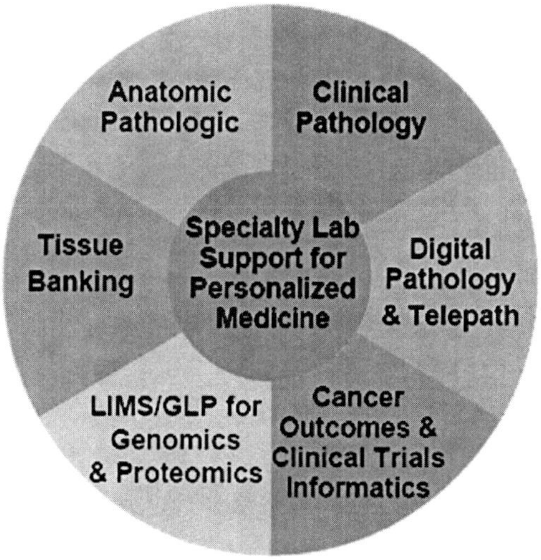

But even considering the great number of standards already established most processes required specialists that also have to deal with *Plug & Play* IEEE 11073 standards from nomenclature to wireless transmission, with integrations such the ones of the IHE (*Integrated Health Care enterprise*) and bioengineering topics including telecommunications or medical device requirements.

UNE: EN 60601-1:2008, THE PESS AND TELECOMMUNICATIONS

Medical devices (MD) containing one or more electronic programmable subsystems (PESS) are controlled by the UNE EN 60601-1:2008 norm. A PESS in any system based in one or more processing central units including the software and interface.

Software programs are systems almost impossible to completely verify, although requirements are specify in the technical report of medical software risk management AAMI-TIR32, it will be an International version in the IEC 80002. In this case software processes have to be considering special and require validation before everyday use is allowed, in order to test possible danger for the patient or the operators (IEC 62304:2006). In fact not only have to follow the medical device norms but also have to assure basic security guarantee and functional guarantee.

This means that not only cannot produce danger, but that they have to demonstrate their efficacy.

In the new European directive of medical devices telecommunications are consider part of the MDDS (*Medical Device Data System)*. In the case of integration together with non-medical products, the integrator have to assure that fulfil the IEC 60601-1 norm.

In brief a MDDS is a device that translates data from one medical device to another.

THE NEW EU DIRECTIVE D-2007/47/CE

The directives applicable to medical devices (MD) are: D 90/385/EEC – RD 634/93, for active implantable MD (i.e.: pacemakers); D 93/42/EEC – RD 414/96, for general MD including active non-implantable MD (i.e.: x-ray equipments); Directive 98/79/EEC – RD 1662/2000, for MD for "in vitro" diagnosis (i.e: kit for blood glucose testing).

The new directive 2007/47/CE include the new definition of **Medical Device** particularly important in the pathology lab, because it defines any instrument, device or computer program, material or any other article used alone or in combination with others as well as any accessory including software produce by a company to be used in humans for: (1) diagnosis, prevention, control, treatment o release of a disease; (2) diagnosis, control, treatment or release or compensation of a lesion or deficiency (3) research, substitution or changes of the anatomy or of a physiological process (4) control or regulation of the contraception, which expected action inside or outsider of the human body is not produced by pharmacological, immunologic or metabolic means, but which function can depend of such products.

For all Medical Devices the CE label is mandatory and therefore not only should be visible in the laboratory devices but also in the software associated to those devices.

Software producers will be responsible during the whole active life of the product. Being a class I or low risk do not require compulsory audits unless there is a formal complain, but being a medical software will be regulated by the IEC 62304:2006 norm.

As soon as the new directive enter into force, around 2010, all software systems should carry a visible CE label and assure warranty of information (no secrecy of how they work and obtain parameters will be possible); of security (have to be previously tested); of functionality (will require a previous validation prior its function in the real world); of quality (the design system should fulfil the ISO-13485 quality design). If this is not fulfil, only could be consider **a demonstrator**.

MICRO-MACRO AND VIRTUAL SLIDE IMAGES

In an environment efficiently managed by the PIMS (*pathology information management system*), all macro-micro and virtual slide images should be stored and annotated at least with the SNOMED code extracted automatically from the pathology report created with an automatic dictation system including voice recognition. (García-Rojo, 1998; Liu, 2005; WIPO, 2008)

According our own definition of what is a Virtual Slide (costumer opinion since it is not yet standardized) <<the goal of a Virtual slide is to get a complete digital image from and histological slide capable to be used for diagnosis and therefore (1) containing metadata for an accurate

colour representation; (2) capable to be used for densitometry and quantification; (3)containing three-dimensional information (Z-plane focus) whenever necessary; (4) supporting digital zoom with diagnostic quality and (5) having quick distance management capable to visualize the ROIs (regions of interest); (6)containing standardized metadata6 for image knowledge mining and (7) occupying the minimum possible space in order to be managed efficiently by the hospital PIS, the HIS and the PACS;(8) being capable to be anonymized depending of whether it is an assistant sample or a bio-sample>>. Following this definition the majority of the market systems would not overpass a quality control check. To get managed by the HIS and PACS virtual slides should have less then 2 GB (maximum allowed in DICOM), for that reason the SSVS (small size virtual slide) technique developed by us has been shown ideal (Ferrer-Roca, 2008).

Obviously images coming from **virtual autopsies** should also be integrated (Thali, 2006; Dirnhofer, 2006) and the autopsy theatre transformed in a place with working flows similar to the ones existing in the ORF (*operating room of the future*), with ceiling suspended monitors voice commanded and touch sensitive screens, together with transportable Magnetic Resonance devices with or without magnetic positioning.

PIMS- ONTOLOGY AND DATA MINING

The PIMS (pathology information management system) (Tobias, 2006; CERNER, 2008; Apollo, 2008) include register, tracking, diagnostic support, speech recognition (CAMT, 2008), automatic extraction of the medical nomenclature (Ruch, 2006; Beckwith, 2006 ; Moore 1994) and classification through ontologies (OBO, 2008).

To provide scientific usability to the huge amount of data managed by each institutional PIMS, data must be anonymised and let them get accessed by the scientific community in private, publicly limited or in worldwide networks. To accomplish this at least three problems have to be faced: How to annotate the data; How to share it and How to find out the information, to finally search and access them efficiently either through CORBA or SOAP.

Annotate

Now a days great number of publicly data sources and services are available on the Internet being necessary to annotate an enormous amount of publicly data in a standardize manner to be interoperable (OBO, 2008). The use of the **ISO/IEC 11179 family** (ISO11179, 2004) of Metadata Registry standards (e.g., ISO/IEC 11179, ISO/IEC 20943, ISO/IEC 20944, ISO/IEC 19763 or MMF) creates **Extended Metadata registries** (XMDR) of the type: *Semantic networks*, that is a graph based representation, nodes are concepts, and directed edges represent binary relationships (is-a, part-of, ...) ie., RDF and the UMLS Semantic Network at NLM (UMLS, 2008); RDF or Resource Description Framework, being a graph-based data model used for encoding metadata on the web. A kind of semantic network; Description logic*(DL)* as a restricted subset of first order logic widely used in knowledge representation applications and in large scale terminology systems, ie., Galen, SNOMED, ect,; OWL-Lite, OWL-DL, OWL-Full Ontology Web Language standardized by W3C Semantic Web working group. Built on top RDF. Semantic Web Rule Language *OWL + RuleML*, allows constraint specifications via RuleML, etc.

Metadata terminology data sets relevant for Medicine and already incorporated in the XMDR are:

- Biomedical Domain, including: NCI (National Cancer Institute) terminology, UMLS (Unified Medical Language System), SNOMED (Systemized Nomenclature of Medicine, GO (Gene

Ontology) and other biological ontologies such as the Open Biological Ontologies

- Chemical Domain such as chemical nomenclature, chemical code sets (CAS registry numbers), chemical reactions, chemical properties. Include: DOE's Collaboratory for Multi-scale Chemical Systems, EPA's Substance Registry System, Material Safety Data Sheets, Enzyme Commission Taxonomy, etc.

Share

The second part is to share the annotated data: DTD´s (Document Type Definition) or XML Schema (also called an XSD or XML Schema Definition) is used to define the grammar and validate the data being shared.

The **ISO/IEC 8825** is the Extensible Markup Language (XML) ideal as a vehicle for interchange of both data and metadata, being the standard for metadata interchange the XMI (XML Metadata Interchange). The family of standards include the ISO/IEC 19501 Unified Modelling Language (UML); ISO/IEC 19502 Meta-Object Facility (MOF) ; **ISO/IEC 19503** XMI ; ISO/IEC 19757 Document Schema Definition Languages (DSDL); ISO/IEC CD 19763-3: MMF-Metamodel for ontology registration; ISO/IEC-9075-14 or SQL/XML related specifications; ISO 10303-28 XML-Schemas, etc.... In fact the SOAP (simple object access protocol) is an XML-based protocol that enables rich and automated web services.

Those ontology-driven information systems for search, integration and analysis take advantage of the **ISO/IEC 13250:2003** or topics maps XML syntax standard (ISO 23485, 2003) that use location address and hyperlinking modules following ISO/IEC 10744, as well as the **ISO-15836:2003** or Dubin Core metadata Element set or the **ISO/IEC 18023** for Synthetic Environment Data Representation using UML.

Query

To access this enormous amount of data it is necessary an efficient ontology query technique that allow to speed-up finding results, diagnosis or annotations among a huge number of samples and related data bases resulting in hypothesis that might inferred new discoveries on aetio-pathology or treatment. These techniques can be accessed at distance in a GRID environment in projects such as the *Shared Pathology Informatics Network* (SPIN) http://spin.nci.nih.gov/ or in the *Cancer Biomedical informatics grid* (Figure 2) containing many *open source* interoperable tools, modular and already validated.

Since bio-medical ontology is very large, **query processing strategies** are essential. Techniques similar to the ones proposed somewhere (Ruckhaus 2008) can be used to efficiently perform the ontology query and reasoning tasks, and thus, facilitate the deduction of new properties of the concepts.

In addition, *Text Mining* techniques have been developed to discover semantic associations between different concepts by traversing publications available in PubMed. Techniques on this area, known as **Literature Based Discovery** or **LBD** (Hristovski, 2006; Srinivasan, 2004), could be used in conjunction with any annotations and data in existing biomedical data sources to discover associations following the Electronic Discovery Reference Model (EDRM, 2008). Similarly *Image Mining* techniques can be developed taking advantage of the standardized image annotation systems and ontologies **ISO 19115/19139** standard on image metadata ontologies, MPEG-7 (MPEG Query Format-MPQF **ISO/IEC 15938-12** an XML based query language), MPEG-21 or **ISO 21000-14**, the **ISO/IEC CD 24800-3** for JPEG query search, the **ISO/IEC 15444-2** for JPX metadata set and DICOM.

This will become an essential element in pharmacopathology and translational research that involve a great number of specialities and research

Figure 2. The old fashion and the modern pathology department. Taken from Cancer Biomedicals informatic Grid. Tissue bank and pathology tools. https://cabig.nci.nih.gov/workspaces/TBPT/tbpt-newcomer/workspaces/TBPT/TBPT_Newcomer_Introduction.ppt

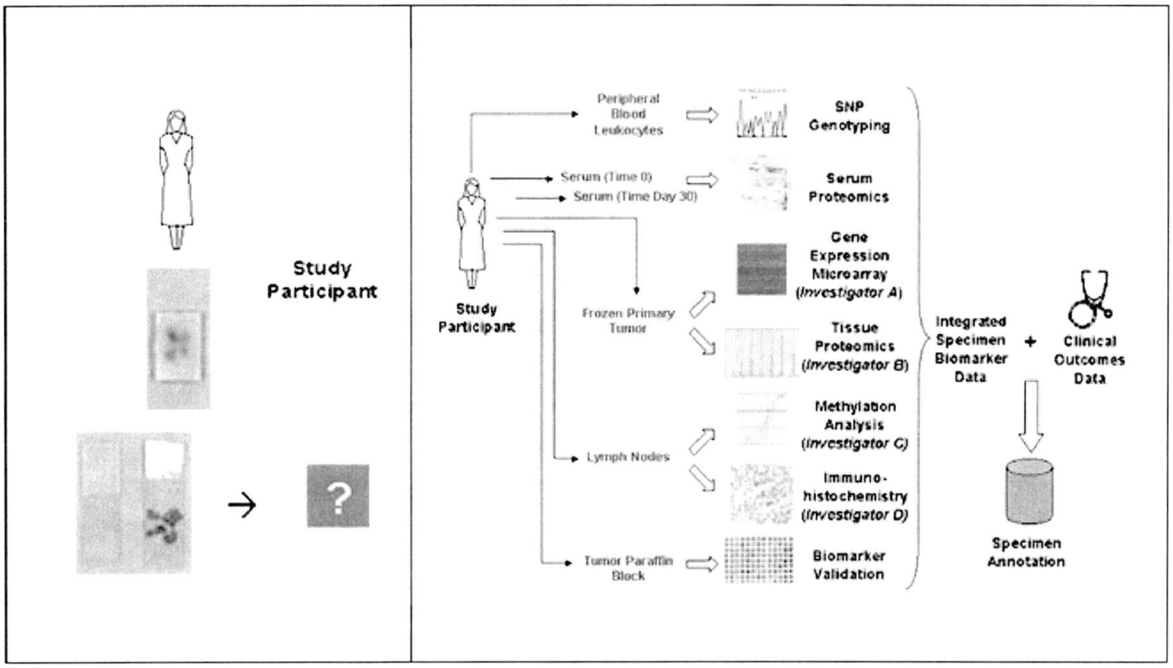

groups (Schmitt, 2007) but require incorporating new technologies together with their associated metadata. The TMA (Tissue Micro Array) techniques as well as the in situ hybridization (Lee, 2006) or the pharmacopathology (Begent, 2008) have already proposed their models. Whereas groups as the Laboratory Imaging digital Project (LDIP)(Berman, 2006) and the cancer GRID (caBIG, 2008) have used extensively metadata annotation agents following the ISO 11179 standard and avoid using DICOM standard due to its complexity.

STANDARDS IN GRID INFORMATION ACCESS

Although several GRID architectures have been proposed to interoperate among dissimilar sources and services (Pollock, 2004; HealthGrid, 2004; Saltz, 2006) the harmonized-standardized flows, data formats, access and annotations techniques will spread the use, improving query results, particularly in pathology. Infrastructures such as *caBIG* (caBIG, 2005) are an example of a federated environment that connects data, resources and users using **ISO/IEC 11179** standard for metadata registries.

In Internet, many metadata frameworks are present ranging from the simplicity of the Dublin Core Metadata Initiative (**ISO 15836**) to the complexity of Machine Readable Cataloguing (ISO 12083 XML-DTD; 12200; 12620; **ISO 16642**-Terminology Markup Language (TML)) and infrastructures of the W3C's Resource Description Framework (RDF) with their SPARQL query language. In semantic web, the open source Ontology Web languages OWL represent the data including the imaginery domain model, and WSDL (web services description languages) and OWL-S describe the pre-conditions, effects and inputs and outputs of the Service Oriented architecture on which the Web Services Agent transforms the sub-queries to XML Protocol (SOAP).

Medicine demands more complex representation then simply ISO 15836 with MeSH as Enterprise Vocabulary System (EVS). Should take advantage of whatever solutions provided by **ISO/IEC 13250** or Topic maps XML syntax with its own **ISO 18048** TMQL or Topics maps query language and its **ISO 19756** or TMCL topic maps constrain language. TM allows modelling and representation of knowledge in an interchangeable form that can be extended by inference rules stored within the topic map.

Furthermore, medical images require even higher complexity taking advantage of their own specific standards such as MPEG Query Format-**ISO/IEC 15938-12**, MPEG-21 or ISO 21000, **ISO/IEC CD 24800-3** for JP-query search or JPEG search-retrieval and of course of the complex DICOM standard (Q/R SCP query-retrieve service class) with a Structured Interpretation Object Message template referencing the SNOMED-DICOM micro glossary and the XML MIRC7-document schema (Gentili, 2008; ORACLE, 2008).

Taking into consideration quality requirements for health care, pathology laboratories should take advantage of collaborative diagnosis and personalized treatment techniques in GRID (Oster, 2007)

Our proposed service can use existing Health-gridded environments, making public the knowledge discover and inferences obtain in image processing and incorporating LBD and JP-query search to help pathologist in "solo-pathology" practice.

In this environment images and virtual slides could be used as a Learning Objects (Ferrer-Roca, 2005) (**ISO/IEC 11404**) having a hierarchically structured metadata (IEEE-LOM) accessed using web services and ontology (Moura, 2005).

CONCLUSION

Robots and distant diagnosis in a patho-informatics driven laboratory face a revolutionary way to practice pathology. This environment together with the translational research require GRID-cooperation allowing data-base access, literature based discovery and knowledge discovery.

Considering that one of the main products in surgical pathology are images, a way to annotate them in natural language will facilitate their diagnostic search by query tools providing a world-wide atlas to support "solo pathology". On this achievement standardization of semantic annotations and specific searching engines are required. This will allow a widespread use of "solo-pathology" supported at distance.

REFERENCES

Apollo Path-PACS. (2008). [Computer software]. Retrieved November 10, 2008, from http://www.apollopacs.com/pathpacs

Becich, M. J., Gilberston, J. R., Gupta, D., Grzybicki, D. M., & Raab, S. S. (2008). Patient Safety and Healthcare Research: The Critical Role of Path Informatics in Error Reduction and Quality Initiatives. *Clinics in Laboratory Medicine*, *24*(4), 913–943. doi:10.1016/j.cll.2004.05.019

Beckwith, B. A., Mahaadevan, R., Balis, U. J., & Kuo, F. (2006). Development and evaluation of an open source software tool for the identification of pathology reports. *BMC Med Inform Decis. Mak.*, *6*, 12-22. Retrieved November 10, 2008, from http://www.pubmedcentral.nih.gov/picrender.fcgi?artid=1421388&blobtype=pdf

Begent, R. (2008). *Developing standards for recording, sharing and integrating data from Antibody Society*. San Diego, CA: The Antibody Society.[Web Site]. Retrieved November 10, 2008, from http://www.antibodysociety.org/data/GIAATE_by_prof_Begent_09March2008.pdf

Berman, J. J., & Moore, G. W. (2006). *LDIP (Laboratory digital image project): RDF data specifications: the simple alternative to complex data standards*. Association for Pathology Informatics. Retrieved November 10, 2008, http://www.pathologyinformatics.org/Resources/jjb_gwm.pdf

caBIG. (2005). *Compatibility Guidelines Revision 2*. Retrieved November 10, 2008, from http://cabig.nci.nih.gov/guidelines_documentation/caBIGCompatGuideRev2_final.pdf

caBIG. (2008). *GRID & metadata with ISO 11179*. [Web Site]. Retrieved November 10, 2008, from https://cabig.nci.nih.gov/

CAMT -computer aided medical transcription. (2008). [Web Site]. Retrieved November 10, 2008, from http://www.escription.com/products/index.htmlhttp://www.nuance.com/dictaphone/products/powerscribe/pathology/

CERNER. (2008). *CoPATHplus solution*. [Computer Software]. Retrieved November 10, 2008, from http://www.cerner.com/public/Cerner_3.asp?id=30881

DIR2007. (2007). *DIR 2007/47/EC - Nueva directiva sobre equipos médicos*. [Web Site]. http://en.wikipedia.org/wiki/Medical_device

Dirnhofer, R., Jackowski, Ch., Vock, P., Potter, K., & Thali, M. J. (2006). VIRTOPSY: Minimally Invasive, Imaging-guided Virtual Autopsy. *Radiographics, 26*(5), 1305-1356. Retrieved November 10, 2008, from http://radiographics.rsnajnls.org/cgi/content/figsonly/26/5/1305

EDRM. (2008). *The Electronic Discovery Reference Model*. [Web Site]. Retrieved November 10, 2008, from http://www.edrm.net/

Ferrer-Roca, O., Figueredo, A., Franco, K., & Diaz-Cardama, A. (2005). Telemedicine Intelligent Learning. Ontology for Agent Technology. *Trans. on Adv. Res, 1*(2), 46-54. Retrieved November 10, 2008, from http://internetjournals.net/journals/tar/2005/TARVol1Num2.pdf

Ferrer-Roca, O., Marcano, F., & Quintana, J. J. (2008). Small Size Virtual Slides in Pathology. *Virchows Arch, 452* (suppl 1), s9-s10. Retrieved November 10, 2008, from http://www.springerlink.com/content/e6721317386258u3/?p=1eff7f89dcc44ce085fc696b4faf4e69&pi=0

Garcia-Rojo, M. (1998). *Management and automation in pathology laboratories*. Retrieved November 10, 2008, from http://www.mcmaster.ca/inabis98/rojo/rojo0500/two.html

Gentili, A., Chung, C., & Hughes, T. (2008). Use of the MIRC DICOM Service for Clinical Trials to Automatically Create Teaching File Cases from PACS. *Radiographics 27*, 269-275. Retrieved November 10, 2008, from http://radiographics.rsnajnls.org/cgi/content/full/27/1/269

Giménez, J. A., Alvarez, R., & Alfaro, J. (2007). *El control interno y externo de la calidad de las técnicas inmunohistoquímicas en relación con la Norma UNE-EN ISO 15189:2003*. Paper presented at the meeting of the XXIII Congreso de la Sociedad Española de Anatomía Patológica, Palacio de Congresos de Tarragona, may 2007. Retrieved November 10, 2008, from http://www.seapcongresos.com/2007/clubes/gestion/gimenez.htm

HealthGrid. (2004). *HealthGrid white paper*. Retrieved November 10, 2008, from http://initiative.healthgrid.org/the-initiative/healthgrids-concept/white-paper.html

Hristovski, D., Friedman, C., Rindflesch, T., & Peterlin, B. (2006). Exploiting Semantic Relations for Literature-Based Discovery. *AMIA ... Annual Symposium Proceedings / AMIA Symposium. AMIA Symposium, 2006*, 349–353.

IEC60601. (2006). *IEC 60601-1:2006 - Seguridad en los equipos electromédicos incluyendo los PESS o subsistemas electrónicos programables*. Retrieved November 10, 2008, from http://www.tecnologias-sanitarias.com/electromedicina/en60601-1.htm, http://www.tecnologias-sanitarias.com/electromedicina/IEC60601-1_ed3-info.pdf

IHS. (2008). *ISO Information/Image technology collection.* [Web Site]. Retrieved November 10, 2008, from http://engineers.ihs.com/collections/iso/information-image-9.htm

ISO11073. (2008). *ISO/IEEE 11073 – Plug & Play Standard.* Retrieved November 10, 2008, from http://www.ieee1073.org/

ISO11179. (2004). *ISO* 11179 - Metadata Standard. Retrieved November 10, 2008, from http://dublincore.org/documents/1999/07/02/dces/, http://www.ukoln.ac.uk/metadata/newsagent/metadata/, http://hpcrd.lbl.gov/SDM/XMDR/overview.html, http://xmdr.org/

ISO13250. (2003). *ISO 13250 - Topic maps.* Retrieved November 10, 2008, from http://www.isotopicmaps.org/sam/sam-xtm/

ISO13485. (2003). ISO 13485:2003. Medical devices -- Quality management Systems. Retrieved November 10, 2008, from http://www.tecnologias-sanitarias.com/calidad/iso13485-2003/

ISO14971. (2007). ISO 14971:2007 Medical devices -- Application of risk management to medical devices. Retrieved November 10, 2008, from http://www.tecnologias-sanitarias.com/iso14971/index.htm

ISO17025. (2005). *ISO 17025:2005. General requirements for the competence of testing and calibration laboratories*. Retrieved November 10, 2008, from http://www.aiha.org/1documents/lab/lqapnews03-0406.pdf

ISO Information/ Image technology collection. (2008). Retrieved November 10, 2008, from http://engineers.ihs.com/collections/iso/information-image-9.htm

Lee, H. W., Park, Y. R., Sim, J., Park, R. W., Kim, W. H., & Kim, J. H. (2006). The Tissue Microarray Object Model A Data Model for Storage, Analysis, and Exchange of Tissue Microarray Experimental Data. *Archives of Pathology & Laboratory Medicine, 130*, 1004–1013.

Liu, K., Mitchell, K. J., Chapman, W. W., & Crowley, R. S. (2005). Automatic clinical annotation in tissue bank specimen. Automating Tissue Bank Annotation from Pathology Reports – Comparison to a Gold Standard Expert Annotation Set. *AMIA ... Annual Symposium Proceedings / AMIA Symposium. AMIA Symposium, 2005*, 460–464.

Moore, G. W., & Berman, J. J. (1994). Performance analysis of manual and automated systemized nomenclature of medicine (SNOMED) coding. *American Journal of Clinical Pathology, 101*(3), 253–256.

Moura, S. L., Coutinho, F. J., Siqueira, S. W., & Melo, R. N. (2005). Integrating Repositories of Learning Objects Using Web-Services and Ontologies. *IJWSP, 1*(1-2), 57-72. Retrieved November 10, 2008, from http://nwesp.org/ijwsp/2005/vol1/6.pdf

OBO. (2008). *The Open Biomedical Ontologies.* [Web Site]. Retrieved November 10, 2008, from http://obofoundry.org/.

ORACLE. (2007). *DICOM XML-Schemes*.[Web Site]. Retrieved November 10, 2008, from http://download.oracle.com/docs/cd/B28359_01/appdev.111/b28416/ap_schemas.htm

Oster, S., Langella, S., Hastings, S., Ervin, D., Madduri, R., Kurc, T., et al. (2007). caGrid 1.0: A Grid Enterprise Architecture for Cancer Research. *AMIA Annu Symp Proc. 2007*, (pp. 573-577). Retrieved November 10, 2008, from http://bmi.osu.edu/resources/publications/cagrid-amia-2007.pdf

Pearson, S., Balis, U. J., Fuller, J., Kowalski, B., Locke, A. P., & Tillman, D. (2006). AUTO8-A Managing and Validating Laboratory Information Systems: Approved guideline. *CLSI (NCCLS). Documents. International Chamber of Commerce*, *26*(36).

PI. (2008). *Pathology Informatics*. [Web Site]. Retrieved November 10, 2008, from http://www.pathologyinformatics.org/

Pollock, J. T., & Hodgson, R. (2004). *Adaptive Information: Improving Business Through Semantic Interoperability, Grid Computing, and Enterprise Integration, (Wiley Series in System Engineering Management)*. Chichester, UK: John Wiley & Sons, Inc.

Ruch, P., Tbahriti, I., Gobeill, J., Baud, R., Lovis, C., & Geissbühler, A. (2006). *Automatic Assignment of SNOMED Categories: Preliminary and Qualitative Evaluations*. Paper presented at the meeting of the Semantic mining conference on SNOMED CT. Retrieved November 10, 2008, from http://www.hiww.org/smcs2006/proceedings/5RuchSMCS2006final.pdf

Ruckhaus, E., Ruiz, E., & Vidal, M.-E. (2008). Query Evaluation and optimization in the Semantic Web. *TPLP*, *8*(3), 393–409.

Saltz, J., Oster, S., Hastings, S., Langella, S., Kurc, T., & Sanchez, W. (2006)... *Bioinformatics (Oxford, England)*, *22*(15), 1910–1916. doi:10.1093/bioinformatics/btl272

Schmitt, F. C. (2007). Image Biobanking: Biomaterial to personalized cancer diagnosis and treatment. In Ferrer-Roca, O. (Ed.), *Quality control in Telemedicine: Biobanking* (pp. 68–72). Tenerife, Spain: Ediciones Catai.

SEAP. (2000). *Catalogo de técnicas y procedimientos*. [Web Site]. Retrieved November 10, 2008, from http://www.conganat.org/seap/informacion/catalogo.htm

SEAP. (2003). CECP - Programa de control externo de calidad en patología. *Rev. Española Patología, 36*(3), 347-349. Retrieved November 10, 2008, from http://www.conganat.org/seap/cecp/index.htm

SNCFP. (2005). Catalogo nacional de calificación profesional. Familia profesional de sanidad. *Anatomía patológica y citología. BOE 238 5*. Retrieved November 10, 2008, from http://www.mepsyd.es/educa/incual/pdf/2/SAN_125_(5).pdf

Srinivasan, P., Libbus, B., & Kumar, A. (2004). Mining MEDLINE: Postulating a Beneficial Role for Curcumin Longa in Retinal Diseases. In Hirschman, L., & Pustejovsky, J. (Eds.), *HLT-NAACL 2004 Workshop: BioLINK 2004, Linking Biological Literature, Ontologies and Databases* (pp. 33–40). Boston: Association for Computational Linguistics.

SRP. (2008). *Speach recognition in pathology*. [Computer software]. Retrieved November 10, 2008, from http://www.escription.com/products/index.html, http://www.nuance.com/dictaphone/products/powerscribe/pathology/

Thali, M. J. (2006). Virtopsy: Virtual Autopsy. In Ferrer-Roca, O. (Ed.), *Personalizad virtual medicine: p-health* (pp. 159–162). Tenerife, Spain: Ediciones Catai.

Tobias, J., Chilukuri, R., Komatsoulis, G. A., Mohanty, S., Sioutos, N., Warzel, D. B., et al. (2006). The CAP cancer protocols - a case study of caCORE based data standards implementation to integrate with the Cancer Biomedical Informatics GRID. *BMC Med Inform Decis Mak, 6,* 25-44. Retrieved November 10, 2008, from http://www.biomedcentral.com/1472-6947/6/25

UMLS. (2008). *UMLS Semantic Network*. [Web Site]. Retrieved November 10, 2008, from http://semanticnetwork.nlm.nih.gov/

VLA. (2006). *Virtual lab automation*. [Computer software]. Retrieved November 10, 2008, from http://www.vmware.com/pdf/virtual_lab_automation_whitepaper.pdf

WIPO. (2008). *World Intellectual property organization: WO/2001/098774. Systems for automated and remote histological analysis and new drug assessment*. [Web Site]. Retrieved November 10, 2008, from http://www.wipo.int/pctdb/en/wo.jsp?gIA=IL2001000561&DISPLAY=DESC

ENDNOTES

1. Now in course the updating ISO 9001:2009
2. LIS= Laboratory Information System
3. PIS= Pathology Information System (AP-LIS in UK)
4. HIS= Hospital Information System
5. PACS= Picture archiving and communication systems
6. Particularly **ISO/IEC 13250:2003** topic maps and **MPEG-7** and **MPEG-21**. and JBIG/JPEG (ISO/IEC JTC 1/SC 29/WG 1- ITU-T SG16) extensions for JPEG query formats
7. MIRC= Medical Imaging Resource Center

Chapter 7
Gridifying Neuroscientific Pipelines:
A SOA Recipe and Experience from the neuGRID Project

David Manset
maatG, France

The neuGRID Consortium

ABSTRACT

In recent times, innovative new e-Infrastructures have materialized all around the globe to address the compelling and unavoidably increasing demand on computing power and storage capacity. All fields of science have entered an era of digital explosion and thus need to face it with appropriate and scalable instruments. Amongst century's cutting-edge technologies, the grid has become a tangible candidate which several initiatives have harnessed and demonstrated the added value of. Turning the concept into a concrete solution for Neurosciences, the neuGRID project aims to establish a grid-based e-Infrastructure providing neuroscientists with a powerful tool to address the challenge of developing and testing new markers of neurodegenerative diseases. In order to optimize the resulting grid and to deliver a user-friendly environment, neuGRID has engaged the process of migrating existing imaging and data mining toolkits to the grid, the so-called gridification, while developing a surrounding service oriented architecture of agnostic biomedical utilities. This chapter reports on a preliminary analysis of the issues faced in the gridification of neuroimaging pipelines and attempts to sketch an integration model able to cope with the several and heterogeneous applications used by neuroscientists.

INTRODUCTION

Over the last decade, innovative new Information and Communication Technologies (ICT) have materialized into concrete e-Infrastructures. In particular, the so-called grid (Foster, Kesselman & Tuecke 2001), born in High Energy Physics, has been massively applied to harness distributed computing resources and thus address the digital explosion faced in all fields of science. Grid computing is an exciting concept promising to

DOI: 10.4018/978-1-61692-010-4.ch007

revolutionise many services already offered by the Internet. This new paradigm aims to provide rapid computation, large scale data storage and flexible collaboration by syndicating the power of a large number of commodity computers. The grid was originally devised for use in computing demanding fields but unsurprisingly was adopted in a number of ambitious medical and healthcare applications.

As of today, several projects around the world have been and still are exploiting grids to support biomedical research. In the US, most notably the caBIG™ initiative (http://cabig.cancer.gov/) founded by the National Cancer Institute (NCI) in 2004 to speed up discoveries in cancer research. In Europe, as key initiatives of the Framework Programmes of the European Commission, e-Infrastructures such as MammoGrid (Amendolia, Estrella, Hassan, Hauer, Manset, McClatchey, et al, 2004), Health-e-Child (Health-e-Child, The EU FP6 Information Societies Technology Project, 2008), @neurIST (http://www.aneurist.org) and many others have also demonstrated their added value.

Coming as a third generation grid, the neuGRID project has been recently launched to establish an international grid infrastructure specialized in the field of Neurosciences. neuGRID (NeuGrid Project, 2008) aims to interconnect major clinical research centres in Europe, ultimately supplying neuroscientists with the most advanced ICT to defeat Alzheimer's disease and neurodegenerative pathologies in general. In neuGRID, the collection and archiving of large amounts of imaging data is paired with grid-based computationally intensive analyses to develop and test new disease markers. Leveraging the grid concept and technology being developed by the Enabling the Grid for E-sciencE (EGEE) project (glite, A lightweight middleware for grid computing, 2008), neuGRID is pioneering an advanced Service Oriented Architecture (SOA) of biomedical research utilities mediating between user applications, backend and other facilities, while empowering them with the grid.

The main objective of this paper is to report on early experiences in the formalisation of an appropriate gridification model to allow neuroscientists from neuGRID to seamlessly run complex, data and computing intensive pipelines of neuroimaging algorithms. To do so, major design goals and underlying concepts are described while the requirements of such pipelines are precisely analyzed.

RATIONALE

Approach to Design

The major goal that guided the present design specification process was to establish a coarse-grained view of the system from the gathered users' requirements. This exercise was useful to identify major software layers, inner constituents and corresponding interfaces, while helping in better splitting the work and responsibilities among collaborators.

Similarly to the Service Oriented Modelling and Architecture (SOMA) (Arsanjani, 2004) process, coworkers aimed at identifying features and gradually grouping them into logical layers for future implementation. Thus, a meet-in-the-middle approach was adopted which reconciled requirements expressed by end-users with the bottom-up grid deployments of existing IT assets. The result of this work is here presented using a Service Oriented Architecture (SOA) (MacKenzie, et al, 2006), as the focal meeting point and federating concept.

In order to give clarity to this manuscript, only a relevant subset of the requirements and design objectives is introduced, with the aim of focussing on the gridification related aspects. The following section therefore briefly presents the service orientation and associated advantages, while progressively describing the retained system architecture, gridification approach and positioning of author's contribution. It is important to note that the latter builds upon former contribution and experiences in the area of gridification (Manset, Pourraz, Tsymbal, Revillard, Skaburskas, McClatchey, et al, in press) and e-health platform developments (McClatchey, Manest & Solomonides, 2006).

Service Orientation

The main characteristics of a SOA are the loose coupling between services, the abstraction from technological aspects and its extensibility; features considered essential to cope with distributed developments, heterogeneous technologies integration and to leverage multi-partners collaborations. SOA provides a simple yet efficient way to reuse software artefacts through the concept of standard services that are not bound to each other. Technological abstraction is obtained from using service contracts that are platform-independent. Extensibility is finally reached through service discovery and composition at execution time. Several definitions of the concept can be found in the literature, however for the remainder of this paper, only the three following are retained, as they are considered most relevant to this work:

- "*A service-oriented architecture is a style of multi-tier computing that helps organizations share logic and data among multiple applications and usage modes*" as stated in 1996 by the Gartner group.
- "*Service Oriented Architecture is a paradigm for organizing and utilizing distributed capabilities that may be under the control of different ownership domains. It provides a uniform means to offer, discover, interact with and use capabilities to produce desired effects consistent with measurable preconditions and expectations*" established in the OASIS reference model.
- "*SOA enables flexible integration of applications and resources by: (1) representing every application or resource as a service with standardized interface, (2) enabling the service to exchange structured information (messages, documents, "business objects"), and (3) coordinating and mediating between the services to ensure they can be invoked, used and changed effectively*".

In spite of the absence of a consensually agreed definition for SOA, three key roles are usually identified: service producers, service brokers and service consumers. The service producer's role is to deploy a service on a server and to generate the description of this service (i.e. so-called the service contract), which defines available operations as well as invocation mode(s). This description is published in a directory of services inside a service broker. Thus, services consumers are able to discover available services and to obtain their description by interacting with the service directory. The obtained descriptions can then be used to establish a connection with the producer and to invoke the desired service operation(s).

Just as for the SOA concept, loose coupling does not benefit from a unique definition. The commonly adopted approach though is to introduce a minimum of dependencies between services in order to better support their reusability. Moreover, these services should be combined in order to quickly and cost-efficiently respond to new demands. To achieve this goal, some engineering rules which are not always specific to SOA, have been identified (Papazoglou,, 2003).

Encapsulation and abstraction principles originally came from the world of object-orientation. The idea was to hide self-contained information of a service to end-users and to propose only one stable interface stressing the details considered to be necessary for handling it. A service is therefore seen as a black box from the outside, which makes it possible to separate its interface (i.e. its external description) from its actual implementation. One can thus modify a service implementation without changing its interface, which turns it into a sustainable entity. The following rules are more specific to SOAs:

- (A) A simple and ubiquitous interface must be provided by any service and must be universally accessible by all suppliers and all customers of services. Thanks to a generic interface, it is then possible to interconnect any services and to forward any messages between the various interfaces. The keyword here is "decoupling" and it can take various roles: (1) to reduce the coupling between modules, for improved reusability, (2) to reduce the coupling with respect to the infrastructure and to the implementation platform, for improved interoperability and (3) to reduce the coupling between a service consumer and a specific implementation of this service, for improved evolution. In Web service architectures, the consensus to achieve this rule is to use the Web Service Description Language (WSDL (Web Service Description Language, n.d.)).
- (B) Messages delivered by a service should not contain business logic. On the contrary, they must be restricted to the transport of, and only of, data structures from one service to another. That makes it possible to modify or to add services without impacting others in the system architecture. These data structures can nevertheless be very complex in order to deal with security management (i.e. authentication, encryption, authorization, etc) or even file transfer. These aspects are addressed thanks to different specifications that strengthen the "standard" Web service architecture (e.g. WS-Security (WS-Security, n.d.), SOAP-attachments (SOAP Attachment, n.d.), etc).
- (C) A well-formed service must be stateless. This rule, which appears very constraining, must be moderated though. It is recommended that the state conservation (i.e. the management of the context) as well as the action coordination (i.e. the management of the transactions) are localised in a specific function of the SOA, such as the orchestration. The application of such a rule facilitates the reuse, the scalability and the robustness of services and thus resulting SOA. Moreover, this rule enforces the loose coupling.
- (D) Cohesion is a difficult rule to define. It translates the degree of operations and functional proximity inside a service. In other words, it aims at facilitating the comprehension and reusability of a service by grouping homogeneous operations belonging to the same functional area.
- (E) A service should be idempotent. That makes it possible to be unaware of multiple receptions of the same request. The idea is that the use of such a service makes it possible to slacken the assumptions of reliability on the communication layer. In Web service architecture, the WS-Addressing (WS-Addressing, n.d.) specification allows among other things to enforce part of this rule.

If some of these rules can or sometimes have to be moderated according to system requirements, i.e. the stateless and the idempotent ones, all of them remain vital to create an open, sustainable and standard SOA. Indeed, these characteristics are mandatory in order to cope with heterogeneous resources ranging from data, to knowledge, to applications, and beyond software, to people. The SOA approach makes it possible for a wide range of collaborators having different backgrounds to develop together a system extensible to different application areas, which is of absolute importance in the case of neuGRID.

Aiming at addressing these challenges, the neuGRID collaborators have therefore started complementing the grid middleware services offering with Neurosciences specific logic following

Figure 1. System Architecture Layer View

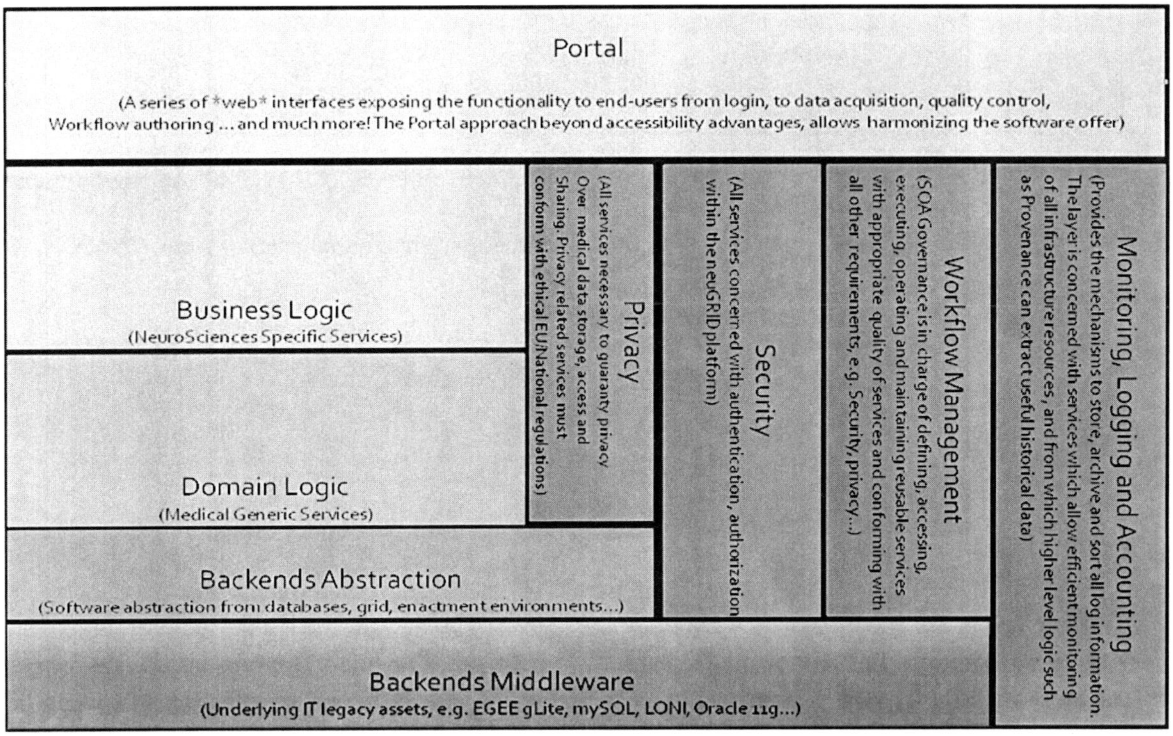

the SOA approach and cornerstones. They have engaged in the development of an upperware stack of facilities ranging from generic middleware services to domain specific interfaces closer to end-users. The latter materializes under the form of a thin layer of software services sitting on top of the grid middleware that wraps up and abstracts from underlying technologies to deliver loosely coupled and adapted functionality to end-users, while respecting the SOA model.

The following section briefly discusses the design of this thin software layer with a special emphasis on the workflow management components, and in what extent it conforms to the introduced rules for delivering a reusable platform. This rather incomplete system architecture description aims to give clarity to the advocated approach, in particular the gridification model.

System Architecture

Turning the requirements analysis into solid technical foundations, a significant effort has been invested at sketching an appropriate system architecture. The following diagram, i.e. Figure 1, thus illustrates the resulting specification in terms of software layers and corresponding functional areas. It introduces the notion of horizontal versus orthogonal layers, where respectively horizontals provide system functionality, whereas orthogonals address non-functional aspects impacting on horizontals.

Starting from the very bottom of the system, i.e. "Backends Middleware", with IT legacy assets such as the grid and database infrastructures, various abstraction levels are then introduced which leverage the loose coupling. The most important one, so-called "Backends Abstraction", wraps up underlying backends and allows partners to develop platform independent software. Above

Figure 2.

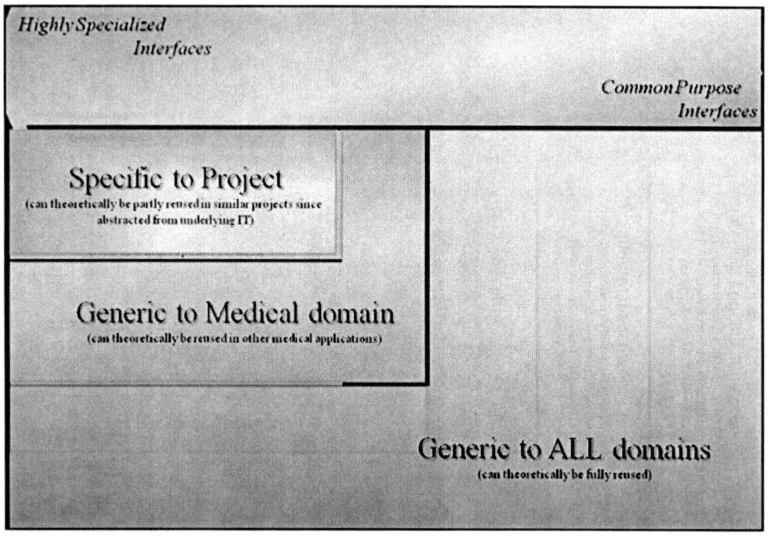

this, further layers are superimposed which deliver more and more specific functions as distance to end-users shrinks. As such, "Domain Logic" aims at grouping medical generic services, e.g. medical querying, medical data acquisition and quality control, whereas "Business Logic" only focuses on Neurosciences applications, e.g. the cortical thickness pipeline (Lerch & Evans, 2005), segmentation/ normalization algorithms etc. The latter is then accessed by end-users through a dedicated web portal exposing specialized presentation interfaces.

Orthogonally, the platform aims to offer various means to trace system activitiy via the "Monitoring, Logging and Accounting" services. Moreover, all applications are delivered within a secure environment implementing a security scheme as dictated by the requirements. This is why the "Security" layer spans from the top business logic, to the bottom abstraction. The same applies for privacy aspects since dealing with sensitive data, though only impacting on business and domain logics. The privacy layer offers facilities ranging from regular pseudonymization to more advanced face scrambling, in order to prevent malicious users from back tracing patient's identity.

This being said and thanks to the enforcement of the cohesion rule (D) as presented in the former section, an additional set of meta-layers can be introduced. Here illustrated on the left of Figure 2, functional and non-functional layers are grouped per estimated levels of reusability. Thus, horizontal layers concerned with backends access/ management, together with orthogonals like monitoring, logging, accounting, workflow management and security can be reused in all other fields of science. Similarly, layers such as domain logic and privacy are reusable in other medical areas, while the business logic, as its name implies has a much lower reusability potential since specialized to Neurosciences.

Figure 3 provides more insights on the identified stateless Web services portfolio per layers. Thus, one can notice the grouping of functionality in, for instance, (1) the "Monitoring, Logging and Accounting" layer where a dedicated service is introduced per aspect. Similarly, (2) "Security" with authentication and authorization services, (3) "Backends Abstraction" with a functional split between components related to databases, grid and Picture and Archiving Communication Systems (PACS) access, (4) "Domain Specific"

Figure 3. System Architecture Component View

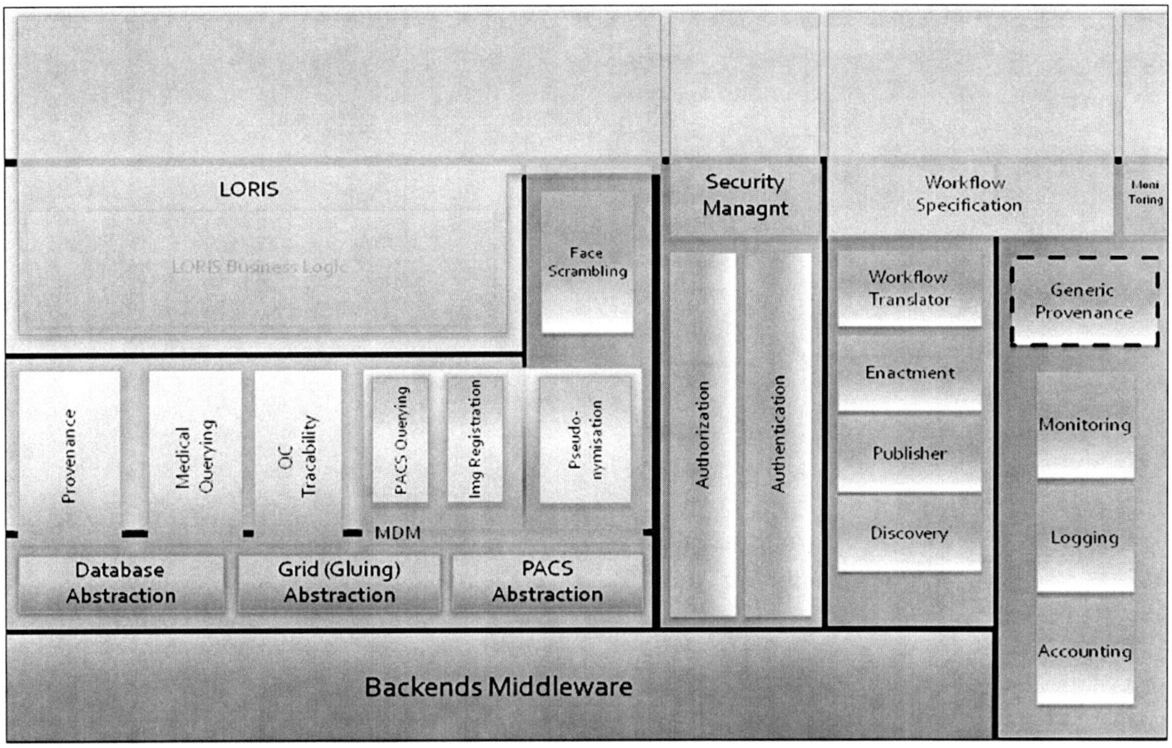

logic with medical querying, data provenance, quality control, image data acquisition and (5) "Privacy" with pseudonymisation and face stripping services.

From a SOA standpoint, the key elements of this architecture lie in (6) i.e. the "Workflow Management", where the necessary logic for publishing, discovering and composing new applications is expected to materialize. Combined with an appropriate gridification model (discussed in the remainder of this paper), such generic low-level mechanisms will demonstrate the benefits of virtualization.

From their experience in similar projects, i.e. EU-funded FP5 MammoGrid (Amendolia, Estrella, Hassan, Hauer, Manset, McClatchey, et al, 2004) and EU-funded FP6 Health-e-Child (Health-e-Child, The EU FP6 Information Societies Technology Project, 2008), the neuGRID technical collaborators intend to make further progress in the field of medical applications gridification. In particular, there has been significant progress made in grid abstraction and web services orchestration within Health-e-Child, which will subsequently be capitalized; the idea being to not reinvent the wheel but rather reuse, consolidate and extend a solid background.

In Pandora, processes can be defined using the Business Process Execution Language (BPEL (Web Services Business Process Execution Language, n.d.)) and then turned into workflows mixing both grid and web resources. The composition service also supports short and long running processes using state-of-the-art technologies. Figure 4 above illustrates the different components of this SOA solution, in particular its three pillars:

- *(1) Service Producer.* Among the most important ones, the Registration Service plays

Figure 4. More specifically, the Publication, Discovery and Composition Services from the Health-e-Child Gateway (Skabuskas, Estrella, Shade, Manset, Revillard, Rios, 2007), so-called Pandora, provide advanced facilities to manipulate the SOA offering, based on the latest World Wide Web Consortium (W3C) standards.

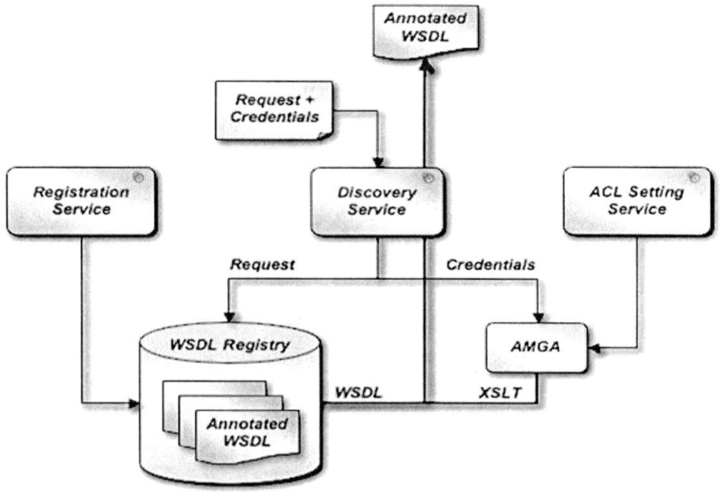

a dual role. It allows uploading and registering new applications in the SOA. Thus, APIs, remote services or even simpler binary applications can be added to the portfolio together with corresponding metadata. Once invoked, the registration service deploys the provided application as a new Web service in the infrastructure. In parallel, the service description is added to the global WSDL repository (so-called Information System Database - ISD).

- *Service Broker*. The Service Discovery is in fact an XPath query service facilitating the retrieval of any functionality deployed in the platform and thus referenced in the ISD database. A query can be performed according to several criteria.One can look for particular operations by navigating through layers, services, functions, functions' inputs or even outputs. Requests can be specified as a string description (i.e. "à la Google"). Behind this query facility, complex registry mechanisms have been implemented to enforce access controls (as shown in Figure 4 through the ACL setting service). After having retrieved the query resultset as an array of WSDL descriptions, an XSLT transformation is performed by the system to filter the resulting list of identified functionality, according to Role Based Access Control (RBAC (Role Based Access Control (RBAC), n.d.)) security policies. Underneath this, an ACL-enabled database abstraction layer, so-called AMGA (AMGA -- the ARDA Metadata Catalogue Project, n.d.), is used.
- *Service Consumer*. Last but not least, the Composition Service provides facilities to use, combine and thus enrich the SOA functionality. It allows defining new BPEL processes to execute workflows of services from within the infrastructure and/or any others from the Web. At the backend of this service, the open-source ActiveBPEL (ActiveBPEL, n.d.). engine is used. ActiveBPEL, in the present case, has been extended to cope with the latest services containers, including Globus (The

Globus Alliance, n.d.) and to run processes either as new Web services or as local processes (i.e. on-the-fly execution). Similarly to all other resources of the system, newly created BPEL processes can be deployed as new services and are ruled by access controls.

Based on this significant asset, the intent is to demonstrate the gridification model as presented in the remainder of this paper. The main assumption made by the author is that all gridification approaches should be supported from low-level batch processing of task-based jobs to more advanced and state-of-the-art Web services composition, thus opening the pathway to wider possibilities.

The next section therefore focusses on preliminary conclusions which can be drawn from end-users needs and a tangible gridification model to be applied to Neurosciences toolkits.

PIPELINE REQUIREMENTS ANALYSIS

Complexity in Neuroimaging

In the study of neuro-degenerative pathologies and more particularly in Alzheimer's disease, various parameters are extracted from imaging that can quantify/ qualify the disease progression and diagnosis. Parameters such as brain volume change over time, regional changes or even white matter lesions can be extracted by applying different image processing techniques onto patients' brain scans. However, in almost all cases, such extractions cannot be fully automated and require the intervention of an expert to clean the data and monitor, refine the subsequent processes.

Let's take as an example the measurement of brain atrophy rates over time (Sluimer, Vrenken, Blankenstein, Fox, Scheltens, Barkhof, et al, n.d.), i.e. the amount of cortical tissue that is lost by Alzheimer's patients over, say, one year. This measure is relevant in that it is the most valid marker of disease activity available to date and is ideal to test the effect of drugs aimed to slow or arrest its progression.

The first step to undertake in its measurement relates to noise reduction and is aimed to decrease random variations in images due to magnetic field changes and scanner calibration. Here, the MRIcro (MRIcro, n.d.) imaging toolkit is used to correct images manually by checking the homogeneity of the signal over the whole brain. This process cannot be automated and requires trained users in that inhomogeneities and other artifacts may not always be obvious to detect.

Still as part of this initial and mandatory data pre-processing phase, the second step involves the digital extraction of the brain through segmentation of brain from non-brain voxels (i.e. volumetric pixels). Here, one of the tools from the fMRIB Software Library (FSL) (FMIRB Software Library, n.d.) is used, namely the Brain Extraction Tool (BET) (MRIco, Brain Extraction Tool, n.d.). The operator manually selects areas to be included (i.e. according to shades of gray, thresholding, etc) and others that should be omitted from the calculation. The obtained brain volume can be compared to a set of reference brains for diagnostic purposes, or can be registered (i.e. aligned in the 3D space) to a follow-up image to compute atrophy rate. The latter is calculated using the SIENA (Structural Image Evaluation using Normalisation of Atrophy (SIENA), n.d.) software. This gives as output the difference of the brain contours between the baseline and the follow-up image in order to compute the actual shrinkage or increase of the brain size in quantitative terms (in cc or ml), giving a volume ratio directly indicative of the disease progression.

This simple and typical example of a process that clinical researchers go through to extract meaningful imaging markers is highly indicative of the toolkits heterogeneity, the interactive nature of pipelines' pre/post-processing, as well as the complexity and high risks of errors intro-

Table 1.

Institute	Pipeline Tools	Analysis Tools
VUmc	fMRIB Software Library (FSL): Flirt, Fnirt, FDT, FAST, Melodic (visualization tool), Siena, XSiena, FEAT, http://www.fmrib.ox.ac.uk • MRIcro, Brain Extraction Tool (BET), http://www.sph.sc.edu/comd/rorden/mricro.html • Montreal Neurological Institute (MNI) (BIC Tools & Software – The Brain Imaging Software Toolbox): N3. http://www.bic.mni.mcgill.ca/software/ • BioInformatics Research Network (BIRN) (Gradiant Non-Linearity Distortion Correction): Gradient non-linearity. http://www.nbirn.net/ • DRG Fluid. • Generic: o Image calculations (adding subtracting, multiplying etc) o Morphological operations on images o File format conversions	Statistical Parametric Mapping – SPM http://www.fil.ion.ucl.ac.uk/spm/software/
KI	• MNI BIC Tool – CIVET Pipeline http://wiki.bic.mni.mcgill.ca/index.php/CIVET, • FSL, • Brainvoyager http://www.brainvoyager.com/ • Matlab http://www.matlab.com, • Analysis fo Functional NeuroImages (AFNI), http://afni.nimh.nih.gov/afni/ • E-prime http://www.pstnet.com/ and • Statistica.	Hermes (Hermes Medical) B-MAP (Pipeline 1 and Pipeline 2) http://www.hermesmedical.com/
FBF	• FSL Tools fMRIB's Diffusion Toolbox FDT 2.0, Melodic • MNI BIC Tools: • Display, register, Brainsuite • LoNI http://www.loni.ucla.edu/Software/ tools: • Dual_warpe_warpcurve, Decoder_blend_all, mk_seg16bit, mk_gray, add_gray_to_inflated_LEFT1, add_gray_to_inflated_RIGHT1, pmap_apeVSctrl, make_UVL_*; 1st_script_tracer_avg_DIAG; 2nd_script_core_test_L_DIAG; 2nd_script_core_test_R_DIAG; Pmap_DistCore_DIAG • MRIcro (MRIcro) (visualization) • BET Function • IdeALab Tools (IdeALab) http://neuroscience.ucdavis.edu/idealab/software/index.php • Image Conversion software • MRIconverter • dcm2nii • New Promising Tools: • 3D Slicer, VTK, Freesurfer, MPIAV, NA-MIC Kit components, MED-INRIA, BrainVoyager, BrainMAP	• SPSS http://www.spss.com/, • Statistical Parametric Mapping – SPM, Matlab, Quanta 6.1 • R (R) http://www.r-project.org • Statistical Parametric Mapping – SPM

Table 2.

	FSL	MNI/ BIC	LoNI	SPM	MRIcro/ BET	SPSS	HERMES	Idealab	Matlab	R	AFNI	E-Prime	Statistica	DRG	BIRN	BrainVoy.	QUANTA
VUmc	X	X		X	X									X	X		
KI	X	X					X		X		X	X	X			X	
FBF	X	X	X	X	X	X		X	X	X							X

duction inherent to data cleaning and algorithms parameterization.

Offering a harmonized environment to run such pipelines therefore suggests a flexible yet powerful gridification model. Such a model should give enough freedom to researchers to tune processes and interact with the system as needed, until a satisfactory version of the pipeline can be massively executed in the grid for clinical assessment of its output.

To do so, it has therefore been necessary to undergo a study of imaging and data mining toolkits being used by clinical researchers within neuGRID. The following of this section attemps to list mostly utilized applications at the three end-user institutions of the project, with subsequent classification according to diverse criteria (e.g. toolkit, software dependencies, imaging features, etc). These classifications then help scoping the nature of such pipelines and algorithms while supporting the formalisation of corresponding use-cases.

Pipeline Toolkits

The following table lists the pipeline tools that are in frequent use by the research centers as expressed by end-users. It aims to give a taste on the faced difficulty and heterogeneity of available imaging/ mining toolkits, whether commercial suites or community software:

This list demonstrates that end-users develop preferences over time from personal experience and projects, which lead them to use various combinations of toolkits/ algorithms to extract complex features. One can notice however that there are a few common ones, as highlighted in the following table.

As a conclusion to this initial comparative table, FSL, MNI/BIC, SPM, MRIcro and Matlab seem to be the most common set of imaging and data mining toolkits being used by our Neuroscientists and thus relevant candidates for gridification. However, the algorithms offered by such

Table 3.

Main Category	Type of Processing	Pipeline / Algorithm	Toolkit
Pre & Intermediary Processing	Normalization	Linear and nonlinear (correction factors)	SPM
		Segmentation (voxels labelling priors-based)	SPM
		Warping (sulci based)	LoNI
		Warping (intensity based)	MNI
	File Conversion	Dicom to MINC	MNI
		Dicom to Analyze	MNI MRIcro
	Anonymization	Face Scrambling	LoNI
		Pseudonymization	--
Research	Segmentation	Cortical Density	SPM LoNI
		Cortical Thickness	LoNI
		Hippocampus Atrophy (shrinkage)	LoNI
		Hippocampus Volume	MNI LoNI
		White Matter Volume and Distribution	IdeALab
		Cortical Thickness	MNI
	Statistics	Cross Population Patterns	--
Diagnostic	Segmentation	Cortical Density	SPM
		Cortical Contour Drawing + Voxels Counting	MNI
		White Matter Age Related Scale (Wahlund)	--
		Regional Brain Metabolism Alterations	HERMES

Figure 5. Pipeline Meta-Process

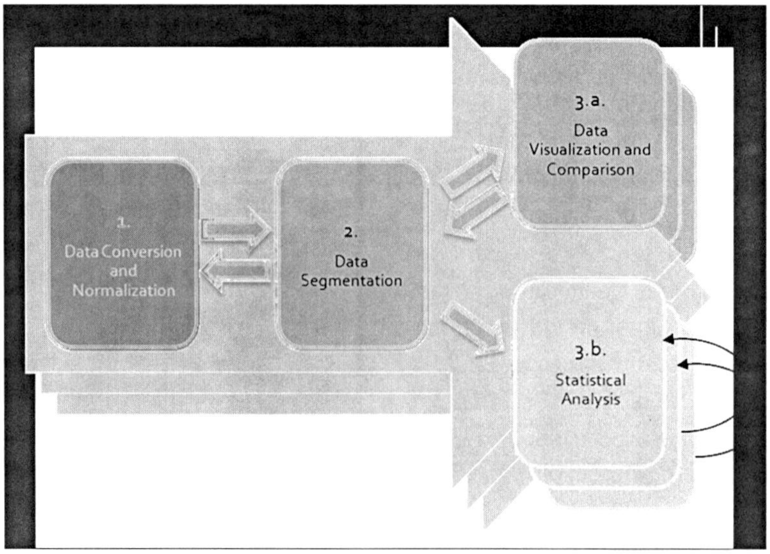

toolkits span a large spectrum of functionality that can greatly differ in scope. The next section therefore intends to define the main categories of such applications to enable their logical grouping in a SOA setting, for the sake of cohesion.

Pipelines vs Imaging Capabilities

The following table gives a list of popular toolkits and corresponding image processing capabilities used to respectively normalize data, convert image files, anonymize data, extract features from within images and process statistics. This classification aims to introduce the notion of categories, that the resulting neuGRID system could use to classify its gridified algorithms portfolio.

From this categorization, it is already clear that algorithms/ pipelines can be classified whether they are used to convert, normalize, anonymize data or to extract meaningful measurements through imaging segmentation and statistical analyses. This wide variety of toolkit utilities also indicates that there is a potentially generalisable pipeline model. Clearly, four steps tend to shape, as illustrated in Figure 5.

(1) *Data Conversion and Normalization.* Before executing any pipelines, the initial step consists in normalizing the data (i.e. making it comparable, homogeneous) and converting it into an appropriate format for further analysis. In some cases, clinical researchers apply a selection of normalization algorithms and then manually trace brain structures or clean images slice by slice to allow for deeper computer aided analyses. Such manual annotation/ quality control processes are time consuming. For instance, when an expert wants to trace brain structures, it takes approximately:
   - For the total brain volume: ¼ hour for 1 patient,
   - For the Hippocampus volume only: ½ hour for 1 patient.

   Normalization algorithms are selected according to the modality and quality of data, which can vary slightly from one imaging device to another due to calibration differences. For this reason, normalization from time to time does not work or outputs wrong results. Neuroscientists therefore have to assess the quality of the output data, thus introducing a human interaction requirement in the loop. Normalization is a "no-return" process; this is the reason why original data must be kept in a separate place. All processing steps are traced and intermediary data also stored in separate folders, for the very same reason. Note: the data acquisition process is not taken into consideration in the present case.

(2) *Data Segmentation.* Once the data has been quality controlled, a concrete measurement is extracted. In the context of neuGRID, researchers usually investigate morphological or functional changes and lesions by measuring for instance how thick the cortex is, from structural imaging. This is done by applying a given pipeline of image processing algorithms onto the brain scan. Such pipelines are either existing/ tested ones that a researcher applies straight away onto his dataset or a pipeline freshly specified from the combination of different algorithms and sometimes fragmented across several toolkits. Once a given pipeline is executed, researchers in almost all cases have to check intermediary data quality, i.e. data produced at the various stages of the pipeline. This assessment is again operated visually and can lead to additional data cleaining or even re-execution of the concerned pipeline step(s), so that subsequent processing is successful. Recalling Figure 5, there is therefore a cycle established between steps (1), (2) and (3) while a given pipeline is running. Also noticeable, the expertize related to pipelines (i.e. algorithms parameters, wokflow/ pipeline description, etc) is stored

in a separate report using an ad-hoc format. In other words, the knowledge associated to a given pipeine is never expressed using a standard notation (nor turned into machine-processable specifications).

(3) *Data Visualization and Comparison.* As formerly introduced, data visualization can occur at various stages of the pipeline. It can be operated at the outset to visualize the resulting extraction or after given steps of the pipeline in order to visually check the output quality. In the latter case, visualization supports the quality control process, whereas in the former it allows end-users to validate measurements or pipelines, as well as to compare obtained measurements with other experiment results or references from the litterature.

(4) *Statistical Analysis.* Recalling the section introductory example, statistical analysis may be applied for interesting measurements onto a large set of patients' scans. In the case of brain atrophy for instance, it would mean running the MRIcro and FSL pipelines several times, as is illustrated in Figure 5 with a series of arrows on the right, onto different patients' brain scans and corresponding follow-ups to obtain an indicative atrophy percentage rate on a given population.

Pipelines vs Software Characteristics

This last table provides detailed information about popular pipeline toolkits in terms of supported Operating System(s) (OS), licensing conditions, programming languages and data formats, while recalling available imaging features. This is useful to understand the potential difficulty which will be faced in gridifying a given toolkit.

This table gives concrete technical hints on the toolkits gridification applicability. Indeed, it shows that most of them are not cross-platform, except SPM. Toolkits accept potentially different file formats although image converters exist and last but not least, toolkits are developed in diverse programming languages. It is noticeable though that in spite of these differences, (almost) all toolkits algorithms materialize under the form of Unix-like binaries/ scripts/ libraries. This simplifies greatly, if not eliminates technically speaking, the problems related to complex SOA data flows between services. Indeed, by doing so, algorithms only have to deal with simple input and output types such as strings of characters, whether being a configuration value for the algorithm itself or a physical path to target image files. This strengthens and confirms the grid relevance and applicability to Neurosciences.

The next section delivers preliminary conclusions by qualifying pipelines and thus introducing possible gridification approaches.

PIPELINE GRIDIFICATION

Pipelines' Nature

By extracting the requirements and findings which are considered to potentially impact on the gridification model, one may generalize intrinsic pipeline characteristics as follows:

1. Pipelines encompass *Significant Added-Value*: pipelines are not just sequences of algorithms. They encompass domain knowledge which is essential to Neuroscientists, and can be considered as intellectual property. Their descriptions thus have to incorporate such knowledge and the latter be kept in a machine readable format, enabling curation and reuse. Solutions may be found in provenance related work (Bunemun, Khanna & Tan, 2001).
2. Pipelines are *Heterogeneous*: pipelines utilize various technologies/ environments and sometimes are fragmented across different toolkits, as demonstrated in the presented

Figure 6. Pipeline Anatomy

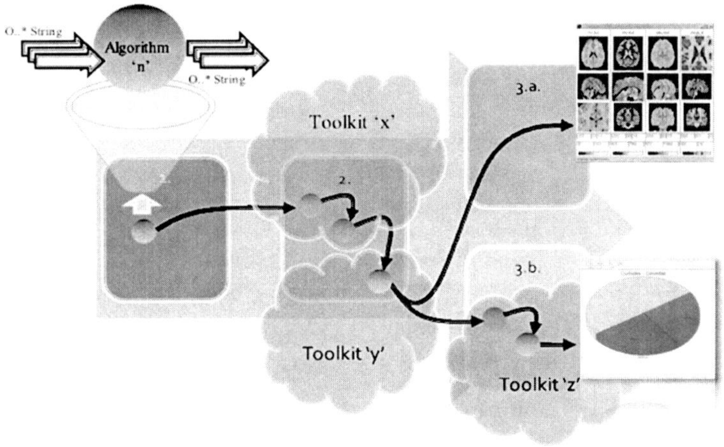

analysis. Toolkits thus have library dependencies which can be difficult to satisfy when mixed.

3. Pipelines and inner stages are *Interactive*: outputs have to be checked in most cases to guaranty successful execution of following ones or even to validate input parameters.
4. Pipelines are *Iterative and Recursive*: in case of incorrect outputs, pipelines or inner steps have to be executed again until a satisfactory output is obtained. Pipelines can also be composite, i.e. pipelines of pipelines.
5. Pipelines are mainly *Task-based*: processing steps are in most cases executable code enacted using ad-hoc or scripting languages describing command lines and associated parameters.
6. Pipelines are mainly *Sequential*: they in most cases consist of a several steps executed in series (especially true for voxel-based image processing) and do not require inter-process communications. Few cases require parallelism (or could be parallelized), taken aside statistical analyses where the same pipeline is run onto a large dataset thus executable in batches over multiple processing nodes to optimize overall runtime.
7. Pipelines are *Computing Intensive*: image processing algorithms used in pipelines usually have short runtimes but are applied to several images and many times, thus making overall pipelines processing times quite long.
8. Pipelines are *Data Intensive*: image processing algorithms usually output intermediary data for inputting in next steps of the pipeline. Pipelines thus tend to produce 'n' times the initial dataset volume, where 'n' is most likely equal to the number of segmentation steps.

Pipelines' Anatomy

From the formerly described nature, Neurosciences pipelines constitute a very good case for gridification. One common characteristic seems to clearly shape, which is the form under which inner algorithms materialize, whatever toolkit they are from. Indeed, imaging algorithms are mainly about Unix-like binaries/ scripts/ Command Line Interfaces (CLI) accepting/ producing simple strings of characters respectively as input parameters and/ or as output values. This is what Figure 6 illustrates below (by recalling the conceptualization as introduced in Figure 5).

In Figure 6, a complex pipeline is illustrated which combines algorithms from three different toolkits, but where algorithms themselves have the same anatomy. From this and former analysis, a number of conclusions can thus be drawn. First, an analysis pipeline corresponds to so-called workflow in computing terminology, where: *"The term workflow is used ... to capture and develop human to machine interaction. Workflow software aims to provide end users with an easier way to orchestrate or describe complex processing of data in a visual form, much like flow charts but without the need to understand computers or programming"* as described in Wikipedia.

The specification of neuroscientific pipelines can imply mixing heterogeneous technologies and data. Such pipelines exhibit a number of intrinsic properties which can be derived into design constraints for underlying workflow engine. Pipelines can involve several stages, each of which materializing in the sometimes iterative, recursive and/or interactive execution of concrete algorithms. The specification of such pipelines is therefore a difficult task, which no workflow environment is able to fully address as of today.

The next section introduces the gridification approach and resulting model that is being brought forward. An initial high-level description of the model is provided to demonstrate in what extent it addresses pipeline specifities but also how it could cope with future extensions. The advocated model builds upon the benefits of the grid and SOA concepts, while bridging the two worlds to satisfy the requirements analysis conclusions.

Design Specifications

Gridification Introduction

Significant work has already been pursued in the area of applications migration to the grid. So-called gridification is concerned with porting or developing applications business logic to software jobs that can further be scheduled in a grid environment. Depending on the application nature and underlying grid technology, this process can become very complex and invasive. While executing non-interactive monolithic Unix-like sequences of CLIs* in grid middleware such as EGEE gLite (glite, A lightweight middleware for grid computing, 2008) or Globus can be straight forward (especially when scheduling optimizations are not considered), it is not the case for modern parallel modular applications involving human interactions and asynchronism. Things are even more complicated when one wants to make full use of the grid capabilities with an application that was not originally designed for it. In this case, reengineering might be needed; gridification may become highly invasive and last but not least introduce execution overheads.

Accompanying today's major fundamental grid paradigms, there are two conceptual approaches distinguishing which address this challenge. On the one hand, so-called task-based job submission relates processing to executable code described as a computation task, hereinafter referred to as "gridification". On the other hand, so-called service-based execution handles processing as workflows of Web services orchestrated in a surrounding SOA, hereinafter referred to as "servitization". While the former applies well to some of the problems faced in neuGRID (i.e. see pipelines' nature, points #2, 5, 6, 7 and 8) and could constitute an interesting short term solution, it does not abstract end-users from the grid specificities nor does it facilitate interactivity.Moreover, depending on the applied scheduling policy, it can introduce considerable overheads (especially when executing multiple short runtime stages such as the ones to be faced in neuroimaging). While gridification and servitization greatly differ in principles – e.g. data input/output, discovery mechanisms, etc, the present design specification argues interesting complementarities, to address neuGRID's objectives. This is what the next section elaborates on.

Figure 7.

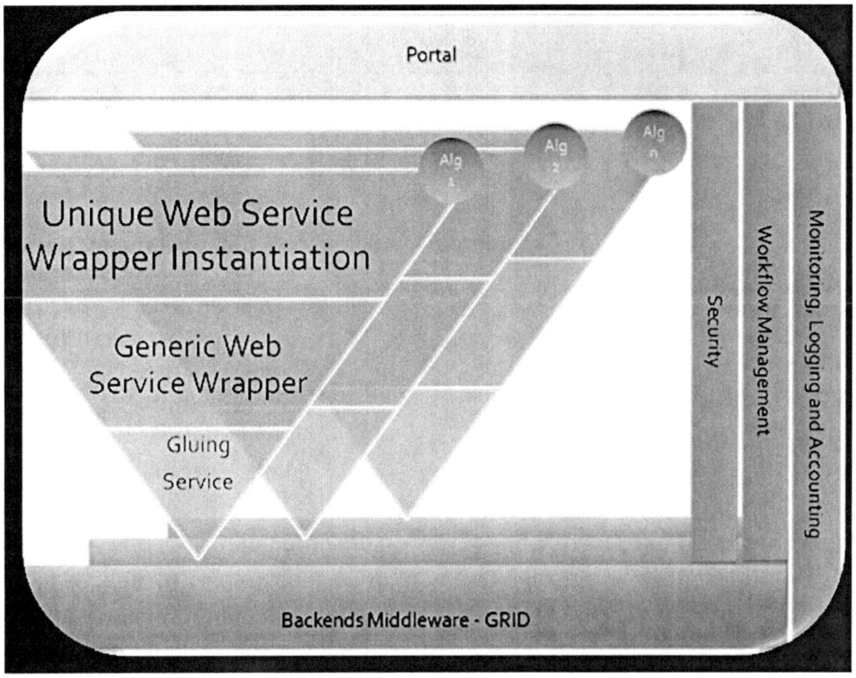

Gridification Approach and Model

The approach chased in this paper is one that advocates a hybrid model sitting in between gridification and servitization of the business logic. Indeed, it is the author's belief that using both concepts jointly would significantly help addressing all formerly raised specificities of neuroscientific pipelines. Moreover, such an approach would introduce enough flexibility to accommodate with new applications integration on the long run, especially thanks to the virtualization/ abstraction dimension brought in by the SOA paradigm.

The model here presented elaborates on former investigations conducted in the Health-e-Child project (The Information Societies Technology Project: Health-e-Child EU Contract IST-2004-027749 Description of Work) and by collaborators involved in the development of the so-called MOTEUR workflow engine (Glatard, Montagnat, Pennec, Emsellem & Lingrand, 2006). The former pionneered a sound SOA framework to efficiently and rapidly create secure simple, ubiquitous, loosely-coupled and stateless Web services (see Service Orientation for detailed explanations of SOA rules). The latter introduced the notion of a generic web service wrapper (Glatard, Emsellem & Montagnat, 2006) embedding legacy codes in service-based workflows (see (Lingrand, Montagnat & Glatard, 2008) for an exhaustive review of legacy code wrapping approaches).

Author's aim is therefore to integrate, extend and complete the above concepts based on respective scientific conclusions.

The survey of neuro-sciences toolkits (and in particular (AMGA -- the ARDA Metadata Catalogue Project, n.d.)), has shed light on interesting practices in the community, which when contrasted with current Web services workflow authoring environments, has opened the pathway to hybrid thinking. This is what Figure 7 illustrates, by recalling the ad-hoc representation used in System

Table 4.

Criteria / Pipelines	OS	Licensing	Prog. Language	Supported Data Format	Features
SPM	OS Independent	GPL*	Matlab	Analyze, NIftTI-1*, MINC*	Images Visualization Segmentation (apriori-based) Registration (linear and affine) Warping (Jacobian) Volumetric Analysis (density and volume) fMRI analysis PET analyses
FSL	MacOS X, Windows NT / 2000, Linux and SunOS / Solaris	FSL* License	C / C++	Analyze*, NIftTI-1*	Images Visualization (FSLview) Segmentation (FAST) Registration (FLIRT) Affine Warp cross-sectional (SIENAX) and longitudinal (SIENA) Volumetric Analysis fMRI analysis (FEAT) Independent Component Analysis (MELODIC) Tractography (FDT) Diffusion tensor voxelwise analysis (TBSS)
LoNI	MacOS X, Windows NT / 2000, Linux and SunOS/Solaris	LoNI Software Licence	Java	AFNI BRIK, Analyze*, bshort / bfloat, DICOM*, MGH/MGZ, MINC*, MINC2, NIftTI-1*	Image conversion (MNI toolkit) Non-uniformity correction (MNI) Segmentation (MNI) Warping (sulci based; flat maps) Image visualization (DISPLAY)
IDeALab	Linux (Fedora core) + SunOS/Solaris	PV-Wave & Quanta license	PV-wave, Shell Scripting	Analyze*, Quanta, Interfile	Image conversion Images Visualization (sv) WMHs Segmentation (Quanta) Linear Registration Warping (Spline)
B-MAP / HERMES	Unix for backend, Windows for frontend	HERMES Commercial Licence	---	---	Image Conversion, Interpolation, Template of reference brains, Masking of extra-cranial tissue, Morphing, Signal Inhomogeneity (Bias field), Tissue Segmentation (Gaussian Estimation, Fuzzy Cluster Analysis), Segmentation with ROI Analysis.
MNI	MacOS X, Linux and SGI IRIX	---	C, Perl, (some Java for visualization)	MINC*	Image Conversion, Images Visualization, Anatomical Regions Labelling, Sulcal Extraction, Cortex Extraction, Image Resampling, Statistical Analysis

Architecture. The proposed approach relies on the following three pillars:

1. Using a so-called generic "gluing service" to submit job execution orders to underlying grids (see JavaGAT/SAGA (A Simple API for Grid Applications (SAGA), n.d.) and

neuGRID's gluing service (Anjum, Bloodsworth, Habib, Lansdale, McClatchey, Mehmood & neuGRID Consortium, 2009) for more information). The gluing service abstracts upper layers of the system from grid specificities and is responsible for actual job submission. Note that this is in line with the conclusions of [34]. The objective here is to address pipeline's characteristic(s): 2, 4, 7 and 8 (see Pipelines' Nature).

2. Using a generic web service wrapper in charge of on-the-fly orchestration and potentially applying scheduling optimization techniques according to specified pipeline content, which is of absolute relevance in the context of neuroimaging toolkits, given their algorithms non-functional similarities. The objective here is to address pipeline's characteristic(s): 3, 4, 5 and 6 (see Pipelines' Nature).
3. Instantiating a unique web service wrapper per algorithm/ pipeline to be published in the SOA, thus allowing (both atomic and composite) processing tasks to be discovered, composed and subsequently published as new ones. See (LONI Software Tools, n.d.) for a similar approach with different implementation and technology. The objective here is to address pipeline's characteristic(s): 1 (see Pipelines' Nature).

Conceptually speaking each of these three substrates, plays a different but key role. While (1) introduces abstraction from grids and thus allows interacting with a wide variety of middleware, (2) takes care of appropriately parameterizing (1), characterizes commonalities of algorithms/ pipelines and opens a broad avenue to job scheduling optimization techniques (e.g. jobs grouping etc). (3) on the other hand and beyond parameterizing (2), turns this ecosystem of virtualized neuro-utilities into a set of publishable, discoverable and composable entities, which are very close to end-users' expertize. Note that (3) slightly differs from the approach undertaken in (Glatard, Emsellem & Montagnat, 2006) both conceptually and technologically, as it is a direct consequence to the strict adoption and application of SOA, as presented in Service Orientation The expected result is a service that can be invoked directly by end-users to execute a given algoritm, and to which neuroscientific knowledge can be attached.

By doing so, the SOA concept is fully exploited and efficiently supports end-users in their pipeline specification work. Indeed, using an advanced WSDL-based service repository such as the one presented in the system architecture (see System Architecture), neuroscientists would be able to query the SOA to discover available algorithms and pipelines which correspond to their needs, in a platform independent manner.

The combined use of these three elements is believed to constitute a tangible solution to address formerly gathered pipelines' characteristics. See the following table for a more detailed mapping (recalling Table 4 and focussing on aspects which are not obvious to tackle in a pure task-based environment):

CONCLUSION AND FUTURE WORK

Turning these requirements and assets into concrete and efficient tools, neuGRID intends to provide end-users with a harmonized and powerful environment to seamlessly create, use, combine and validate new image processing and data mining algorithm pipelines. Since early 2009, the online neuGRID infrastructure (http://neugrid.healthgrid.org), as illustrated in Figure 8 below, already offers interesting capabilities. As such, it exposes data acquisition and control interfaces (see left screenshot of Figure 8), grid access (see middle screenshot of Figure 8) and last but not least, a promising algorithm pipeline created at the Montreal Neurological Institute (MNI), i.e. the analysis of Cortical Thickness (Lerch & Evans, 2005), see screenshot on the right of Figure 8. This

Table 5.

1. ***Added-Value***	Pipelines can be specified as workflows of Web services, in spite of having concrete algorithms published in the grid. Current W3C standards allow describing such complex workflows and encompassing semantics/ annotations to store and machine-process associated knowledge/ expertize (see WSBPEL - http://www.oasis-open.org/committees/tc_home.php?wg_abbrev=wsbpel, and SAWSDL - http://www.w3.org/2002/ws/sawsdl/) for more information.
2. ***Heterogeneity***	Exposing algorithms and pipelines as Web services makes them virtualized/ abstracted and thus allows composing new pipelines with algorithms coming from potentially different toolkits and running in different environments.
3. ***Interactiveness***	Web services are naturally indicated for satisfying such requirements as they act as blackboxes triggered by an orchestration entity within the SOA. The orchestration entity and underlying workflow capability are the ones basically offering such interactiveness. Engines such as ActiveBPEL allow handling human interactions with the inclusion of dedicated services in the resulting workflow.
4. ***Iterativeness and Recursiveness***	In addition to virtualizing algorithms through Web services, the introduction of a generic web service wrapper allows applying scheduling optimization techniques. In the case of highly recursive pipelines of short runtime algorithms, optimization could be obtained by grouping jobs prior to submission to the underlying grid.

early prototype demonstrates underlying computing engine capacity and expects to gradually enrich its portfolio to enter into larger exploitation by beginning of 2010.

Using neuGRID, European neuroscientists and algorithm developers will have a powerful testbed to use, develop or even test their own products, making faster progress in their research while potentially raising the interest of pharmaceutical industries, which may be interested in such imaging markers to study the effect of drugs on chronic brain diseases, potentially speeding up their drug design and development cycles.

Actively pursuing collaboration with other projects in the field such as the French NeuroLOG, the Canadian CBRAIN and the American LONI initiatives, neuGRID aims to become the "Google" for Brain Imaging, offering a grid-based, easy-to-use and interoperable set of tools with which scientists can transparently perform analyses and collaborate internationally.

This paper presented an analysis of neuroscientific pipelines requirements as discovered in the neuGRID project, with the aim of formulating a set of preliminary design objectives, constraints and conclusions. By doing so, a survey process was engaged, which helped better understanding the faced issues. Following this, a significant effort of conceptualization and formalization was invested (and still is ongoing) to produce a relevant analysis conclusion as well as a first gridification model which can be applied to neuroscientific pipelines.

Part of the proposed model has been inspired by past but similar experiences as well. It consti-

Figure 8. Online neuGRID Portal

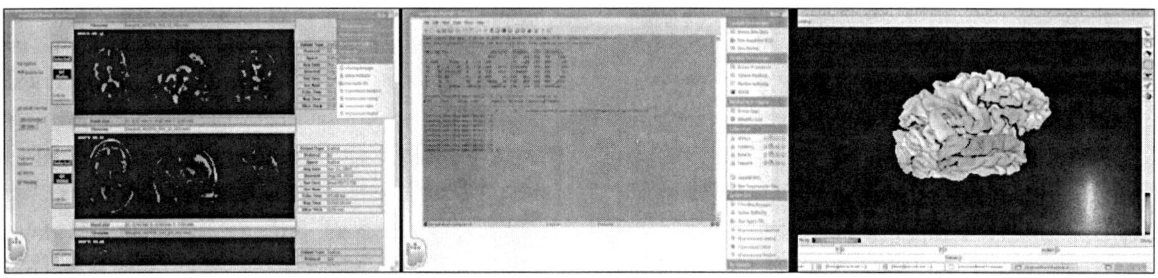

tutes an interesting mix of existing technologies and approaches while attempting to bring the SOA benefits closer to end-users. The model is expected to evolve as further prototyping tests are undergone. This work is also anticipated to open the pathway to interesting new research in the use of model driven engineering (MDE) techniques (see (Manset, McClatchey, Oquendo & Verjus, 2005), (Manset, Verjus & McClatchey, 2007) for insights on its application to grid architectures modelling and refinement), in particular within the generic Web service wrapper to dynamically change scheduling policies (e.g. grouping optimization vs isolation, middleware selection, etc), as well as within the orchestration entity to address non-functional aspects such as Ethical, Legal and Socio-Economical (ELSE) constraints.

ACKNOWLEDGMENT

The author would like to acknowledge the efforts of the complete neuGRID Consortium. Particular thanks go to colleagues who have been working on the SOA and grid aspects of the project.

The author would like to also acknowledge the support of Giovanni B. Frisoni, the neuGRID Project Coordinator and Prof. Richard McClatchey, the neuGRID Project Technical Coordinator.

The neuGRID project is funded by the European Commission's Seventh Framework Programme under grant agreement no 211714 and thanks are extended for this support.

REFERENCES

A Simple API for Grid Applications (SAGA). (n.d.). Retrieved from http://saga.cct.lsu.edu/index.php?option=com_content&task=view&id=71&Itemid=158

ActiveBPEL. (n.d.). Retrieved from http://www.activevos.com/community-open-source.php

Ad-Dab'bagh, Y., et al. (2005). Native space cortical thickness measurement and the absence of correlation to cerebral volume. In K. Zilles, (ed.), *Proceedings of the 11th Annual Meeting of the Organization for Human Brain Mapping*, Toronto, NeuroImage 2005.

Amendolia, S. R., Estrella, F., Hassan, W., Hauer, T., Manset, D., McClatchey, R., et al. (2004). MammoGrid: A Service Oriented Architecture Based Medical Grid Application. In *Proceedings of the 3rd International Conference on Grid and Cooperative Computing – GCC'04*. Wuhan, China, (LNCS Vol. 3251, pp 939-942). Berlin: Springer-Verlag.

AMGA – the ARDA Metadata Catalogue Project. (n.d.). Retrieved from http://amga.web.cern.ch/amga/

Anjum, A., Bloodsworth, P., Habib, I., Lansdale, T., McClatchey, R., Mehmood, Y. & The neuGRID Consortium. (2009). *Reusable Services from the neuGRID Project for Grid-Based Health Applications*. Accepted as Poster at the International Healthgrid'09 Conference.

Arsanjani, A. (2004). *Service-oriented modeling and architecture*. IBM technical article. Retrieved October 20, 2008, from http://www.ibm.com/developerworks/library/ws-soa-design1/

Buneman, P., Khanna, S., & Tan, W. C. (2001). A Characterization of Data Provenance. In *ICDT, 2001* (pp. 316–330). Why and Where.

EGEE. *Enabling the Grid for E-sciencE, 2007 Conference, Live Demo Competition*. (2007). Retrieved October 20, 2008, from http://indico.cern.ch/contributionDisplay.py?contribId=174&sessionId=23&confId=18714.

FMRIB Software Library. (n.d.). Retrieved from http://www.fmrib.ox.ac.uk

Foster, I., Kesselman, C., & Tuecke, S. (2001). The Anatomy of the Grid. *International Journal of High Performance Computing Applications, 15*(3). doi:10.1177/109434200101500302

Glatard, T., Emsellem, D., & Montagnat, J. (2006). Generic web service wrapper for efficient embedding of legacy codes in service-based workflows (workshop). In *Proceedings of the Grid-Enabling Legacy Applications and Supporting End Users Workshop (GELA '06),* (pp. 44--53), Paris, France, June 2006.

Glatard, T., Montagnat, J., Pennec, X., Emsellem, D., & Lingrand, D. (2006). *MOTEUR: a data-intensive service-based workflow manager.* Research Report I3S, number I3S/RR-2006-07-FR, (pp. 37), Sophia Antipolis, France, Mar 2006. *glite, A lightweight middleware for grid computing.* (2008). Retrieved October 20, 2008, from http://glite.web.cern.ch/glite/

Health-e-Child. *The EU FP6 Information Societies Technology Project.* (2008). Retrieved October 20, 2008, from http://www.health-e-child.org/

Lerch, J. P., & Evans, A. C. (2005). Cortical thickness analysis examined through power analysis and a population simulation. *NeuroImage, 24,* 163–173. doi:10.1016/j.neuroimage.2004.07.045

Lingrand, D., Montagnat, J., & Glatard, T. (2008). Estimating the execution context for refining submission strategies on production grids (workshop). In *Proceedings of the Assessing Models of Networks and Distributed Computing Platforms (ASSESS / ModernBio) (CCgrid'08),* (pp. 753 – 758).

LONI Software Tools. (n.d.). Retrieved from http://www.loni.ucla.edu/Software/

MacKenzie, C. M., et al. (2006, 2 August). *Reference Model for Service Oriented Architecture 1.0, OASIS Committee Specification 1.*

Manset, D., McClatchey, R., Oquendo, F., & Verjus, H. (2005). A Model-driven Approach for Grid Services Engineering. In *Proceedings of the 2005 International Conference on Software Engineering and their Applications - ICSSEA '05, (France), ICSSEA 2005.* (Vol 1. pp 135-142).

Manset, D., Pourraz, F., Tsymbal, A., Revillard, J., Skaburskas, K., McClatchey, R., et al. (in press). Gridifying Biomedical Applications: Experiences of the Health-e-Child Project. In *Handbook of Research on Computational Grid Technologies for Life Sciences, Biomedicine and Healthcare.* Hershey, PA: Information Science Reference.

Manset, D., Verjus, H., & McClatchey, R. (2007). *Managing Separation of Concerns in Grid Applications Through Architectural Model Transformations,* (LNCS Vol. 4758, pp. 308-310). Berlin: Springer-Verlag.

McClatchey, R., Manset, D., & Solomonides, T. (2006). Lessons learned from MammoGrid for integrated biomedical solutions. In *19th IEEE Int. Symposium on Computer-Based Medical Systems, CBMS 2006.*

Miles, S., Groth, P., Branco, M. &, Moreau, L. (2005). *The requirements of recording and using provenance in e-Science experiments.* Technical Report, Electronics and Computer Science, University of Southampton, UK.

MRIcro, Brain Extraction Tool (BET). (n.d.). Retrieved from http://www.sph.sc.edu/comd/rorden/mricro.html

MRIcro. (n.d.). Retrieved from http://www.sph.sc.edu/comd/rorden/mricro.html

NeuGrid Project. (2008). Retrieved October 20, 2008, from http://www.neugrid.eu/.

Papazoglou, M. P. (2003). Service-oriented computing: concepts, characteristics and directions. In *Proceedings of the 4th International Conference on Web Information Systems Engineering, WISE 2003, Roma, Italy.*

Role Based Access Control (RBAC). (n.d.). Retrieved from http://en.wikipedia.org/wiki/RBAC

Skaburskas, K., Estrella, F., Shade, J., Manset, D., Revillard, J., Rios, A., et al. (2007). Health-e-Child: A Grid Platform for European Paediatrics. In *Proceedings of the 2007 Computing in High Energy and Nuclear Physics International Conference - CHEP07, (USA), 2007 Publication in Journal of Physics: Conference Series.*

Sluimer, J. D., Vrenken, H., Blankenstein, M. A., Fox, N. C., Scheltens, P., Barkhof, F., & van der Flier, W. M. (n.d.). *Whole-brain atrophy rate in Alzheimer disease - Identifying fast progressors. SOAP Attachment.* (n.d). Retrieved from http://www.w3.org/TR/SOAP-attachments

Structural Image Evaluation using Normalisation of Atrophy (SIENA). (n.d.). Retrieved from http://www.fmrib.ox.ac.uk/fsl/siena/index.html.

The Globus Alliance. (n.d.). Retrieved from http://www.globus.org/

The Information Societies Technology Project: Health-e-Child EU Contract IST-2004-027749 Description of Work

Web Service Description Language (WSDL). (n.d.). Retrieved from http://www.w3.org/TR/2007/REC-wsdl20-primer-20070626/

Web Services Business Process Execution Language (WSBPEL). (n.d.). Retrieved from http://www.oasis-open.org/committees/tc_home.php?wg_abbrev=wsbpel

WS-Addressing. (n.d.). Retrieved from http://www.w3.org/TR/2006/REC-ws-addr-core-20060509/.

WS-Security. (n.d.). Retrieved from http://www.oasis-open.org/committees/tc_home.php?wg_abbrev=wss

Chapter 8
Computational Grids:
An Introduction to Potential Biomedical Uses and Future Prospects in Oncology; Neuro-Oncology Applications as a Model for Cancer Sub-Specialties

Ribhi Hazin
Harvard University, USA

Ibrahim Qaddoumi
St. Jude's Children's Research Hospital, USA

Francisco Pedrosa
Instituto Integrado de Medicina Prof Fernando Figueira - IMIP, Brazil

ABSTRACT

A network of interconnected computers, or "computational grids," can facilitate the ability of users to complete complex computational tasks that would be virtually impossible with a single computer. By leveraging the computational strength of grids, individual users can efficiently disseminate, exchange, and retrieve information as easily as if it were stored locally. As the authors found in this study, the possibilities computational grids present for highly specialized medical fields such as neuro-oncology are limitless. By harnessing the power of grids, neuro-oncologists can link to sophisticated interactive medical images around the world, perform complicated statistical analyses, create larger collaborative research projects, and improve delivery of care to patients around the globe. Thus, utilization of grid computing modules will inevitably lead to marked improvements in clinicians' ability to detect, manage, and prevent complications associated with brain tumors.

BACKGROUND

Computational grids are networks of interconnected computers that are linked in a manner that enables users to carry out very large or complicated computational tasks that could not be performed on a single computer or a small group of computers alone. By linking thousands of computers via high-speed networks, grid systems enable thousands of interconnected

DOI: 10.4018/978-1-61692-010-4.ch008

computers (or "computer farms") to be accessed on demand to meet the varying needs of many users (Hernandez, Blanquer, Solomonides, Breton & Legre, 2006). This pooling of computational resources in grids facilitates the ability to share and aggregate computational capabilities and thus allows greater efficiency in performing tasks. In perspective, each grid serves dozens to hundreds of independent user communities with each user community consisting of hundreds or thousands of users. Table 1 provides an overview of a sample computational grid implemented to deal with national public health concerns. Similar grids have been proposed in fields ranging from ecology and economics to business management and industrial engineering (Hernandez, Blanquer, Solomonides, Breton & Legre, 2006), (Ahmed, Lenz, Liu, Robinson & Ghafoor, 2008). By distributing the workload among large numbers of computers, users are able to speed up response times for many applications (Toffler & Toffler, 2007), (Breton, Blanquer Hernandez, Legre & Solomonides, 2006). Three primary forms of grids currently have widespread use and reflect the preferences and needs of the users:

a. **Computational grids:** using computing power from multiple linked computers to enable users to solve complex computational problems.
b. **Data grids:** harnessing the strength of interconnected computers to enable the exchange of data among users, primarily those engaged in data mining and decision support. Data grids do not share computing power as computational grids do.
c. **Collaborative grids:** harnessing the power of computational grids to enable users to cooperatively conduct and monitor ongoing collaborative projects.

Given the rapid dissemination of information in the Internet era, many researchers in business, academia, and other spheres of society have become increasingly dependent upon the ever-expanding amount of computational and electronic data available (Ahmed, Lenz, Liu, Robinson & Ghafoor, 2008), (The University of Washington School of Public Health's Center for Public Health Informatics, n.d.). Accessing grid systems can provide shared resources that transcend geographic boundaries and thus improve their productivity as researchers (Hernandez, Blanquer, Solomonides, Breton & Legre, 2006), (Goble, 2001). Although primarily used in business and academic applications in the past, grid technology has increasingly become useful in healthcare in a variety of ways, including genetic linkage analysis, determination of protein structures, molecular sequence analysis, data mining, and biomedical image processing, to name a few (Table 1) (Hernandez, Blanquer, Solomonides, Breton & Legre, 2006), (Toffler & Toffler, 2007), (Weiss, 2001). The pooling of computers allows individual users to disseminate, exchange, and retrieve information as easily as if it were stored locally (Goble, 2001), (Camarasu, Benoit-Cattin, Montagnat, & Racceanu, 2008), (Swedlow, Goldberg, Brauner & Sorger, 2003). Instructive scenarios on how grids can be used in biomedical experiments are described in Table 2.

The "excess computing power" (Toffler & Toffler, 2007) that grids offer has emerged as a platform to address the computational, storage, and information management requirements of large-scale biomedical applications (Ahmed,

Table 1. Healthcare applications for grid technology (Ammen & Versweyveld, 1998)

Genetic linkage analysis
Molecular sequence analysis
Determining structural patterns of proteins
Biomedical image processing and analysis
Information retrieval
Data mining of medical information databases
Text mining of medical information databases

Table 2. Sample scenarios for using a computational grid (Ammen & Versweyveld, 1998; Scotch, Yip, & Cheung, 2008; Zou, Miller, & Schmidtmann, 2007; Alonso, Ferrero, Hernandez, Molto, Saiz, & Trenor, 2008).

* **Robert the Biologist:** *Robert was a biologist working with a team of other biologists to determine yeast gene expression. Before conducting a microarray experiment, he checked to see whether any other similar experiment had been conducted and whether the data from such an experiment were already available. The system recommended a set of parameters for the machine. A sample was logged into a database and labeled. The microarray machine, recognizing Robert from the log, set parameters to those he had used on previous runs. The parameters were recorded with the output results, which were stored in his personal database alongside the image results.* *The results were immediately accessible from Robert's office, where he analysed them with specialized statistical computations and a complex interactive time-series visualization, both of which dynamically exploit multiple computational resources to get better performance. The visualization was examined collaboratively with a colleague at a remote site. Online personal notes were attached to the results by both scientists. Several products with upregulated expression looked interesting. A search using the SRS database portal identified a gene as encoding a transcription factor. Papers, in free text, quoted in the database entries and extracted online from the Medline digital library revealed that, in certain circumstances, this gene could control other genes related to the yeast gene of interest. The system recommended other scientists who had published work or experiments that were related.* *adapted from Goble C (2001)
Zou the Epidemiologist: *After years of working for a renowned medical school in the northeastern United States, Zou was asked to join a national health organization to develop novel techniques for predicting epidemics. Only a few months after he began his new job, the media were abuzz with stories of the West Nile Virus (WNV), which is a mosquito-borne viral infection that was originally described in New York City in 1999. If left unchecked, WNV can cause widespread mortality in both humans and animals, particularly during summer months, when the mating and activity of the mosquito vector peaks.* *Zou established a computational grid with regional partners that combined temperature data from environmental biosensors to create a WNV "surveillance system" that monitored infections in humans, birds, and mosquitoes. His surveillance system successfully identified high-risk WNV areas and was instrumental in the implementation of important public health measures to curb the spread of the deadly disease.*
Ahmed the Cardiologist: *Ahmed was an accomplished invasive cardiologist with a thriving research laboratory at a teaching hospital. For years, he had employed dozens of research technicians, summer medical students, and resident physicians to partake in various aspects of research projects he supervised. Although the high attrition rate associated with hiring medical students and residents was at times unbearable, his overwhelming workload made this pattern virtually unavoidable. One particular project he had been unable to complete since its inception 9 years ago was one that attempted to analyze the action potential propagation on cardiac tissues.* *The completion of this project would likely never have seen fruition had Ahmed not decided to incorporate high-performance computational grid technology into his laboratory. With the help of the grid system, Ahmed was able to formulate mathematical models of the electrical behavior of excitable cardiac cells, which ultimately enabled him and fellow researchers to quantitatively describe various characteristics of ventricular and atrial action potentials. The discoveries Ahmed's research achieved through computational grids has been heralded as a harbinger for the reduction of heart disease, the leading cause of death in many developed countries.*

Lenz, Liu, Robinson & Ghafoor, 2008), (Weiss, 2001), (Ammen & Versweyveld, 1998), (Scotch, Yip & Cheung, 2008), (Zou, Miller, & Schmidtmann, 2007), (Alonso, Ferrero, Hernandez, Molto, Saiz & Trenor, 2008), (Singh, Chen, Liu, Mitchell & Schmidt, 2008). For instance, the role of image analysis has long played a critical role in various aspects of basic research and clinical studies. Researchers using high-resolution scanners and sensors can, through sophisticated image analysis, amass detailed measurements of various molecular and biochemical entities rapidly (Goble, 2001), (Singh, Chen, Liu, Mitchell & Schmidt, 2008), (Kumar, Rutt, Kurc, Catalyurek, Pan, Chow, Lamont, et al. 2008), (Muller, Michoux, Bandon, & Geissbuler, 2004). Information synthesized from such measurements can be used to improve the diagnosis of rare diseases, to assess the efficacy of treatment paradigms, and to analyze the relevance of various scientific hypotheses (Goble, 2001), (Kumar, Rutt, Kurc, Catalyurek, Pan, Chow, Lamont, et al. 2008). The potential this technology represents has not been overlooked by leading radiologists, who have recently developed programs that capitalize on a computational grid's ability to perform complex and computationally demanding applications in medical imaging, such as computer-aided detection (CAD) (Pan, Gurcan, Langella, Oster, Hastings, Sharma, & Rutt, 2007), (Farag, El-Baz, Gimelfarb, El-Ghar & Eldiasty, 2005). Radiologists from around the world are in the process of creating software that would allow users worldwide to use CAD software in a collaborative manner to enhance the performance and accuracy of detecting potentially malignant lung nodules (Pan, Gurcan, Langella, Oster, Hastings, Sharma, & Rutt, 2007), (Gurcan, Sahiner, Petrick, Chan, Kazerooni, Cascade, et al., 2002). In this system, lung lesions that meet certain criteria specified in a grid-supported CAD program would be isolated via a composite automated reading and combined or compared by one or more users for research purposes or clinical imaging interpretation (Pan, Gurcan, Langella, Oster, Hastings, Sharma, & Rutt, 2007), (Farag, El-Baz, Gimelfarb, El-Ghar & Eldiasty, 2005), (Gurcan, Sahiner, Petrick, Chan, Kazerooni, Cascade, et al., 2002). After preliminary testing of the system, researchers have begun suggesting that a substantial percentage of clinically significant lung lesions that are overlooked during routine clinical interpretation of thoracic computed tomographic studies might be detected with the use of grid-supported CAD systems (Pan, Gurcan, Langella, Oster, Hastings, Sharma, & Rutt, 2007), (Peldschus, Herzog, Wood, Cheema, Costello, & Schoepf, 2005), (Brown, Goldin, Rogers, Kim, Suh, McNitt, Shah, et al. 1999). Similar grid-dependent computer-aided diagnosis programs are currently being used to hasten the early detection of suspicious colonic polyps, signaling an evolving trend in medicine that favors increasing the use of grids in various clinical applications (Giger, Doi, MacMahon, Metz, & Yin, 1990), (Summers, Jerebko, Franaszek, Malley & Johnson, 2002), (Krauter, Buyya, & Maheswaran, 2002).

Various forms of grid computing systems have been used by scientists and researchers for "researching smallpox, cancer, AIDS," (Toffler & Toffler, 2007) and other significant medical and non-medical problems globally (Camarasu, Benoit-Cattin, Montagnat, & Racceanu, 2008), (Collins, Morgan & Patrinos, 2003). The anthrax scare that gripped the United States in 2001 is perhaps the best known public health application of grids thus far. In an effort to avert a national panic, the National Foundation for Cancer Research teamed up with Oxford University, Microsoft, and Intel to create a massive grid that enabled them to screen more than 3.5 billion suspected compounds in less than 24 days (Toffler & Toffler, 2007). By establishing a virtual supercomputer that allowed scientists from around the globe to solve complex computational problems, researchers were able identify suspicious compounds in a manner that would have been virtually impossible otherwise (Hernandez, Blanquer, Solomonides, Breton & Legre, 2006), (Camarasu, Benoit-Cattin, Montagnat, & Racceanu, 2008), (Roure, Jennings & Shadbolt, 2005). A similar scenario played out in 2002 with the severe acute respiratory syndrome outbreak, which many feared would take on pandemic proportions. Many healthcare and medical institutions worldwide have since capitalized on this technology by using it as a means of managing databases and improving access to important diagnostic information (Hernandez, Blanquer, Solomonides, Breton & Legre, 2006), (day, Dagtas, Iino, Khokhar, & Ghafoor, 1995).

The *Neurobase* project, which is supported by the government of France, is perhaps the best-known example of this. Due to the rapid increase in the amount of data generated by the neurosciences community following the advent of the Internet, many in the science and medical community deemed it necessary to devise a method for sharing data and knowledge. *Neurobase* is a consortium of various experimental, clinical, and research centers that have utilized a computational grid to improve the dissemination of and access to neuroimaging data from around the world (Temal, Dojat, Kassel, & Gibaud, 1995). This collaborative research is essentially an all-purpose program for the acquisition, storage, and digital processing of images, audio and visual data, and other documents (Barillot, Benali, Dojat, Gaignard, Gibaud, Kinkingnéhun, 2006). *Neurobase* has been instrumental in allowing neurologists to undertake a task that has long been deemed impossible: construction of functional cerebral maps under normal and pathologic conditions.

Neurologists and neurosurgeons interested in developing these maps of the brain were often unable to internally manage large quantities of data and to compare the data and the programs they developed from the data with the programs and research findings developed in other centers (Barillot, Benali, Dojat, Gaignard, Gibaud, Kinkingnéhun, 2006), (Bidgood, Horii, Prior, & Van Syckle, 1997), (Olive, Rahmouni, & Solomonides, 2007), (Mazziotta, Toga, Evans, Fox, & Lancaster, 1985). Furthermore, researchers involved in this gargantuan undertaking were often unable to conduct the large-scale experiments that the ambitious project warranted due to lack of manpower and technological capabilities (Hernandez, Blanquer, Solomonides, Breton & Legre, 2006), (Barillot, Benali, Dojat, Gaignard, Gibaud, Kinkingnéhun, 2006), (Fost & Kesselman, 1999). By compiling experimental data through their virtual supercomputer, researchers at *Neurobase* were able to broaden the scientific achievement of individual neurologic research sites as well as increase the number of people involved in neuro-imaging studies. This development led to *Neurobase*'s success in finding functional relationships between anatomic structures in the brain where neuronal activations and cerebral functions occur. This advanced understanding of the nervous system would not have reached fruition without the formation of brain maps, which were created by pooling thousands of neuro-images into one. This mapping of various magnetic resonance, functional magnetic resonance, positron-emission tomography, magneto-encephalography, and electroencephalography images into one distinct set of maps proved to be a critical step toward discovering the relationship between anatomic structures in the brain and cerebral function (Hernandez, Blanquer, Solomonides, Breton & Legre, 2006), (Camarasu, Benoit-Cattin, Montagnat, & Racceanu, 2008).

This collaborative approach toward biomedical informatics was duplicated by the *Cancer Biomedical Informatics Grid (caBIG)*, which was created by the National Cancer Institute's Center for Bioinformatics. The *caBIG* computational grids focus on enhancing the cancer researcher's ability to recognize and treat as well as provide novel preventive approaches to various cancers (Breton, Blanquer Hernandez, Legre & Solomonides, 2006), (Bidgood, Horii, Prior, & Van Syckle, 1997). Similarly, a consortium of private and public organizations recently launched the *FightAIDS@Home* initiative, which relies on a computational grid system to develop creative molecular and biochemical strategies to effectively treat individuals infected with human immunodeficiency virus in light of the many drug-resistant strains of the virus. Table 3 provides a succinct overview of other recently launched biomedical applications that are dependent on deploying the massive computer power offered by computational grids.

POTENTIAL TARGETS FOR COMPUTATIONAL GRIDS IN ONCOLOGY

Despite the benefits, many areas of biomedicine have yet to tap into the vast repository of informational wealth computational grids can offer. Although cancers in general have been the focus of the *caBIG* grid, no grids have been tailored to fit the emerging needs of specialists in rare subspecialties such as neuro-oncology and ocular oncology, especially in children. Medicine in gen-

Table 3. Biomedical applications using Computational Grids

Discipline	Project	Goal/Objective	Web site	Ref
Neuroscience	*Neurobase Project*	Mapping of cerebral functions	http://www.irisa.fr/visages/demo/Neurobase/index.html	29
Oncology	*Cancer Biomedical Informatics Grid (caBIG):*	Early detection, consolidation of preventative measures	https://cabig.nci.nih.gov/	4
Infectious Disease	*FightAIDS@Home*	Tailor current treatment paradigms to the drug-resistant strains of the HIV virus	http://fightaidsathome.scripps.edu	31,4
Biology	*TeraGrid Bioportal*	Provide researchers and students unfettered access to biological data and applications.	http://www.teragrid.org/	6
Epidemiology/ Infectious Disease	*Smallpox Research Grid Project*	Identifying various drug molecules and linked them with cellular protein targets to isolate important targets for future drug and vaccine development.	http://www.chem.ox.ac.uk/smallpox/	1, 4
Cancer Pharmacology	*Cancer Research Project*	Links over 400,000 users and computers to share processing power in a manner that focuses on improving the search for effective cancer drugs.	http://www.nfcr.org/	4, 33
Public Health	*Grid-Enabled Medical Simulation Services (GEMSS):*	Provides physicians and other healthcare workers access to sophisticated simulation and imaging processing applications at levels unattainable via smaller systems used by local hospitals. Although this application is currently unavailable, a prototype application is planned for European hospitals in the near future.	http://www.it.neclab.eu/gemss/	10
Virology	*Virolab*	Virolab uses the power of computational grids to establish a 'virtual laboratory' that facilitates the discovery of novel treatments for resistant HIV strains.	www.virolab.org	1, 31
Pediatrics	*Health-e-Child Consortium*	Utilizes a network of computers to promote the optimal delivery of care for various pediatric hospitals and healthcare facilities throughout Europe.	http://www.health-e-child.org/links/health-e-child-consortium-members	1, 31
Neuropsychiatry	*BIOPATTERN Grid*	Describes a program designed to use computational grids as a means of biologically profiling individual patients to improve detection of dementia and brain injury.	www.biopattern.org	28, 32,1
Radiology & Oncology	*MammoGrid Project*	Established as a means of examining the results of thousands of grid-based medical images to improve early detection of breast cancer	http://mammogrid.vitamib.com	1,7

continues on following page

Table 3. continued

Discipline	Project	Goal/Objective	Web site	Ref
Public Health & Epidemiology	*Africa@Home Project*	A conglomeration of volunteer researchers, physicians, and humanitarian aid workers who have relied on grid computing to develop a revolutionary epidemiological computer model that provides the team with optimal strategies for delivering mosquito nets, anti-malarial medications, and vaccinations throughout endemic areas of Africa.	http://africa-at-home.web.cern.ch/africa-at-home	33
Cancer Genomics	*Advancing Clinico-Genomic Clinical Trials on Cancer (ACGT)*	Established to create an infrastructure that would facilitate the identification of patients' characteristics that would determine the most appropriate treatment for individual patients	www.eu-acgt.org/	35

eral often addresses clinical needs by examining experimental and clinical precedents. That is, using antibiotics to treat a certain disease is an action that results from years of trial and error, numerous research and clinical studies, and very certainly, numerous analyses of empirical data pointing to the benefits of such an action (Breton, Blanquer Hernandez, Legre & Solomonides, 2006), (Kumar, Rutt, Kurc, Catalyurek, Pan, Chow, Lamont, et al. 2008). Clinical treatments in modern medicine have benefitted from this system and stand to benefit still further from the continuation of such a meticulous process. Unfortunately, certain medical disciplines such as neuro-oncology simply lack the large patient populations needed to conduct the large-scale studies such as those that have been done with more commonplace diseases such as the common cold or bronchitis (Hernandez, Blanquer, Solomonides, Breton & Legre, 2006). Given the fact that medicine relies heavily on established precedents for improving future treatment paradigms, it stands to reason that disciplines focused on the treatment of rare diseases could benefit immensely from the establishment of a computational grid. The ability of neuro-oncologists to develop reasonable conclusions on treatment or detection of various brain cancers is often limited by the relative paucity of cases.

Using a computational grid system that harnesses the power of numerous computers around the world could permit neuro-oncologists to establish a standardized method for the exchange of valuable data among clinicians. This could be valuable for clinicians in that it would allow various physicians to collaborate with one another on difficult or atypical cases and could encourage the sharing of rare cases in clinical studies that were previously impossible due to the small numbers of cases seen at individual institutions (Hernandez, Blanquer, Solomonides, Breton & Legre, 2006). A virtual neuro-oncology department could foster such research by maximally utilizing the sophisticated tools for statistical analysis and image modeling and simulation that computational grids provide. This can have important clinical implications for tele-oncology and other forms of telemedicine. Given the complexity of brain and spinal cord tumors, the subspecialty of neuro-oncology will serve as an example to illustrate how a grid system such as *BIOPATTERN* can be dedicated to studying brain injury. The possibilities for the neuro-oncologist are endless, with grids providing the possibility of the following:

a. Establishing a parametric mapping analysis that would allow for early detection of neurologic tumors in a manner similar to the way the *BIOPATTERN* grid identifies brain injury. *BIOPATTERN* can be also helpful in neuro-oncology for evaluating brain injury that is due to treatments such as surgery, radiation, or chemotherapy (Hernandez, Blanquer, Solomonides, Breton & Legre, 2006), (Mazziotta, Toga, Evans, Fox, & Lancaster, 1985).

b. Using computational grids to link sophisticated interactive medical image processes with pharmacokinetic modeling processes to combat various forms of brain cancers. Similar programmatic combinations have been successfully used in fighting various liver cancers (Hernandez, Blanquer, Solomonides, Breton & Legre, 2006), (Breton, Blanquer Hernandez, Legre & Solomonides, 2006).
c. Using sophisticated tools for statistical analysis that would allow neuro-oncologists to analyze existing data on the genetic basis of certain tumors and make educated predictions about clinical outcomes
d. Providing a grid-based collaboration that would enable the sharing of patient data, research findings, and digital images around the world
e. Developing novel ideas to use grids to monitor brain tumor patients equipped with biosensors that would regularly interact with computational grids to alert neuro-oncologists of anatomic changes that often precede or are associated with metastasis. Although this technology has yet to be developed, harnessing the power of grids to analyze the combination of mapping and advanced anatomic responses to metastasis could allow physicians to predict such clinical outcomes in the near future
f. Providing a valuable data resource that could improve clinical outcomes for patients with brain tumors in remote locations around the world
g. Sharing the processing power of thousands of computers to enable neuro-oncologists to create a virtual cadaver that could provide current and future neurosurgeons and neuro-oncologists with valuable resources for teaching and practicing complicated neurologic surgeries and invasive techniques for treating brain tumors.
h. Implementing new imaging techniques to study brain tumors such as spectroscopy magnetic resonance imaging and diffusion tensor imaging. Grid technology may be useful in analyzing and interpreting the data from such studies in a timely fashion. In addition, it can help in advancing such imaging technologies.
i. Implementing targeted therapy, which is a promising new frontier in oncology that relies on the analysis and utilization of millions of small molecules, many of which have yet to be studied. By facilitating the selection of potential small molecules to target for therapy, grid technology can significantly improve current approaches to this cutting-edge field.
j. Advancing new, complex techniques in radiation therapy such as intensity-modulated radiation therapy and proton beam therapy, which require numerous complex calculations involving of dosages and targeted field evaluations. Grid technology can dramatically improve the efficiency of such techniques.
k. Analyzing central nervous system toxicity due to the tumor, chemotherapy, or radiation therapy. Computational grids similar to *BIOPATTERN* can be designed to help in analyze this oft-revisited issue in clinical neuro-oncology and design strategies to reduce future toxicities.

FUTURE RESEARCH DIRECTIONS

Clinicians and researchers involved in the study of neuro-oncology should be encouraged to create investigative committees to identify potential uses for a computational grid system in their individual institutions. Given the importance of including large numbers of users in a grid system, clinicians and researchers should also work to identify other institutions with similar research or professional interests that would agree to the collaborative approaches inherent in the grid system (Breton, Blanquer Hernandez, Legre & Solomonides, 2006). Once this has been established, a meeting could provide participants with an overview of recent literature on computational grids, provide insight into launching a pilot program, assign a reliable person the task of being coordinator of the grid, and identify ways to secure funding and support for the grid system (Table 4). Given the promise offered by smart grid computing, the European Union has actively promoted interest in and provided funding for research and applications involving grid computing systems. Keeping the patient abreast of many aspects of grid technologies can ensure that increased reliance on technology does not lead to a deterioration of doctor-patient relationships in institutions using grid technologies. Furthermore, increased public awareness campaigns involving patients and patient advocates can increase patient compliance with such initiatives, increase funding for grid systems and, ultimately, improve public understanding of the benefits of this technology.

Continued governmental support will likely facilitate the future use of grid technologies in a broader sense than that in which they have been traditionally used.

CONCLUSION

Computational grids hold enormous potential for the healthcare industry. Whether grids are used for enhancing recognition of potentially deadly lung nodules or simply for storage or data mining purposes, it is clear that this new technology offers a valuable resource that remains largely untapped. Select communities in the healthcare and medical fields have already embraced grid computing systems and have reaped tremendous benefits in terms of saved time and resources as well as improved delivery of care to their patients. Nonetheless, most medical professionals and healthcare workers remain uninformed of the limitless possibilities grid computing offers and the myriad of ways it can improve various aspects of their work. This is particularly true of highly specialized fields such as neuro-oncology, where adoption of grid computing modules would almost certainly lead to marked improvements in the ability of clinicians to detect, manage, and prevent complications associated with brain tumors.

Table 4. Five easy steps for establishing a computational grid (Breton, Blanquer Hernandez, Legre & Solomonides, 2006)

1) Create Committees to identify potential uses
2) Identify institutions with similar ideological and professional values
3) Establish colloquium for brainstorming and ensuring the essential dialogue and interaction necessary for establishing a mission with a set of clear goals
4) Identify a coordinator to monitor the implementation of the grid and ensure its users' adherence to the expected goals
5) Secure funding

REFERENCES

Ahmed, W., Lenz, D., Liu, J., Robinson, P. J., & Ghafoor, A. (2008). XML-Based Data Model and architecture for a knowledge-based grid-enabled problem-solving environment for high-throughput biological imaging. *IEEE Transactions on Information Technology in Biomedicine*, *12*, 226–237. doi:10.1109/TITB.2007.904153

Alonso, J. M., Ferrero, J. M., Hernandez, V., Molto, G., Saiz, J., & Trenor, B. (2008)... *IEEE Transactions on Information Technology in Biomedicine*, *12*(2). doi:10.1109/TITB.2007.907982

Ammen, E., & Versweyveld, L. (1998). Virtual Medical Worlds Magazine - A Euromed on-line information building block for HPCN related telemedicine. *Future Generation Computer Systems*, *14*(1-2), 131–136. doi:10.1016/S0167-739X(98)00015-6

Barillot, C., Benali, H., Dojat, M., Gaignard, A., Gibaud, B., & Kinkingnéhun, S. (2006). Federating distributed and heterogeneous information sources in neuroimaging: the NeuroBase Project. *Studies in Health Technology and Informatics*, *120*, 3–13.

Bidgood, W. D., Horii, S. C., Prior, F. W., & Van Syckle, D. E. (1997). Understanding and using DICOM, the data interchange standard for biomedical imaging. *Journal of the American Medical Informatics Association*, *4*, 199–212.

Breton, V., Blanquer, I., Hernandez, V., Legré, Y., & Solomonidés, T. (2006). Proposing a roadmap for HealthGRIDs. *Studies in Health Technology and Informatics*, *120*, 319–329.

Brown, M. S., Goldin, J. G., Rogers, S., Kim, H. J., Suh, R. D., & McNitt-Gray, M. F. (1999). Computer-aided lung nodule detection in CT: results of large-scale observer test. *Academic Radiology*, *12*, 681–686. doi:10.1016/j.acra.2005.02.041

Camarasu, S., Benoit-Cattin, H., Montagnat, J., & Racoceanu, D. (2008). Content-based medical image indexing and retrieval on Grids, First International Symposium on ICT for Health, Ateneo de Manila University, Manila, Philippines. *Philippine J Info Tech. 1*, 46.

Collins, F. S., Morgan, M., & Patrinos, A. (2003). The human genome project: Lessons from large-scale biology. *Science*, *300*, 286–290. doi:10.1126/science.1084564

Day, Y. F., Dagtas, S., Iino, M., Khokhar, A., & Ghafoor, A. (1995). Object-oriented conceptual modeling of video data. In *Proc. 11th Int. Conf. Data Eng.* (pp. 401-408).

Farag, A. A., El-Baz, A., Gimelfarb, G., El-Ghar, M. A., & Eldiasty, T. (2005). Quantitative nodule detection in low dose chest CT scans: new template modeling and evaluation for CAD system design. *Med Image Comput Assist Interv*, *8*(pt1), 720–728. doi:10.1007/11566465_89

Fost, I., & Kesselman, C. (1999). *The Grid: Blueprint for a future computing infrastructure*. San Francisco: Morgan Kaufmann Publishers, Inc.

Freund, J., Comaniciu, D., Ioannis, Y., Liu, P., McClatchey, R., & Morley-Fletcher, E. (2006). Health-e-child: an integrated biomedical platform for grid-based paediatric applications. *Studies in Health Technology and Informatics*, *120*, 259–270.

Giger, M. L., Doi, K., MacMahon, H., Metz, C. E., & Yin, F. F. (1990). Pulmonary nodules: computer-aided detection in digital chest images. *Radiographics*, *10*, 41–51.

Goble, C. (2001). The low down on e-science and grids for biology. *Comparative and Functional Genomics*, *2*, 365–370. doi:10.1002/cfg.115

Gurcan, M. N., Sahiner, B., Petrick, N., Chan, H. P., Kazerooni, E. A., Cascade, P. N., & Hadjiiski, L. (2002). Lung nodule detection on thoracic computed tomography images: preliminary evaluation of a computer-aided diagnosis system. *Medical Physics*, *29*, 2552–2558. doi:10.1118/1.1515762

Hernandez, V., Blanquer, I., Solomonides, T., Breton, V., & Legre, Y. (Eds.). (2006). *Challenges and Opportunities of HealthGrids: Proceedings of Healthgrid 2006,* (pp. 407.). Washington, DC: IOS Press, Washington, DC.

Krauter, K., Buyya, R., & Maheswaran, M. (2002). A taxonomy and survey of grid resource management systems for distributed computing. *Software, Practice & Experience*, *32*, 135–164. doi:10.1002/spe.432

Kumar, V. S., Rutt, B., Kurc, T., Catalyurek, U. V., Pan, T. C., & Chow, S. (2008). Large-scale Biomedical Image analysis in Grid environments. *IEEE Transactions on Information Technology in Biomedicine*, *12*(2). doi:10.1109/TITB.2007.908466

Mazziotta, J. C., Toga, A. W., Evans, A. C., Fox, P., & Lancaster, J. L. (1985). A Probabilistic Atlas of the Human Brain: Theory and Rationale for its development. *NeuroImage*, *2*(3), 89–10.

Muller, H., Michoux, N., Bandon, D., & Geissbuler, A. (2004). A review of content-based image retrieval systems in medical applications-clinical benefits and future directions. *International Journal of Medical Informatics*, *73*, 1–23. doi:10.1016/j.ijmedinf.2003.11.024

Olive, M., Rahmouni, H., & Solomonides, T. (2007). From HealthGRID to SHARE: a selective review of projects. *Studies in Health Technology and Informatics*, *126*, 306–313.

Pan, T. C., Gurcan, M. N., Langella, S. A., Oster, S. W., Hastings, S. L., & Sharma, A. (2007). GridCAD: Grid-based computer-aided detection system. *Radiographics*, *27*(3). doi:10.1148/rg.273065153

Peldschus, K., Herzog, P., Wood, S. A., Cheema, J. I., Costello, P., & Schoepf, U. J. (2005). Computer-aided diagnosis as a second reader: spectrum of findings in CT studies of the chest interpreted as normal. *Chest*, *128*, 1517–1523. doi:10.1378/chest.128.3.1517

Roure, D. D., Jennings, N. R., & Shadbolt, N. R. (2005). The semantic grid: Past, present, and future. *Proceedings of the IEEE*, *93*, 669–681. doi:10.1109/JPROC.2004.842781

Scotch, M., Yip, K. Y., & Cheung, K. H. (2008). *Development of Grid-like Applications for public health using Web 2.0 mashup techniques*. Journal American Medical Informatics Association.

Singh, A., Chen, C., Liu, W., Mitchell, W., & Schmidt, B. (2008). A Hybrid Computational grid architecture for comparative Genomics. *IEEE Transactions on Information Technology in Biomedicine*, *12*, 218–225. doi:10.1109/TITB.2007.908462

Summers, R. M., Jerebko, A. K., Franaszek, M., Malley, J. D., & Johnson, C. D. (2002). Colonic polyps: complementary role of computer-aided detection in CT colonography. *Radiology*, *225*, 391–399. doi:10.1148/radiol.2252011619

Swedlow, J. R., Goldberg, I., Brauner, E., & Sorger, P. K. (2003). Informatics and quantitative analysis in biological imaging. *Science*, *300*, 100–102. doi:10.1126/science.1082602

Temal, L., Dojat, M., Kassel, G., & Gibaud, B. (2008). Towards an ontology for sharing medical images and regions of interest in neuroimaging. *Journal of Biomedical Informatics*, *41*(5), 766–778. doi:10.1016/j.jbi.2008.03.002

The University of Washington School of Public Health's Center for Public Health Informatics. (n.d.). Retrieved on October 14, 2008 from http://www.cphi.washington.edu/research.html.

Toffler, A., & Toffler, H. (2007). *Revolutionary Wealth: How it will be created and how it will change our lives*. New York: Doubleday Business.

Wegener, D., Sengstag, T., Sfakianakis, S., Ruping, S., & Assi, A. (2007, December 10-13). GridR: An R-Based Grid-Enabled Tool for Data Analysis in ACGT Clinico-Genomics Trials. In *IEEE International Conference on e-Science and Grid Computing,* (pp. 228 - 235).

Weiss, T. (2001, November 29). Grid computing to aid breast cancer research. *CNN news*. Retrieved October 3, 2008 from http://archives.cnn.com/2001/TECH/industry/11/29/grid.cancer.research.idg/

Zou, L., Miller, S. N., & Schmidtmann, E. T. (2007). A GIS tool to estimate West Nile Virus Risk based on a degree-day model. *Environmental Monitoring and Assessment*, *129*(1-3), 413–420. doi:10.1007/s10661-006-9373-8

Chapter 9
Grid for Post Operative Care through Wireless Sensor Networks

N.P Chowdhry
Mehran University of Engineering and Technology, Pakistan

Adnan Ashraf
Mehran University of Engineering and Technology, Pakistan

B.S Chowdhry
Mehran University of Engineering and Technology, Pakistan

A.K Baloch
Mehran University of Engineering and Technology, Pakistan

A.W Ansari
University of Sindh, Pakistan

H. De Meer
University of Passau, Germany

ABSTRACT

To address the solution for problems of e-health systems, the various new algorithms are developed. Today, the parallel and distributed programming concepts have motivated the doctors and technology experts for the development of e-health grid systems. This e-health grid system is expected to provide more efficient patient care system, better security and more dedicated links among patients, pharmaceutical companies and their experts. The chapter discusses the project significance of grid computing with its past, present and future in the perspective of e-health. The interdisciplinary research and development in the field of biochemistry, health care, information technology and biomedical engineering has enabled technologists to develop equipments and systems for patient monitoring at distances. The pharmaceutical companies, doctors and technology experts have been working for platforms with continuous connectivity for the treatment and post operative care for patients in homes and in hospitals. The practical significance of such developments shall be discussed in the Chapter including the exponential growth and exploration

DOI: 10.4018/978-1-61692-010-4.ch009

of new areas in post operative care systems where Wireless Sensor Network (WSN) is playing a vital role. Moreover, the chapter explains that 'how video conferencing or face to face examination of patient can be performed in the preview of e-learning'. Since, this e-health grid system contains varied parametric input and output and there is a need of data fusion system. The last, but not least, we discuss here the challenges and process of acquisition and retrieval of the abstract data types (medical images and different sonic beats) using web-portal and MIS e-health care systems.

GRID COMPUTING FOR E-HEALTH SYSTEMS

The Grid Computing is an interaction of computing networks, communication and information systems. It has applications in government, businesses and medical sciences where a useful data excerpts are gathered from different data locations.

In fact, the Grid Computing is an advance form of distributed data system which was termed with different names in the past such as operations research, distributed database management and parallel processing. The Grid Computing is popular because it is secure, flexible and helps in data sharing among the experts. With the time, the Grid Computing has got boost with the application of e-Health in the fields of biosciences, medicine and genomics.

This Chapter discusses e-Health Grid in community services to develop a Community Grid. The Community Grid is a term that should exhibit system security, automation, and end-to-end recovery during disaster management. The Chapter enlightens the extraction of useful information from e-Health Grid using some web-portal. This approach shall help doctors to provide contact their patient from remote locations. This Chapter focuses on recent developments in e-Health and share a discussion on it, with its reader. It debates on latest concepts and developments of e-Health Grid and its optimization with the use of new technologies like Wireless Sensor Networks for Post Operative Care.

Overview of Grid Technology: From the Perspective of Technology and Scope

In the mid of 1980s, multiple users concept was developed for parallel processing. The procedures were then run on the priority queues. The searching techniques were implemented through the area of statistics and engineering known as operation research by using matrices to solve the problems. The network techniques were introduced at some limited nodes of local area networks with data transfer rate of 56 Kilo bits/sec. Then, the concept of wide area networks evolved but, restrained to metropolitan cities at speed of 155 Mega bits/sec globally. Later on, the sharing data was extended by scientists with the speed of penta bytes to Giga bits/sec. Thus, the process of parallel computing was utilized -to make advantage of OOP- to solve parallel processing problems. With the passage of time, emergence of internet, complex and global networks, speedy computing and large memory demanded to introduce a new concept of Grid Computing.

The use of Grid Computing in e-Health is viable as multiple resources are shared in the form of distributed data. In an e-Health System, doctors give consultancy to patients remotely and can access the distributed information if it is supported by e-Health Grid. This patient related information is recorded as history in the hospital MIS.

The advantage of Grid Computing is the extraction of real-time patient specific data from a huge data repository. This is achieved through Grid planning and scheduling for parallel processing of e-Health Grid. The concept of e-Health Grid

Figure 1. e-Health Grid and Data Fusion (Hospital MIS)

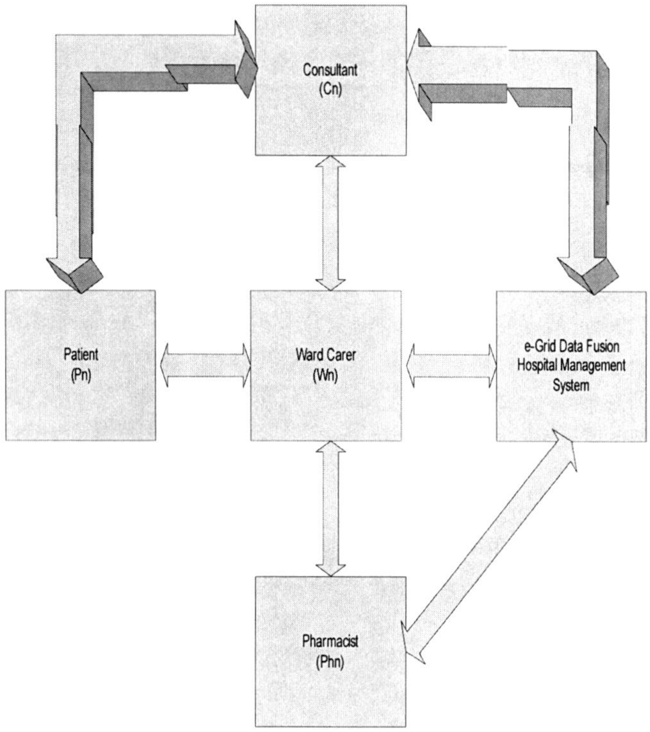

can be thought as an enhanced Hospital MIS, as illustrated in Figure 1. Every patient, ward attendant, consultant and the pharmacist are building blocks of an e-Health Grid.

In the following scenario, the patient is denoted with Pn, the ward attendant with Wn, the corresponding consultant with Cn, and the particular pharmacists with Phn. In this figure, there is always an alternative route in case of non-availability of node parameters.

The Past, Present and Future of e-Health Systems

Though, modern telecommunication technology has made remote consultation between doctors and patient easy, the telemedicine has evolved from the era of Air-mail, Telephony and Telegraph, and Internet. These means have been in use by a large mass since last many decades. When the induction of internet implanted for the consultation, the Local Area Networks (LAN) was extended to the Global Area Networks (GAN). Today, the Wireless Sensor Networks (WSN) is being used by pharmaceutical companies and psychologists to monitor the physical and behavioral acts in their patients.

In the following, we spotlight a few of current projects in the field of e-Healthcare for the information and interest of our readers.

Tele-Home HealthCare System for Patient with Chronic Diseases

This project has been successfully completed in Italy, to monitor the chronic patients with cardiopulmonary and diabetic patients with problem of retinopathy, provide healthcare facility for all people from home to general practioners or specialist from hospital [Sicurello, F., 2008]. This continuous monitoring of vital sign method is very much useful for old people, who fell unconscious in moving from one place to another place.

Best Practice of Mobile E-Health in the Netherlands

This project is launched by European Institute of HealthCare Information to analyze the use of mobile communication in HealthCare system in Netherlands [Ketelaar P., 2008].

Clinical Efficiency of Telemedicine in Trauma and Orthopedics

In Ukraine, telemedicine project for managing the trauma and orthopedic patients is on progress, for further details; please refer to [Vladzymyrskyy A.V., 2008]. This project is also useful in case of earthquake or any disaster aftermath, many of the patients get psychological problems. In this regard, they can be better treated form distance with the use of telemedicine and Tele-HealthCare system.

e-Health Networks

Medical specialist and clinician's can exchange their views with native communication languages over the countries. In this project, world health organizations (WHO) are providing funds for 53 commonwealth countries [Richardson R., 2008]. This project will provide facility to 1.8 billion world citizens through the launch of these e-Health networks.

Benefits of Grid Computing, and Network Technologies in e-Health Development

Earlier technologies solved problems sequentially or hierarchically. These solutions of data in form of tables or ledgers was solved on the data structure of tree structure programming or graph theory.. In the early 1980s, the concept of parallel programming emerged as new paradigm. In the presence of internet the structural programming using Java paved the way for the initiation of the Grid Computing. The optimal use of dedicated networks programming supports Grid Computing.

The Grid Computing is the consequence of the use of previous techniques of programming such as operations research, graph theory and distributed data processing. Similarly, latest network technologies have been benefitted by Grid Computing of which, the Wireless Sensor Networks have become prominent in e-Health Monitoring System.

Procedures and Protocols in Grid Computing

A simple Grid protocol contains a number of Grid computers on the internet using transmission control protocol (TCP) and user data gram protocol (UDP). Here, unused CPU resources are utilized in Grid form. In this technique, the local jobs are solved at user's side, while web-portal based jobs are handled at remote side. The other protocol is SABUL, which is an application level data tranfer protocol. This is used at high bandwidth delay in networks over the UDP. The features of this protocol are relibility, high performance, fairness and stability [Yunhong & Robert, 2003]. However, the TCP is used for getting messages back. The third type of protocol is known as the anonymity protocol, to maintain the secrecy and degradation in the system, when un-authorized intruders attack the system. [Souvik & Zhang, 2004]. The procedures in Grid Computing are written to enhance the performance in computing. For this purpose strategy in domain decompositions and task scheduling is pre-planned. Also, if needed, additional procedures are specified and written in advance. Thus, in the data fusion system having multiple sources discussing various characters of errors and level of generalization are carefully understood [Wang et al., 2002].

Protocol Integration with Wireless Sensor Networks

For wireless sensor networks, a protocol DPEG algorithms is available that gathers and aggregate the data. It also solves cluster coverage problems. The author of the reference [Liu et al, 2005] claims that it increases sensors network life time by 1800% and 300% as compared with other data algorithms protocols such as LEACH and PEGASIS. This Grid system provides a sensing environment through an open Grid Computing system. In case of multiple sensor networks web service resources frame work is used to support interoperability among multitude sensor networks. The other Grid Computing techniques are radio frequency identification (RFID) used in the field of WSN. In case of service oriented it provides architecture model that defines modem, virtual organization based on resource limited technologies.

GRID COMPUTING MODELS

In Grid Computing resource sharing defines problem status. This provides coordination, manageability, and high performance in distributed data system. Thus, we can study simple file transfer to complex and collaborative problem solving in the form of Grid Computing. Whenever large Grid Computing is involved on service sharing then resource collaborative models are created with the help of open standard platform for dynamic applications. The following models are taken from reference [Josef et al., 2004].

Grid Architecture and Programming Model

In this model, the first requirement is the involvement of open architecture model; alignment with existing programming models and standards. The next requirment is to study use cases and find interopertable best solutions. The standards of this model are services architecture, web programming and java semantic Grid.

Grid Management Model

This is used, when heterogeneous resources and standards are based on monitoring system. The Grid management models consist of common management model, Grid monitoring architecture and web services distributed management.

Grid Data Management Model

This model provides integration of structured and semi-structured data across Grid. Also, it performs the discovery and storage of multitude of data. Further it provides enhanced data mining for global information exchange. In its developed form the Grid management model standards are Grid access and data integration.

USE OF GRID COMPUTING FOR POST OPERATIVE CARE

The patient needs very intensive care after operation. Although, surgeons are available onsite but in emergency, there is need for expert opinion from distant. In this area of technology, e-Health has widened very large, the setup works from local area networks (LAN) to wide area networks (WAN), so e-Grid works for multiple patients and experts through a WAN. However, medical is a huge field and it has many fields for surgery such as heart surgery, eye surgery, kidney surgery, so, there are dedicated experts who can monitor critical situations of the patient. That's why web-portal system is developed, thus for patient monitoring wireless sensor networks are used. In this way patient information is distributed from LAN to WAN passing through many intermediate networks forming a Grid networking system. The essential form of Grid Computing is data collection and analysis, preventive care and instant measures to help patient to avoid the danger of possible critical situations. In this part of post operative care, the ward staff, physicians, experts are made alert to face any emergency conditions locally or remotely. The wireless sensor networks through wide area network using web-portals have provided a facility to look aft the patient after surgical operations. Since the information is distributed and moves from Local area network to wide area network using many intermediate networks form a Grid networking system for communication data collection, data collection, data analysis, and preventive care and instant measures to help patient to avoid possible un-avoidable circumstances. In this part of the postoperative care, the ward staff, physicians and the experts is made alert to face any emergency conditions locally or remotely [Pallikonda, et al., 2008].

Requirements of Post Operative Care

The remote care becomes necessary when a patient is under observation in hospital or at home. The telemonitoring system provides information about the after effects of operation in terms of pain, injury, trauma and physical conditions, biological and physical aspects of the patient to the drug reactions are ready rescue in case of emergency.

Instant, Post Operative Care Strategy

There are various ways of instant post operative strategy.

1. Analog communication, for example telephone lines, interactive TV systems at the local site.
2. Digital communication system, here we can use mobile and satellite communication by using internet and managing the arrangement for PC to PC, video conferencing or chatting with the patient or staff available at the patient site.
3. The other aspects of instant monitoring is biological and chemical test of the patient information sent through local or satellite communication system.

It is required that both IT and medical expert should be available to monitor to patient response to drug or post operative complications to get response immediately.

Web-Portal System for Post Operative Care

Since, global areas networks are best from metropolitan networks connected with other networks and thus become a huge network of networks. In this system a search engine is connecting networks through domain IP addresses along with Mac addresses. As there is group system to make subnetworks through dedicated or hotlines to make a distributed particular group of users. This way of using networks for a particular group is know as web-portal. This is useful because of security reasons and fast communications systems. It become more useful then we are using a particular web-portal for patient monitoring and healthcare connected through the pharmaceutical networks. As illustrated in Figure 2 Data Fusion e-Grid model for tele-consultation for multiple patients and experts interaction [Chowdhry et al., 2008].

Data Fusion e-Grid Patient Monitoring System

The condition of patient mainly depends on clinical Laboratory tests such as- Blood CP, Urine DR, Kidney function test, Liver function test, X-rays and pathological reports. In patient monitoring

Figure 2. Data fusion e-Grid model for tele-consultation for multiple Patients and expert interaction

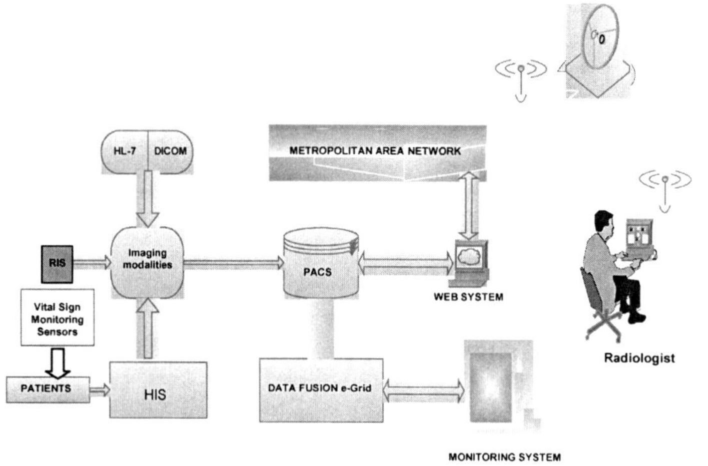

system the pre-monitoring and post monitoring test are compare to examine the physical condition of the patient. In every hospital, there are testing laboratories are near to share data for local and remote experts in concerned area of patient's health. When a large number of patients are involved, we make a data fusion and Grid monitoring system to analyze multiple parameters of patients for distribution for particular expert available for consultation from many concerned doctor in the similar area. The Figures 3 (a) and (b), illustrates the scenario, that how a patient can be monitored remotely from diagnostic laboratory or micro laboratory for reports or information from the patients and experts in case of emergency through tele-diagnsotic devices.

Distributed Data System or Grid Computing

In the early days of computing, a program was run through a single processor and as well as through sub-routines in a procedural computing manner. It was found that there lays, a difficulty in computing, when the program is too large. Then, on priority basis the program parts were run, called queuing system based on first come first serve basis. This gave a birth to parallel processing system, in which the programs were stored in buffer and the parts were simultaneously run on the priority basis with a single or multiple processing. This method of computing is known as distributed computing. At highest level the distributed computing can be thought of hardware, software using multiple processors for computing in a distributed manner that is computing the program in parts in a paradigm or parallel programming. The distributed system connect user, resources in a transparent manner to make benefits of fault tolerant system in a better way as compared to standalone computers [Ref. book Distributed Computing].

The advantages of distributed system are open system, Monotonicity, Pluralism and unbounded Nondeterminism. The disadvantages of distributed systems are reliability, troubleshooting, computation, synchronization, bandwidth and latency, if the system is not managed properly. The Leslie Lamport pointed out that the distributed system fails, if a single computer is not working properly and this failure is unknown to a system instantly [Wikipedia, January 9, 2009].

Figure 3. (a)Remote Diagnosis of Patient through Micro Lab and (b) eGrid Patient Monitoring System through Tele-Diagnostic Devices

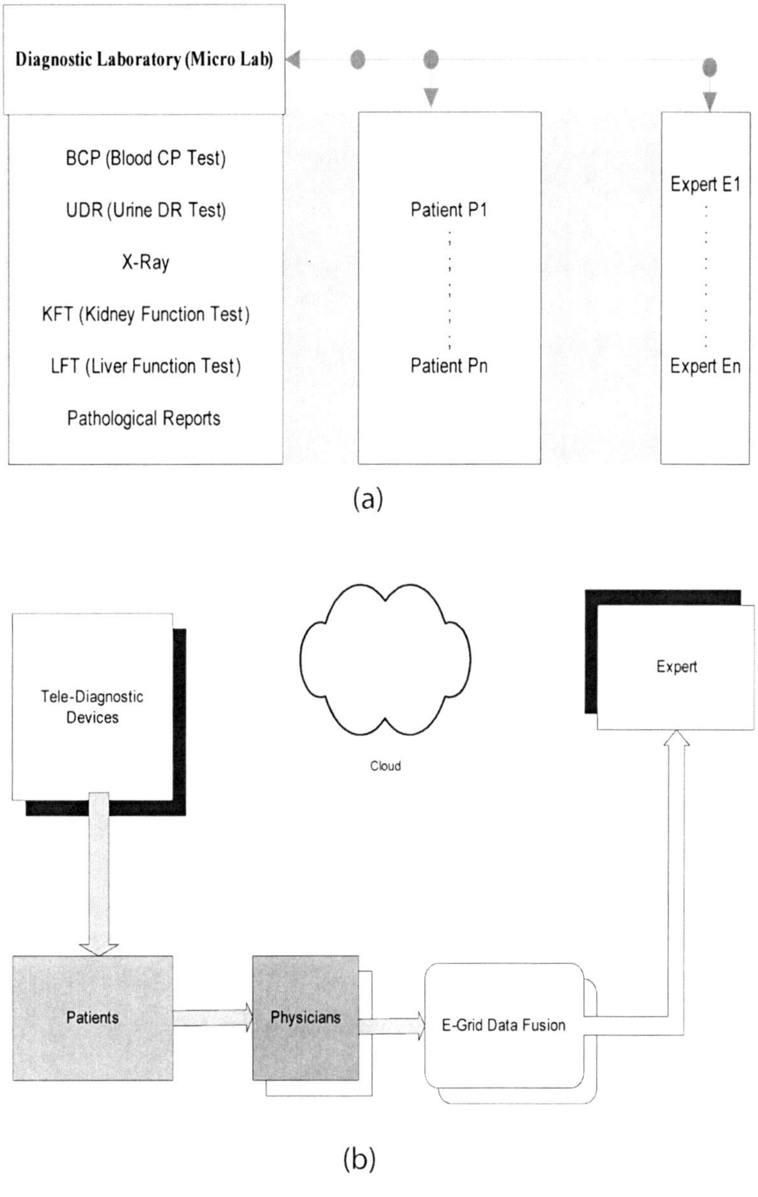

ELECTRONIC COMMUNICATION SERVICES IN E-HEALTH

The electronic communication in olden days was done through analog communication systems such as using telephone and TV channels for local and remote consultation and healthcare. With the advent of digital communication has change their scenario and has made record keeping and instant communication particular in health care to make available diagnostic reports and remotely monitoring patient through various ways. The present state of art is the use of drug delivery and study after effects of drug can be monitored remotely.

e-Clinic, e-Health and e-Learning through Telemedicine

The e-Health in general can be viewed from two perspectives, one from medical side and other from information technology side. The telemedicine specialist should have both information but we see generally that they are not properly trained in both aspects of e-Health. There is always need of learning and up gradation the weakest knowledge amongst the experts using video-conferencing. The communication system has made it possible to train the persons through video conferencing using teaching software tools.

There are many institutes which provide training on various subjects that can be available through web-portal communication or becoming the member of the sites on the subject by paying subscription on subsidized payments. The educational networks on national hookup for examples are, Pakistan Educational and Research Network (PERN), IEEE Educational Networks and Science online.com etc. Similarly, the e-Health can be categorized into two parts, one in hospital and other private clinics. In both the cases, at the first step to acquire vital sign monitoring such as, blood pressure, heart beat, pulse oximetry, and ECG. The telemonitoring devices [Ash A., 1997] that help to acquire various patient data, this includes stethoscope, dermoscope, otoscope, echocardiogram, laparoscope, duodenoscope and endoscope.

Wired and Wireless Clinical Networks

Electronic networks may be categorized in e-Health in two parts. One type of electronic communication is tightly bounded called wired network. On the other hand, loosely electronic communication system is known as wireless networks. The first one system is used for onsite monitoring consultation and treatment of the patient to acquire the target of online e-Health System onsite. While the second one, is used from a remote site for expert's opinion and connection is made from a pharmaceutical companies for service of drugs from distance. The devices used in this wireless communication system is laptop, palmtop, cell phone or PDA, and radio modem communication system along with wireless sensor networks are used [Andrew, D., et al, 2008]. In short, satellite communication plays its important role in wireless communication system, while in its analog communication system TV and telephone system also plays its vital role in healthcare delivery and services.

METHODOLOGIES AND ALGORITHMS USED IN E-HEALTH GRID

Fast Fourier transform (FFT) has applications in digital computation to analyze signals. In e-health care, while monitoring from distance, we are dealt with numerous number of analog and digital signals generate from Grid of computers. A butterfly method is one method to carry out such a data in un-certain environment. In such a Grid data is complex in its nature, so Fast Fourier Grid Computing is used. For further details refer to [Robert D Kent, et al].

Cluster Grid Computing

When data is in form of small or large chunks in distributed data system then tribology techniques of FFT are used. Tribology is a science that talks about the surface and its relative motion can be studied by studying convolution of FFT.

Feasibility, Functionality and Objectives of Patient Monitoring System

Feasibility

Feasibility of a system starts from the study of the system and writing of the pseudo code, to achieve the overview of e-Health System. Then, cost for building petrol oil and logistic (POL) is calculated. After that electrical, mechanical system cost is calculated along with gas supplies. After that the cost of the hardware used along with software's is calculated. The main item is people and expert, their pay scales and pays is calculated. Since no hospital is complete without furniture, so its cost is included. Since remote patient monitoring needs wide area networks, so their cost and engineers payment are calculated. Lastly, the drugs fast availability and environmental issues are calculated.

Functionality

This way of monitoring the patient requires high technology. So in this field always experts at local area should be available every time so that without delay information should be exchange from remote. In every time there should be standby equipments to replace the faulty equipment within healthcare environments. MIS should be available to avail the experts in the relevant field through internet. It is advisable that video conferencing equipment should be available for instant advice and recovery of the patient.

The main objective of the remote monitoring is to avail the patient for medical doctor/surgeon advice after post operative care and quick availability of the drugs at their door steps or community centers, hospital, clinics.

Expert System Design in e-Health

An expert system is a technique that behaves the working of a computer instead of relevant human expert. For example, an expert system for general practioner is available that makes curies from the patient and record the related information through interactive method, then on the basis of symptoms, sign and history of patient the disease is diagnosed and then treatment is suggested. There are so many expert systems in e-Health; one of the examples is the mycin for the experts in the e-Healthcare system. The expert system for remote monitoring should have the following features:

1. Health Level 7 systems, where history of patient is recorded, then physical and medical checkup are recorded.
2. On the basis of tests, patient may be advised to go at home and take the drugs as advised by local physicians to go for certain operation.
3. The patient needs more care after surgery that is why vital sign monitoring devices are provided to collect patient data instantly through wireless sensors networks.

By looking at the requirements of hospital for the patient, the local area networks and web-portals should be available. Thus, database system based on oracle and Java is designed. It should be noted that monitoring patient's data through robots is also involved. So, in designing the expert system, all the above mention expects of the design should be well studied and the data management, data processing and data collection and data analysis are critically viewed. So, that the remote experts gets data easily for experts opinion and its interaction.

PHARMA GRIDS AND COMPUTING

Without the existence of pharmaceutical companies the worth of e-medicine and e-Health becomes bleak. Basically pharmaceutical companies have three major roles.

1. Drug preparation
2. Drug Research
3. Balance of demand and supply of drugs

The pharmaceutical companies are the best example of Grid of Grids, because nationally and internationally they have very close interaction and information exchange to meet the challenges of invention of new drug by research. We have discussed the trica relationship among medical experts, pharmaceutical companies and patient itself. This cyclic relationship provides better care and e-Health services in the society. On the other hand it has got three aspects in terms of Grid Computing.

Drug Discovery

Research and development programs globally can develop a Grid for demand and supply for e-Health Systems. These scientists exchange their information to avoid any repeatability of research but quickly provide instant information to carry out research in an easiest way and save time and money. The national international seminars, conferences have made this pharma Grid attractive at site monitoring, by becoming the member of e-Grid professional society.

Academic Pharmaceutical Discovery

The scientists and researchers are the backbone for the development of economy of any country. The academicians of various fields such as physics, chemistry, toxicology, pharmacology, genomics, proteomics and pharmacy genomics are in action to contribute their knowledge in designing and modeling of the simulated proteins or genes for making computer simulation to achieve their actions at particular target, reaction the drug to confirm their required achievements.

Drug Discovery and Computing

The drug discovery can be viewed in three ways of treatments and investigations such as vivo, vitro and silico. The role of IT has many services in pharmaceutical industries. At first through computer simulation modeling and various structure of proteins, DNA structure, compound, tissues and complicated muscle structure even whole body of living creature can be simulated for pharmaceutical computing tests. The 3D computing modeling can be used to re-model and make computer colorful model using x-rays, ultraviolet rays and magnetic resonance interface.

SERVICES AND SECURITIES ISSUES IN GRID COMPUTING

In Grid Computing, security and services are very challenging issues, when ever patient is monitored from a distant. The security becomes essential, particularly, when personal data of regarding medical care is to be secure to the satisfaction of the patient. One way of securing data is creating a web portal or hotlines for dedicated field of experts and the other way is to provide protection from the hackers and viruses to protect patient data from stealing and disintegration. The cryptography is a field that handles such data through software and hardware called Intruder Detection System (IDS). Also, data can be protected by using firewalls made of software and hardware. Recently, a new data protection system has been developed in e-Health is called a photon computing.

GCM in Terms of Services, Security and Delivery

The Grid Computing model (GCM) has three components; these are services, security and delivery. The expanding global network system has made communication itself as complex system. Thus huge data transfer in communication has a major role to take security measures and medical services and delivery.

Firewall, IDS, Hardware and Software Connectivity

In healthcare system, patient's personal data, examination reports and conversation about patient health between the consultant and GP needs higher security alerts. So, in transferring data of patient for collection, analyzing and diagnosing, through Grid Computing needs proper attentions to satisfy the confidence and trust of patient in healthcare. In this context, Intruder Detection System (IDS) is more feasible with hardware and software connectivity at both ends. As for as software control security system is concerned, there are two ways of handling security, one is photon computing and secondly is Grid Computing, facing the security issues and are known as intruder detection system, firewall and kernelling systems.

GRID COMPUTING AND BIOLOGICAL ISSUES

Since, the Grid Computing is more useful for technologists, having experience in computing but for the common user, there should be an easy interactive method such as web-browsing for this purpose iGrid portal is more easy to use.

Grid Computing Issues

Grid Computing is a technique, which is specifically helpful to the programmers for computing purpose, where as users are less familiar with this technique and is not necessary essential to go for understanding this technology. But through training users may be made skillful to use this technology. This technique has more effect and usefulness in biological sciences, particularly and generally for browsing data from internet architecture and infrastructure. For a common people web-portal links are easy to use that uses Grid Computing techniques. Since, Grid computation in biological sciences has wide scope; therefore, various issues arises in the different field of biological sciences, such as data mining, DNA assembly, clustering of molecules and data, mapping, gene expression and micro array, protein structure prediction and Grid infrastructure tool for bio data [El-Ghazali Talbi, 2008].

Anatomical, Physiological and Surgical issues

In case of accidental or disaster cases, there are anatomical issues involved for remote consultation. Here, orthopedics experts and surgeons would like to have required instant data for consultation. In this issue, ultrasound and x-rays are commonly used, but in case skull injury radiological images and magnetic resonance interfaces images are sent for expert opinion. In this manner, the higher the resolution of images, better the quality of image transfer, since high resolution images takes more memory and faces difficulty in transmission of images, so lesser resolution is used on transmission time and at the receivers end the resolution is increased to enhance the quality of image. Secondly, in case of physiological issues, the intensity of the radiation is set to get muscular images and the blood flow attributes could be acquired to study the patient effects of drugs and rate of recovery. For local expert to identify the cause of failure in the improvement of patient health during surgical difficulties, it is required that remote experts of dedicated area using web portal to form e-Grid for doctor's consultation can be helpful.

Bioinformatics and Biological Issues

The bioinformatics provide information about genomes, which can be exploited with fields of natural sciences including computer science, mathematics, physics and biology [Chowdhry, et al., 2008]. This area of science that collects molecular information at the levels of genes and genome to identify the characteristics of universal stem cells to build and creates 220 basic cells from the human body [Liebman, 2005]. This needs scholars in the field of molecular biology such as physicist, computer scientists, engineers, pharmacists and medicine peoples to develop the database for the care of general public use in the perspective of e-Health [Chowdhry, et al., 2007].

Grid Model for Biological information Networks

The Grid model presents biological information networks, as illustrated in the Figure 4. This model consists of three layers; first biological information system layer, consists of four sub-links: the science & technology, medical, bioinformatics tools. Also, the model presents stem cell therapy for disease diagnosis and providing genomic data in the form of sequence database. This information helps medical experts to diagnose diseases, and the pharmaceutical companies to develop new drugs. The left side of model uses bioprocess that collects e-Health data for clinical and medical use. The scientific knowledge layer provides Grid based mathematical models by using Mat Lab and Lab View software.

Wireless Sensor Networks and Data Distribution System

As human have five senses to identify the changes in environment, so scientist have developed sensors to feel the presence of abrupt change in the environment in form of energy. Sound, light, heat is some form of energy. We can categorize sensor in two categories, one which feel the energy are called pure sensors and secondly those device which converts one from of energy to another form is called transducers. In recent development the science and technology has produced miniaturized form of sensors to collect data patient monitoring system. The sensor can be integrated and wirelessly be connected to remote information centre called data fusion centre. Wireless sensors have ability to feel the heart beat, respiration, blood flow, speech and many other physical aspects along with medical images to be transmitted for expert's opinion. Mostly, these sensors convert potential energy of the body into electrical or magnetic energies which on the other hand are modulated signals sent for communication for remoter area. These wireless sensors have made easy to monitor patient from home to local dispensaries to the big hospital from metropolitan areas.

WEB-PORTAL WITH MIS SYSTEM

With the increase huge networks it was thought to make communication domain wise but still there was need to serve communication among dedicated group of networks. For example, Business, doctors, pharmaceutical companies and specific government organizations to provide confidential secure and fast communication network. In Pakistan, the education and research network (PERN), this provides fast communication among researchers from distance. These networks also provide IT we-portal between medical university for exchange of information for discussion and consultation. It is also used to manage information databases, where ever needed. The information of this category can be divided into top-level management information, medium and low level management information. The sequential data of e-Health System like HIS, MIS etc.

e-Health's System for Different Countries

E-Health System has wide scope, so locally or internationally different regions have different e-Health System, especially when dedicated web-portal is decide for a special group of users. For example: different radiologists are connected with a hotline to exchange and consult different radiological images such as x-rays, computed

Figure 4. e-Grid Model for Biological information Networks

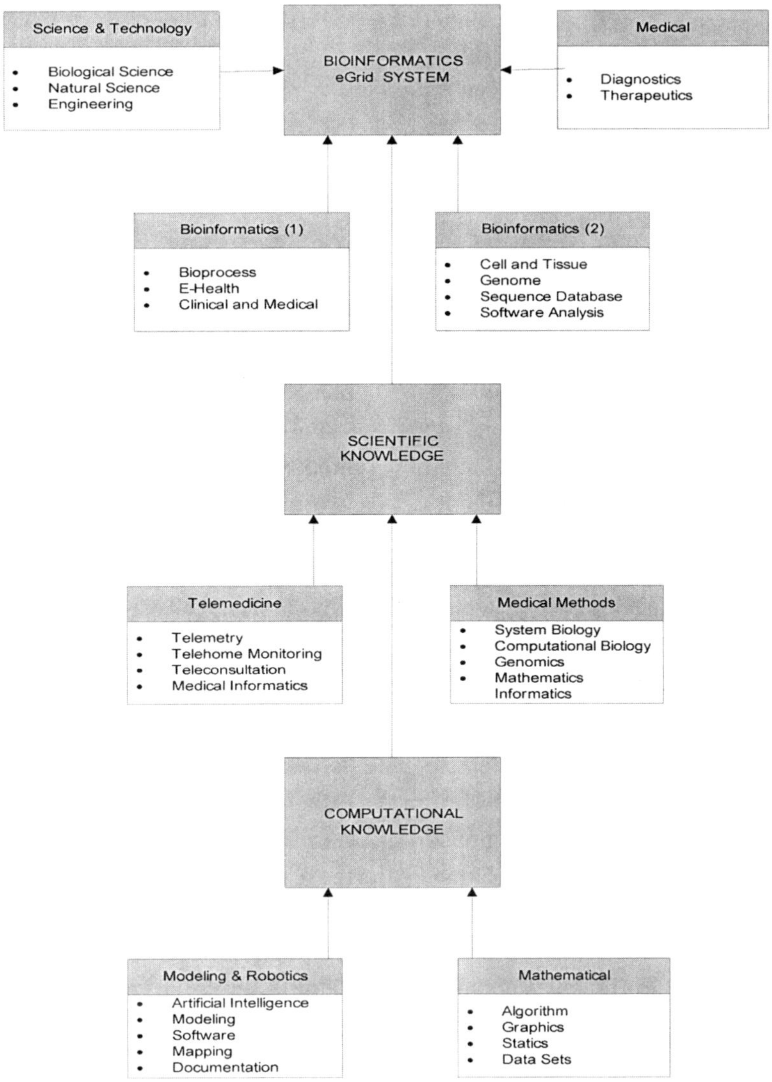

tomography, magnetic resonance imaging, and single photon emission computed tomography.

Australian Quest for e-Health

In this news, the Philip Davis Deputy Secretary of Department of Health, and Ageing, Australia, is delighted to claim that in 1997 the 15% of general practioners through wide area network could successfully transmit prescriptions through e-Health web-portal network [Jianggan, 2008].

African e-Health Program

The view of author [Boakai, 2008] is that, in the e-Health program various diseases could be investigated and treated after the diagnosis. For example: HIV, TB, and Malaria patient can be connected through e-Health web-portal.

Web-Based e-Health Portal System

The importance of e-Health based web-portal is due to patient trust and communication and secures the privacy and data security of the patient, when monitored from distance. One other factor is data flow on rule based system which is already available in web-portal system [Quin, 2008]. For the security purpose, biometric system hierarchies of trust are followed according to the requirements. Also, in this reference, the details about the development of access control method for workflow based tele-Health services are discussed.

Web-Portal Grid and Management Information System

In medical services, a Grid is a huge system, where Grids of Grid are connected for data distribution in dedicated way as in web portal system. For example, specialist group of physicians may be categorized as eye specialists have their own web-portal and management system. On the other hand, heart specialists have their own web-portal and MIS system for exchange of data through video conferencing to discuss patient's cases by specialists as a panel of board of examiners. It may happen when accidental cases come under investigations, for example, wounds on head, infected eyes and broken legs. In such cases, if we have a Grid of Grids, it is easier to consult an expert from remote, as if we are calling a board of examiners onsite. In this case hospital management system is also required, so to have closer interaction between web portal and MIS, we should have collective interactive system to respond instantly.

FUTURE RESEARCH DIRECTIONS

In the future, private sector, government agency and researchers will make a group through health grid association to make grid computation, information research and awareness programs for general public to make advantage of the new emerging technologies in the society.

SUMMARY

The Grid technologies have paved the path for sharing of the information and provide facility for the fast recovery of post operative patients. Wireless Sensor Networks transforms physical information and vital signs from patients to doctors for interpretation and the treatment advice. The Chapter explains the usefulness of micro/mobile laboratories to get real time patient-data. The Chapter also features benefits of e-Health Grid in such laboratories for post operative care of the patient. The e-Health Grid helps to timely extract the valuable information of the patient. Development of e-Health Grid serves remote medical stations as a repository and can embed logics for extraction of information quickly about patient, disease, its diagnosis, past-references and expert opinions. This gives a leverage to operate patient in time as a post operative care solution.

We emphasized on the use of web-portals in e-Health Grid applications as a compact solution. This will make an easy user interface and help to provide public information or warnings online. Using web-portals the patient from the same disease or treatment cycle can form groups and share valuable healthcare tips. To invoke future thought process among the readers, the issues of Grid and Biological Computing Models have been discussed to elaborate that how GCM services and avoidance of intruder entrance in the healthcare network is achieved. In the last, but not least, the anatomical, physiological and surgical issues in terms of bioinformatics are discussed here. In short, the Chapter develops a Global HealthCare System (for Post Operative Care) using e-Grid Web-Portal backed by Hospital-MIS and Wireless Sensor Networks to give a seamless connectivity.

REFERENCES

Andrew, D., Jurik, & Alfred, C.W. (2008). Remote Medical Monitoring. *Computer Magazine*, 96-99.

Ash, A. (1997). Telemedicine: Technology and Equipment Enabling New Models of HealthCare Delivery. *Informatics in HealthCare Australia*, *6*(3), 90–96.

Boakai, M. Fofana. (2008). The African e-Health program. *All Africa's Boakai Fofana blogs on a Rockefeller Foundation conference on how to use information technology to improve access to health care*, Italy.

Chowdhry, B. S., Rajput, A. Q. K., & Chowdhry, N. P. (2007). *Major challenges and opportunities in the practice of research and development in the area of bioinformatics. In 5th annual international conference, "Role of medical universities in promotion of research", at Liaqat University of Medical & Health Sciences, Jamshoro, PK* (p. 70).

Chowdhry, N. P., Ansari, A. W., & Baloch, A. K. (2008). Diagnostic image archive system for rapid web based access to the consultant through metropolitan area networks. In *proc. of the Med-e-Tel, the international educational and networking forum for E-Health, Telemedicine and Health ICT, Luxembourg,* (Vol. 1, pp. 300-306).

Chowdhry, N. P., Ansari, A. W., Memon, A. A., & Fatima, M. (2008). Bioinformatics awareness system for skin diseases using stem cells therapy in the perspective of e-Health. In *Handbook of communications in Computer and information Sc* (pp. 261–267). Berlin: Springer Verlag.

El-Ghazali, T., & Albert, Y. Zomaya. (2008). *Grid Computing for bioinformatics and computational biology*. Chichester, UK: Wiley InterScience.

Holger, K., & Andreas, W. (2006). *Protocols and Architectures for Wireless Sensor Networks*. Chicester, UK: Wiley & Sons.

Jianggan, L. (2008). An Australian quest for e-Health. *Future Gov, free weekly newsletter.*

Josef, J., Ernest, M., & Fellenstein, C. (2004). Evolution of Grid Computing architecture and Grid adoption models. *IBM Systems Journal*, *43*(4), 624–645. doi:10.1147/sj.434.0624

Ketelaar, P. (2008). Best practices of mobile e-Health in the Netherlands: The lessons learned. In *proc. of the Med-e-Tel, the international educational and networking forum for E-Health, Telemedicine and Health ICT, Luxembourg*, (pp. 1818 9334, 228-229).

Kincade, K. (1999). Wireless hits the ground running. *Telemedicine and Telehealth Networks*, *5*(6), 14–18.

Liebman, M. N. (2000). Bioinformatics. In *proc. of the 23 Annual EMBS International Conference, Istanbul, Turkey*, (pp.7211-7215).

Liu, M., Cao, J., Gang, G., Li-Jun, C., & Li, X. (2005). A distributed power efficient data gathering and aggregation protocol for wireless sensor networks, parallel and distributed processing and applications. *international symposium,* (3758, 743-756).

Mohammad, I., & Imad, M. (2004). *Handbook of Sensor Networks: Compact Wireless and Wired Sensing Systems*. Boca Raton, FL: CRC Press.

Nirupama, B., & Sanjay, J. (2005). *Wireless Sensor Network A Systems Perspective*. Boston: Artech House.

Pallikonda, M., Radhakrishan, S. & Subbaraj, P., (2008). *Remote monitoring of post operative patients using wireless sensor networks*, (9) 247-257.

Pileggi, S. F., Palau, C.E. & Esteve, M. (n.d.). *Integrating wireless sensor networks with Grid Computing and RFID technology for products monitoring into airports.*

Price, H. (2007). Delivering Tele-Health in kent England, Best practices of European E-Health Expertise, proc. of the Med-e-Tel, the international event and conference for E-Health. In *Telemedicine and Health ICT,* Luxembourg, (pp. 1818-9334, 291).

Quin, L., Shuo, L., Yuan, H., et al. (2008). *Securing tele-Health applications in a web-based e-Health portal,* (pp. 3-9).

Rajeev, S., Ananda, A., & Mun, C. C., Wei, T, O., (2006). *Mobile, wireless, and sensor networks: Technology, Applications, and Future Directions.*

Richardson, R. (2008). E-Health Networks, International Telemedicine and E-Health initiatives. In *proc. of the Med-e-Tel, the international educational and networking forum for E-Health, Telemedicine and Health ICT,* (pp. 224).

Souvik, R., & Zhang, Z. (2004). An efficient anonymity protocol for Grid Computing. In *Proc. of the 5th IEEE/ACM, international workshop on Grid Computing,* (pp. 200-207). Washington, DC: IEEE computer society.

Sucurello, F. (2008). A Tele-homecare System for patients with chronic diseases. In *Proc. of the Med-e-Tel, the international trade event and conference for E-Health, Telemedicine and Health ICT,* Luxembourg (1818-9334, pp. 41-42).

The distributed computing. (n.d.). Retrieved January 9, 2009, from Wikipedia: http://en.wikipedia.org/

Vladzymyrskyy, A. V., et al. (2008). Clinical efficiency of telemedicine in trauma and orthopedics. In *proc. of the Med-e-Tel, the international educational and networking forum for E-Health, Telemedicine and Health ICT,* Luxembourg, (pp. 224).

Wang, S., Armstrong, M. P., & Bennett, D. A. (2002). Conceptual basics of middleware design to support Grid Computing of geographic information. In *Proc. of International Conference on Geographic Information Science,* September, 25 - 28, Boulder, CO, (pp. 197-200).

Yujie, Y. Shu, Wang (2005). The key research on integration wireless sensor network with Grid. In *Proc. Wireless communication networking and mobile computing,* (pp. 1477-1480).

Yunhong, G., & Robert, G. (2003). SABUL: A transport protocol for grid computing. *Journal of Grid Computing, 1*(4), 377–386. doi:10.1023/B:GRID.0000037553.18581.3b

KEY TERMS AND DEFINITIONS

e-Health Grid: Parallel or distributed acquisition / retrieval of patient related information by means of e-Technology for HealthCare and Monitoring.

Telemedicine: The remote monitoring of patients by experts for diagnosis and treatment and postoperative care.

Post Operative Care: To monitor problems at a distance created after the surgery and solve it locally or remotely.

Data Fusion: It is a centre, where multiple data is embedded, before processing in a buffer memory and data is called when processing, when ever it is needed.

Health- Web Portals: It is dedicated communication parallel processing system for a particular area under investigation. In this system the experts are grouped in a particular area of e-Health for consultation.

APPENDIX

List of Abbreviations

OOP: Object Oriented Programming

e-Health Systems: Electronic Health Systems

LAN: Local Area Network

MAN: Metropolitan Area Networks

GAN: Global Area Networks

e-Communication: Electronic Communication

Chapter 10
Data Security in Electronic Health Records

Stefane M. Kabene
Ecole des Hautes Etudes en Sante Publique (EHESP), France

Raymond W. Leduc
University of Western Ontario, Canada

Candace J. Gibson
University of Western Ontario, Canada

ABSTRACT

Traditionally, patient information has been recorded on paper and stored in file folders at healthcare facilities and within physicians' offices. The implementation of electronic health records (EHRs), the lifetime record of an individual's health and health services delivered, allows for information to be stored on computers and offers the opportunity to store considerably more data, in much less space, with new efficiencies and value added as information is easier to access, legible, timely, non-redundant and readily available. However, there are many issues to consider with the implementation of a fully shared EHR. The protection of the information contained in the record is of the utmost importance as individuals stand to become quite vulnerable if that personal health information is compromised or accessed by unauthorized users. Therefore, one of the goals of this chapter is to uncover ways in which personal health information is being protected in EHR systems. The second objective, a broader one, examines what regulations, legislation and policies are in place that remove some of the uncertainty and risk and make the use of shared information safe and secure. Many of the techniques and technologies used so far are adopted from the corporate world, where data security has been an issue for some time. Current legislation in the United States and Canada at both the federal and state/provincial levels has addressed the general principles of data security and privacy but are still lacking in specifics with regard to cross-jurisdictional sharing of health information and the implementation and use of EHRs. Many of the researchers and studies on the subject find this to be one of the most important areas of concern moving forward. The opportunities for EHR implementation and use are exciting as they have the strong potential to improve both individual health care and population health, but without proper regulation and policies in place it is possible that the risks may outweigh the benefits.

DOI: 10.4018/978-1-61692-010-4.ch010

INTRODUCTION

It is undeniable that the rapid pace of technological advancement has had an impact on every facet of modern society. Old ways of doing things are often transformed overnight and society is left to catch up. It is also our responsibility to take a step back occasionally and analyze the direction our new technology is taking us, and decide if it is leading us down the path initially intended. One of the most important areas where technology is being applied is in the healthcare industry where advancement and new developments alter people's lives on a daily basis and can quite literally mean the difference between life and death. Yet as the medical field races ahead with nanotechnology, genome mapping, telerobotic surgery and countless other projects (Anvari, 2007; Godman, 2008), it is imperative that we take a closer look as to where we might end up, and more importantly, what we must be wary of not leaving behind. The subject of this paper is electronic health records (EHRs) that allow patient health information from multiple sources to be stored electronically as opposed to the traditional pencil and paper method. More specifically, we will examine the issue of privacy rights and take a closer look at what technology is being employed to ensure the security of health data.

The objective of this paper is to look at ways in which EHRs are currently being used in the healthcare industry. It will focus on the key issues involved in discussions of privacy rights, what different methods are currently employed to ensure data security, and what needs to be fixed, or kept in mind, with regard to its future potential. EHRs provide an interesting facet of modern health care as the potential benefits are significant (reduction of medical errors, reduction of test duplication and cost savings, accessibility of the record anywhere, anytime, disease surveillance, resource planning and management), but in many ways the technology is proceeding faster than the policies and regulations required to ensure its safe and secure use.

CONCEPTUAL FRAMEWORK

With the ability to store large amounts of data from multiple sources in a small space and relatively inexpensively, EHRs are becoming a desired goal in the healthcare industry. The electronic health record, the longitudinal record of an individual's encounters with the health system and various health providers, is the goal of the ultimate multi-user, multi-facility, multi-purpose record. The EHR is envisioned as connecting institutional or facility-based electronic paper records (EPR) and the physician-provider electronic medical record (EMR) to provide a comprehensive lifetime record of care. The EHR will include information from different healthcare providers and in different formats, for example, text, voice, and digital images. This information, including demographic and clinical data, diagnostic results, alerts, reminders, and evidence-based decision-making support, should be accessible only to authorized users. A truly integrated electronic health record facilitates data linkage and data sharing among a number of different users in geographically different locations. The EHR supports care by multiple providers, and the use of health data for secondary purposes such as research, planning, management and administrative decision making. It provides value well beyond the capabilities of the current paper record. It also presents challenges in sharing information across jurisdictional boundaries and the maintenance of privacy and confidentiality (Crook, Gibson, Adam, Levesque, O'Reilly-Brunelle & Hwee, 2009; Dick, Steen & Detmer, 1997).

Potentially, patient information including everything from family medical history, laboratory results, medication information, and even a genomic map of the individual could be stored for access to anyone who might have an interest in the information and is authorized to access it. Patients would be able to look up lab results from home, or have prescriptions refilled and delivered (Wiljer et al, 2008). A Health Canada review (EXOCOM Group, 2001) of privacy technology stressed the benefits for healthcare professionals as faster access to health records, facilitation of better care, reduction of costs, accommodation of future developments and support of clinical and health services research.

However, this new technology is not without its risks. With the enhanced ability to store and share large volumes of information in cyberspace comes the increased threat of that data being compromised. Kaelber, Jha, Johnston, Middleton and Bates (2008) found that "91% of people [in the US] are very concerned about the privacy and security of personal health information." This suggests that many patients are cautious about providing information to professionals who use EHRs. An estimated 1.2 million Canadians have withheld personal information from a health care provider because of concerns over how it might be used or with whom the information would be shared (EKOS, 2007).

There is some evidence to illustrate that the risks associated with EHRs are not based purely on speculation. Meingast, Roosta and Sastry (2006) identifies risks such as "access rights to data, how and when data is stored, security of data transfer, data analysis rights, and the governing policies." These are only some of the issues that recur in the literature on EHRs. It is important to recognize that security issues are in reference to both internal and external threats. There are no easy answers to these issues and they have been the topic of much debate. There is also evidence to show that in the short time of limited EHR implementation these risks have resulted in legitimate losses or breaches of security (Office of the Information and Privacy Commissioner, 2002).

In October 2001, physicians in the Chatham-Kent Primary Care Network agreed to participate in the first information technology transition pilot project (Office of the Information and Privacy Commissioner, 2002). The purpose was to test different forms of information technology and to identify weaknesses or vulnerabilities before the technology was used province-wide. Patient information was recorded on computer touch screens, then sent to a docking station in the physician's office and transmitted across the Internet to a central server to be stored. The then Smart Systems for Health agency (SSH) (superseded by eHealth Ontario), provided the security for collection, storage, transmission and exchange of information. In December of the same year that the project went "live" a reporter for the national newspaper the Globe and Mail informed the Information and Privacy Commissioner (IPC) of Ontario that he had received internal documents stored by SSH from an outside source. Further, three separate companies had received access to patient information that was supposed to be confidential.

Clearly there was initial reason to be concerned with the ability of institutions to protect patients' confidential information. Dr. Paul D. Clayton of Columbia Presbyterian Medical Center in New York and chair of the National Research Council's Committee on Healthcare Privacy and Security (Burke and Weill, 2000) has stated that "sharing of information within the health care industry is largely unregulated and represents a significant concern to privacy advocates and patients alike because it often occurs without a patient's consent or knowledge."

It is clear that patients are concerned about having the information contained in their EHRs compromised. The information that might be contained in an EHR could easily be used for a number of unethical or even criminal reasons. The Federal Trade Commission estimated that 10 million Americans reported being victims of some form of identity theft in 2003 (Diamond, Goldstein, Lansky & Verhulst, 2008). Identity theft can lead to enormous financial losses, not to mention the hardship and violation that is common to most victims. Yet, this is only one of the potential challenges. Others include government misuse of the information, data quality issues, potentially harmful medical and social consequences, and commercial misuse of data (Diamond et al., 2008).

Advancements in this field must be approached carefully. Deapen (2006) summed it up by stating that "achieving a proper balance between measures to protect privacy and the ability to guard and improve public health requires careful consideration and development of appropriate policies, regulations and use of technology." Before we examine what measures are being taken to achieve this balance, it is necessary to have a closer look at what privacy really means.

Privacy is defined as the "the right of individuals to be left alone and to be protected against physical or psychological invasion or misuse of their property. It includes... the right to maintain control over certain personal information" (Deapen, 2006). Both the UN Declaration of Human Rights and the International Covenant on Civil and Political Rights recognize the right to privacy (Diamond et al., 2008). It would not be unreasonable to consider a breach of privacy to be a violation of one's basic human rights. Data security, on the other hand, is the process of assessing and countering threats and risks to information, and implementing the technical and administrative safeguards necessary to protect personal information. Technical safeguards include mechanisms for data back-up (hardware and software); anti-virus protection; intruder alerts; secure networks and the means of providing safe and secure remote and wireless access and transmission of data; the layout and location of workstations; authentication (that may include level of access determined by the user's role); and the use of audit trails that can provide transaction logs and track inappropriate use (Rindfleisch, 1997). Administratively, organizations and facilities should have clearly defined policies and procedures for confidentiality and privacy that set out and define access rights (for example by professional status or by the relation between the user and patient, by type of data, and/or intended action) that are consistent with current legislation or policies of professional organizations.

The lack of proper data security and clearly articulated privacy policies can lead to 'privacy-protective' behavior where patients engage in measures to shield themselves from potential harmful uses of their personal health information (CHCF, 2005; Deapen, 2006). This behavior ranges from disguising one's name to remain anonymous, to disclosing untrue, or refraining from disclosure of information due to their fear of its use within EHR systems. Roughly 50 million Americans, engage in privacy-protective behavior to shield themselves from misuse of their information (CHCF, 2005). These behaviors included asking a physician not to report a health problem or to record a less serious (or less embarrassing) diagnosis, avoiding their regular physician for certain health conditions, avoiding certain diagnostic tests due to anxiety that others might find out about the results, or paying out of pocket for procedures to avoid submitting a claim (CHCF, 2005; Deapen, 2006). Negative consequences from this type of behaviour can lead to increased risk of missed diagnosis or poor quality care. It is therefore extremely important that however EHRs are implemented, privacy be of the utmost importance, and more importantly, that patients recognize this initiative.

This also poses important questions for human resources management (HRM) as many companies have considered providing employees with access to their EHRs. HR managers must decide who will have access to the data, who will have the ability to alter the information, how data will be protected from unwanted view or use, and how to get employees to trust in the system enough in order to use it properly. Purdy (2000) found that "61% of Americans felt that too many people have access to their medical records." This is troublesome not only when it leads to privacy-protective behavior, but also when it leads to underutilization of the EHR program and distrust of the company.

Thus, in order for EHRs to be successful in the future it is imperative that not only protective measures take place effectively, but also patients/individuals must be informed and made aware of such protection and who they can speak to about privacy concerns.

Two other issues should be considered before moving on. The first is in regards to who owns the data contained in the EHR, and second, whether there are sufficient laws and regulations in place that allow institutions the means to provide the needed security. At first glance, it seems rational to assume that the patient owns the information and would allow him/her the opportunity to decide what should be done with the information, who should have access, and grant them the power to alter it. On the other hand, much of the information is the product of medical tests and examinations stored by medical institutions for their reference and other future purposes, such as research, i.e. the medical record is 'created' by the health provider(s). Physicians are not required to seek permission to make notes in a patient's paper file or to simply look it over. Why should electronic records be any different? This calls for several considerations, for if it is deemed that the individual owns the information, then consent must be sought for each and every activity involving one's record. Yet, as Burke and Weill (2000) point out, the majority of computer frauds and security breaches are committed internally by authorized employees, therefore restricting access to the patient alone and requiring written consent for its use may be the most prudent option. The second relates to external powers and their effect on assisting or hindering health institutions in providing consistent health data security. There need to be strong national regulations or policies as data often passes beyond individual state or provincial or regional boundaries. Without regulation as a guideline for EHR implementation it will be difficult to ensure security across different institutions and will be almost impossible to integrate information from multiple sources properly.

METHODOLOGY

A selected review of the current peer-reviewed literature on issues of implementation, success and failure of EHRs was conducted. Given the fact that the fully integrated EHR technology is still in its preliminary stages, many of the implementations, revolve around feedback from pilot studies such as the Chatham-Kent project. Articles chosen for analysis were those that conducted a review of such projects, along with related privacy issues. Given the nature of the topic, the majority of the information is of a qualitative manner. Information on the techniques employed for data security examined literature from both pilot projects, what methods were used and literature on the devices/techniques used for data protection in general. Given that the nature of data security is very similar to that of businesses that seek to ensure security of their corporate and personnel information, it is assumed that many of the same methods could be used in the healthcare industry. This provided insight into some of the latest and most robust technologies for information protection.

Current legislation and regulations in North America that deal with personal health information and the EHR specifically (the latter relatively sparse) were also reviewed. Articles and white papers that provided an account of the current efforts to produce policy and regulations for the future were also reviewed.

RESULTS

The results are separated into two categories. The first illustrates a number of the methods that are currently used to implement and maintain the security of EHRs. According to Kaelber et al. (2008) "many patients already see physicians with the proper program for EHRs." The simplest electronic record systems generally include basic personal computers and other electronic devices such as those used in the Chatham-Kent project

(OIPC, 2002). Despite its suspected and reported failures, the IPC did a thorough investigation of the project and discovered five stringent measures that proved to be necessities for EHR implementation. These five measures were: the use of secure servers, physical security such as security guards and video surveillance, secure network services such as firewalls and encryption technology, encrypted email between people in the group, security and user authentication, and 'privacy-enhancing technologies' or PETs. The security authentication included measures such as the use of key fobs to carry passwords, i.e. small key chain sized displays that show a different sequence of numbers every 60 seconds that complemented other measures such as user names and role-based access. The privacy-enhancing technologies were mainly focused around public key infrastructures that will be discussed later. These techniques are important in maintaining the security of information and/or restricting access to only approved personnel.

Trust Management Systems (TMS) are another security measure that is employed in the use of EHRs. These systems watch over the general collection of information and monitor potentially dangerous operations by analyzing who is requesting the operation, what the local security policy is, what the credentials of the requester are, among other factors. They also provide a standard language for writing policies and credentials that control what is allowed and what is not. Along with the common language for describing how operations are to be handled, TM systems have four other beneficial characteristics, including a mechanism for identifying principles of the system, a language for application policies, another for specifying credentials and a compliance checker. They are gate keepers of the medical information in the sense that they take into account a number of factors in determining which operations are legitimate and which are not. It can be an effective way to ensure the privacy that is so vital to successful implementation of EHRs.

Other technological methods of privacy control also warrant recognition. The first is "smart cards" which contain stored values that are transmitted when the card is inserted into a reader, or more recently, when the card is within a certain range of a receiver. The card stores information about the holder including the amount of access and privileges he is offered with respect to accessing the confidential information. Biometrics is another method of identification that incorporates unique features of the individual. These include features such as retinal scans, fingerprints and/or voiceprints. This is a more difficult method to duplicate. Smart cards are open to theft or duplication, whereas physical features are much harder to fake or replicate.

Finally, public key infrastructure sums up the most potentially beneficial technological privacy control measures. Public key infrastructure involves encryption based around a mathematical formula that takes information and scrambles it or changes it into an unintelligible form. In order to convert it back to its original form an individual must have access to a decryption key. There are generally two keys involved in encryption. The "public key" is available to everyone and is used to scramble the information that is stored. In order to access the information in its proper form a person must have a "private key" which would only be given to authorized personnel. This method is most useful with regards to information transfers, specifically between two or more locations or persons.

While all these methods are effective tools for guarding against unauthorized access they fail to solve the issue discussed previously, the fact that a large percentage of fraud cases or security breaches result from authorized individuals. However, it is also important to recognize that as the (EXOCOM Group, 2001) stated, "there is not one simple solution, but only a combination of techniques will provide optimal privacy, and consistency within the EHRs."

The other area to be examined regards the laws and regulations that govern the EHR landscape. In the Canadian context, the Supreme Court ruling of McInerney versus MacDonald, a case involving a request by a patient for access to her complete record, states that while not an absolute right, patients have a right to access their personal health information in all but a few circumstances and the information contained in the health record belongs to the patient (Frelick & Jovellano, 2009, p. 319). However, as Wiljer et al. (2008) point out, this ruling came before the widespread use of EHRs and the courts have yet to clarify many of the issues that are raised by sharing of information in the electronic record. Harris, Levy and Teschke (2008) point out that while Alberta, Saskatchewan, Manitoba and Ontario have separate legislation that governs health information, many other provinces do not and there is currently no separate federal law regarding health information. Humayun et al. (2008) conducted a review of studies performed in Canada and discovered that quite a few family physicians do not fully understand their obligations towards patient privacy and confidentiality. In an attempt to meet this need, the Canadian Committee for Patient Accessible Electronic Health Records was formed. It is a group of researchers, clinicians, and information specialists who work to promote patient access to, and involvement with, EHRs. They have taken on a two part project to scan the country for hospital readiness for implementation of EHRs, and to assemble a workshop of stakeholders in the field of EHR (Wiljer et al., 2008). While attempts are being made to create regulation and standards for implementation and use of EHRs, a specific federal regulation has not yet been established.

The US situation is very similar to that of Canada's regarding regulations for EHRs. The Health Insurance Portability and Accountability Act (HIPAA) enacted in 1996 outlines the procedures to be followed by doctors, hospitals, and other health care providers to ensure that all medical records, medical billing and patient accounts comply with certain consistent standards for documentation, handling and privacy (Meingast et al., 2006). Each state also has its own laws for disclosure of information. Much of the literature tends to agree that the HIPAA does not contain strong enough regulations to solve many of the current issues. It is also widely believed that the problem is multiplied by having each state governed by its own laws. This makes it difficult to apply regulation to information that is shared beyond state lines. Rosenbaum, MacTaggart, and Borzi (2006) examined Medicaid's budget (the federal program that provides medical insurance coverage to low income and low resource families) and showed it has historically spent little on information technology, yet it has always contained provisions to ensure the security of collected data. As a system that is built on being interoperable, by combining medical records with education records, income information, child welfare system information, among others, it has been debated as to whether Medicaid's regulations for privacy should mirror those of the HIPAA.

The US is making strides with the Certification Commission for Healthcare Information Technology. Founded in 2004, the commission was created to rigorously test software developed by companies to establish whether or not their systems can support and perform required functions, exchange information with other systems, and maintain data confidentiality and security (Glaser, Henley, Downing & Brinner, 2008). The American Health Information Community has also done its part by creating the Public Health Workgroup (PHC) which works to inform policy makers on developments in EHR standards. In March 2007, the PHC group identified four priority areas moving forward, one of them being privacy and security. So while ground is being made and there are those who are working to see that regulations to EHR use are established, we have still not reached a fully integrated and longitudinal electronic record in either country

DISCUSSION

From these privacy and security reviews, a number of conclusions become apparent. The ability to record, store and use an increasing amount of personal information has continued to grow with the boom of the information age. As long as this ability has existed, so too has the necessity to ensure protection of sensitive personal health information from unauthorized use and prying eyes. While IT implementation is still fairly new in the healthcare industry, it has been rapidly progressing in the business world for some time. Much can be learned from the world of business, and as EHR system providers continue to improve their programs they are starting to borrow some of the ideas used in the business world for information protection. Public key interfaces, secure servers, authentication techniques, and trust management systems have been used with success in the corporate world. However, one clear message is that the issue of in-house fraud has yet to be addressed. As noted before, the majority of computer fraud cases or security breaches come from authorized users, not outside hackers. Much of the privacy protection techniques involve ensuring that the only people who need to have access to the information are the only ones who will truly see it. Yet, if these people in some cases are part of the problem what is really being solved? This will be a challenge for HR managers and privacy officers going forward, as the solution to this problem will likely depend on the ability to properly screen and train employees, particularly those who are to have access to the stored information. This could include integrity testing, employee monitoring, confidentiality agreements, and certainly the development of corporate cultures in both hospitals and software companies that value the ethical and moral imperative of privacy protection.

Kaelber et al. (2008) provide another interesting implication of the EHR environment. They acknowledge the fact that in many ways the techniques being used for data security create a safer environment for the information. Yet they also point out the fact that by storing the information on a giant network (the Internet) the information is now everywhere as opposed to the paper based forms which would be kept in folders, locked away in cabinets. Some of the main advantages of the EHR system can also be seen as weaknesses as it is possible for people anywhere in the world to hack in and access the information stored on servers. Also, by making attempts to integrate the information so that similar or linked information is grouped together for easier retrieval it is easier to get a greater amount of information. With a paper record an unauthorized party would potentially have to break into numerous filing cabinets and search through many stacks of paper to obtain the complete record; with an integrated EHR server a hacker could access information from any number of sources making misuse of the information much more attractive as the information would be more valuable. Certainly if the data could be safely secured, the benefits of an integrated record (for public health surveillance, accessibility of the record in an emergency, etc) would likely outweigh the risks, but currently there is a strong debate that much of the data cannot be secured, and until security can be ensured it would be wise to consider, and attempt to minimize the risks.

Perhaps the most recurring concern when one studies EHRs is the issue of inadequate regulation. The absence of federal regulation or international treaties that govern the broad use of EHRs is holding the advancement of the technology use in the health care industry back. There appears to be a general consensus amongst researchers who have examined this issue that one of the most important areas moving forward is the need for regulation that will address cross-jurisdictional use of and sharing of health data. The fact that it has taken this long is an indication of the relative difficulty that is faced in coming to a conclusion on the issue. Not only must the regulations govern what information is to be collected, by whom, who owns it, who may access and edit the information, and a limitless other number of issues, it is also likely that there will be exceptions to the rule. Deapen (2006) suggests that there needs to be exceptions that address times when the need to access personal health information for government purposes may supersede any personal privacy rights, such as in times of epidemic outbreaks and disease control. The variations between state and provincial legislation illustrates the need for consensus and harmonization of existing laws and work to be done to generate effective federal legislation that covers all jurisdictions.

Perhaps the delayed process to generate such regulations for EHRs can be viewed as a positive sign. There may be a general consensus after all; the importance of the dilemma is well understood and those charged with creating the regulations want to be sure to do it right. There are few things more sensitive than an individual's personal health information and when integrated with a great deal of other personal information, there are few things more valuable. The information age has offered a wealth of new opportunities, yet it is important not just to take them at face value; as society changes and evolves old norms, customs and legislation becomes outdated. New technology is often produced and introduced faster than we are able to govern its use. So perhaps instead of viewing the lack of regulation as a deterrent to advancement it should be viewed as an opportunity to take great care in a matter that can have a dramatic effect on people's lives, beyond the simple gains that are often thought of as being the main outcome of EHRs.

Another important point to consider is that with attempts to discover ways to spread EHRs across the country, the new technology is being forced on many in the healthcare industry who may not champion the idea. Wiljer et al. (2008) discuss the need for a strong cultural shift in many healthcare institutions that must accompany the adoption and increased integration of advanced technologies. Many have become so used to the ease of use of having patient information stored at hand in a manilla folder and may not be comfortable entering it into computers and having it stored on a server off the hospital or facility site. As a result, it is just as important to convince the provider as well as the patient of the importance of securing health data, as it is to actually do so. Further, healthcare professionals will have to adapt to the idea of 'custodianship' of personal health information rather than 'ownership' (Wiljer et al. 2008). The fostering of such a cultural shift may take time and patience, but will be instrumental in the ultimate success of the EHR. This will have an impact on the field of human resources management as it may be HR managers within health organizations that are faced with orchestrating this cultural shift and supervising the transition to optimum electronic record use.

RECOMMENDATIONS

Given that there is still limited deployment of EHRs much of the literature on the subject focuses on recommendations for the future, and not one, but a number of published recommendations, needs to be considered. Deapen (2006) suggests five steps in implementing any EHR software. First, he suggests the development of technical standards for privacy protection. He then suggests a focused dialogue and documentation of best practices, use and release of information. A centralized repository could be developed and instances of privacy breaches as well as instances of interference or hampering of research or public health surveillance collected. This would allow for the collection of information that would aid in further debates about the adaption of regulations to further the efficient use of information. Finally, he suggests creating a board of experts from among several different stakeholders to whom policy makers would send suggestions for proposed regulations and the board would offer advice. These steps would not only allow for a clear set of regulations agreed upon by all relevant stakeholders, but also allow for the continuing collection of information for the purpose of review and to see if new changes would need to be made.

Diamond et al. (2008) offers a slightly different perspective for the future that should also be considered to increase EHRs' future success. They are strong advocates of having patients involved in each step of the collection and use of their EHRs. They offer nine principles for the successful implementation of an integrated information network. The first is openness; this ensures that information is readily available to patients and what is contained in the record is easy to access, they are aware of how it is being used and their informed consent is sought before anything is done with the information. The second step is purpose specification; data will never be collected without the knowledge of the patient and it will be used for the original purpose for which it was gathered. Collection and use limitation are the third and fourth principle. Individual participation and control should be used where patients are seen as key participants in the process, data integrity and quality principles should be developed, along with security safeguards and controls. The final two principles are accountability and appropriate remedies for infringements. They suggest that a Chief Privacy Officer (CPO) position should be created wherever EHRs are used whose task it is to oversee the continued security of the information and to see that best practices are followed. Employee training is also an important part of accountability. Finally remedies need to be established for those who are victims of privacy breaches. Many of these suggestions have been incorporated into both federal and provincial privacy legislation and within Canada reflect the CSA's model code for the protection of personal information (Q830) that sets out ten principles (of accountability; identifying purposes for data collection; consent for collection, use and disclosure of information; limiting collection; limiting use, disclosure and retention; accuracy; safeguards; openness; individual access; and challenging compliance) that balance the privacy rights of individuals and the information requirements of private organizations (http://www.csa.ca/cm/privacy-code). Both Canada's Personal Information Protection and Electronic Documents Act (PIPEDA) and the US Health Insurance Portability and Accountability Act have used these principles as the basis of their respective laws.

Yasnoff (2003, p. 202) offered further suggestions, some relating to potential regulation of the collection of information. They suggest that any regulation regarding the collection of information should be based on the principles of relevance, integrity, written purpose, need-to-know access, capacity for correction and open consent. The use of confidentiality agreements and authentication procedures is proposed to ensure that information is restricted to those who truly need to see and/or use it. These agreements would be signed upon initial hiring and each year thereafter. These agreements would also specify clear disciplinary action if the confidentiality agreement is breached. They also suggest that intrusion detection software be used that looks for unusual access patterns and the implementation of statistical techniques to examine usage patterns. For instance, "most work systems have a peak use in mid-morning and mid-afternoon, and a rare surge in activity in the middle of the night might illustrate potential misuse" (Yasnoff, 2003). These suggestions may also assist in the detection of fraud or breaches generated by internal authorized personnel. These could be important considerations in moving forward as internal misuse is still a major concern in the field of data protection.

The current landscape with each province or state creating its own privacy laws is not sufficient to cover the widespread potential of EHR in which information may be shared across multiple jurisdictions each with its own set of regulations and legislation. One of the main benefits of EHRs is the centralization of large amounts of data, but this advantage can only be realized if all steps, from collection to final use, are conducted consistently, nationwide. Although a long term initiative and goal is a global EHR system, the preliminary process of implementation can only be controlled locally or domestically. Although this paper focuses on the implementation of EHRs, and specifically the effect on data security and privacy, it is important to note that much of the delay in implementation is due to inconsistencies at the local level. Differences in data collection, data standards and interoperability, even at the lowest level - from hospital to hospital within a given city - are causes for much of the delay. Therefore, although the call for federal legislation is necessary for addressing privacy issues, it can also be beneficial for policies that relate to consistent record keeping and data standards. Within Canada health delivery and hence health policy, to a certain extent, is a provincial mandate, but with regards to the long term effectiveness of EHRs it is important to instigate a nationwide policy to ensure consistency in both privacy issues, and record keeping and data standards, to speed the process of implementation. There is still debate over what minimum information should be collected, how it should be collected, who owns the information, who has the right to use/edit the information, how it should be secured and stored, within a nation-wide electronic health record. These issues need to be resolved and federal legislation must apply to all uses of the EHR that contains information from different systems, different organizations, different providers, and in different formats.

All of the above suggestions will also have an impact on and help improve the field of HRM. Those in the field of human resources must develop new standards for employees with regards to who is given access to important information, who will be given control to perform different operations with the information, and what types of information will be recorded. Ensuring the security of information will also become an important task for HR managers as they will likely be dealing with information that is personal to each employee/patient and their consent and input will need to be sought before the information can be used. HR managers will also need to find creative ways to use this information to the advantage of their company or institution (e.g. planning fitness programs, provision of personal health records). There is great potential for this new technology, but due to the delicate nature of its content, challenges are on the horizon for the field of human resources.

CONCLUSION

In conclusion, there are a number of developments in the field of electronic health records, yet there is still much to be accomplished. There are many different ways and methods in which developers and implementers of EHRs are approaching the issues of security of personal health information. These methods include the use of:

- Secure servers
- Physical security measures
- Security authentication
- Privacy enhancing technologies, including encryption, trust management systems, smart cards, biometrics, and public key infrastructure.

These methods are all important in ensuring that stored personal health data is not subject to potential misuse. A combination of methods, not a single method is necessary, as pointed out in our privacy technology review - "the most promising technology combination for EHRs appears to be a combination of trust management and public key infrastructure, possibly enhanced with smart cards and biometrics" (EXOCOM Group, 2001). Trust management is the best known technological tool for controlling internal threats, while the latter three address outside threats. Most of the available methods of control are directed at outside threats. The assumption is made that human resources management will be the best suited tool for ensuring confidentiality, through training, disciplinary policies, and other initiatives directed at internal users and minimizing internal threats to security.

The other facet of EHR that was examined was the area of regulation and legislation enacted to govern the use of the technology. In both Canada and the US it was found that there is federal legislation to govern private information (through PIPEDA and HIPAA) but that it is often subject to, or superseded by, individual state or provincial law. This will be inadequate for the future as much of the information may travel beyond state or provincial lines, creating uncertainty with respect to the relevant legislation. While both countries have formed a number of committees with the focus of establishing principles of best practice, they have yet to do so and the lack of regulation has hindered the development of EHR systems. So while progress is being made and the opportunities associated with EHRs are still very real, there is much work yet to be done before the full potential is to be realized.

It is through a combination of recommendations and privacy principles, the use of privacy enhancing technologies, progressive legislative action, and human resources management that EHRs can be expected to be successful in the future. There is no single solution, and it will take a collaborative effort of all those involved, at all levels, to ensure progress in the secure implementation of the EHR, with minimal drawbacks and restrictions. Once these initiatives are realized, the full benefits of electronic health record systems can be realized.

REFERENCES

Anvari, M. (2007). Impact of information technology on human resources in healthcare. *Healthcare Quarterly, 10,* 84-88. Retrieved November 9, 2008 from <http://www.longwoods.com/product.php?productid=19320&cat=513&page=1>

Burke, L., & Weill, B. (2000). *Information Technology for the Health Professionals*. Upper Saddle River, NJ: Prentice-Hall Inc.

California HealthCare Foundation. (November 2005). *National Consumer Health Privacy Survey 2005*. CHCF Org. Available at: http://www.chcf.org/topics/view.cfm?itemID=115694

Crook, G., Gibson, C. J., Adam, C., Levesque, L., O'Reilly-Brunelle, B., & Hwee, J. (2009). Chapter 7: Towards an Electronic Health Record. In CHIMA (Ed.), *Fundamentals of Health Information Management.* Ottawa: CHA Press.

Deapen, D. (2006). Cancer surveillance and information: balancing public health with privacy and confidentiality concerns (United States). *Cancer Causes & Control*, *17*, 663–637. doi:10.1007/s10552-006-0002-1

Diamond, C., Goldstein, M., Lansky, D., & Verhulst, S. (2008). An architecture for privacy in a networked health information environment. *Cambridge Quarterly of Healthcare Ethics*, *17*, 429–440. doi:10.1017/S0963180108080559

Dick, R. S., Steen, E. B., & Detmer, D. E. (1997). *The Computer-Based Patient Record: An Essential Technology for Health Care*. Washington, DC: National Academy Press.

EKOS Research Associates. (2007, August). (Submitted to). Electronic Health Information and Privacy Survey [Canada Health Infoway, Health Canada, and the Office of the Privacy Commissioner of Canada, Ottawa.]. *What Canadians Think*.

EXOCOM Group. Business Strategy and Consulting IT Division for Office of Health and the Information Highway, Health Canada. (2001). *Privacy Technology Review*. Retrieved November 14, 2008 from http://www.hc-sc.gc.ca/hcs-sss/pubs/ehealth-esante/2001-priv-tech/index-eng.php#anne

Frelick, K. M., & Jovellano, J. (2009). Chapter 13: Legal Aspects of Health Information Management. In CHIMA (Ed.), *Fundamentals of Health Information Management*. Ottawa: CHA Press.

Glaser, J., Henley, D. E., Downing, G., & Brinner, K. M. (2008). Advancing personalized health care through health information technology: An update from the American Health Information Community's Personalized Health Care Workgroup. *Journal of the American Medical Informatics Association*, *15*(4), 391–396. doi:10.1197/jamia.M2718

Godman, M. (2008). But is it unique to nanotechnology? Reframing nanoethics. *Science and Engineering Ethics*, *14*, 391–403. doi:10.1007/s11948-008-9052-y

Harris, M. A., Levy, A. R., & Teschke, K. E. (2008). Personal privacy and public health: Potential impacts of privacy legislation on health research in Canada. *Canadian Journal of Public Health*, *99*(4), 293–296.

Humayun, A., Fatima, N., Naqqash, S., Hussain, S., Rasheed, A., Imtiaz, H., & Imam, S. Z. (2008). Patients' perception of actual practice of informed consent, privacy and confidentiality in general medical outpatient departments of two tertiary care hospitals of Lahore. *BMC Medical Ethics*, *9*(14), 1–8.

Kaelber, D. C., Jha, A. K., Johnston, D., Middleton, B., & Bates, D. W. (2008). A research agenda for personal health records (PHRs). *Journal of the American Medical Informatics Association*, *15*, 729–736. doi:10.1197/jamia.M2547

Meingast, M., Roosta, T., & Sastry, S. (2006). Security and privacy issues with health care information technology. In *Proceedings of the 28th IEEE EMBS Annual International Conference,* New York, August 30- September 3, (pp. 5453-5458).

Office of the Information and Privacy Commissioner. (2002). *Privacy Review: Chatham- Kent IT Transition Pilot Project*, (pp. 1-32). Toronto: Ontario. Available at http://www.ipc.on.ca/images/Resources/up-042202.pdf

Pedersen, C. A., & Gumper, K. F. (2008). ASHP National Survey on Informatics: Assessment of the adoption and use of pharmacy informatics in U.S. hospitals-2007. *American Journal of Health-System Pharmacy*, *65*(23), 2244–2264. doi:10.2146/ajhp080488

Purdy, J. (2000, July). An Intimate Invasion [Electronic Version]. *USA Weekend Magazine*. Retrieved November 3, 2008 from http://www.usaweekend.com/00_issues/000702/000702privacy.html

Rindfleisch, T. C. (1997). Privacy, information technology, and health care. *Communications of the ACM*, *40*(8), 92–100. doi:10.1145/257874.257896

Rosenbaum, S., MacTaggart, P., & Borzi, P. C. (2006). Medicaid and health information: Current and emerging legal issues. *Health Care Financing Review*, *28*(2), 21–30.

Wiljer, D., Urowitz, S., Apatu, E., DeLenardo, C., Eysenbach, G., & Harth, T. (2008). Patient accessible electronic health records: Exploring recommendations for successful implementation strategies. *Journal of Medical Internet Research*, *10*(4), e34. doi:10.2196/jmir.1061

Yasnoff, W. A. (2003). Privacy, confidentiality and security of public health information. In *Public Health Informatics and Information Systems*. New York: Springer. doi:10.1007/0-387-22745-8_10

Chapter 11
A Secure Teleradiology Grid

Robert Rudowski
Medical University of Warsaw, Poland

Michal Dzierzak
Medical University of Warsaw, Poland

Bartosz Kaczynski
Medical University of Warsaw, Poland

ABSTRACT

A modern secure teleradiology grid consists of several important parts. The first part is to ensure the highest security of storing the medical data. At present time the old fashioned storage solutions are replaced by Grid Storage and Content Addressable Storage (CAS) infrastructure of archiving medical records in a flexible and secure way. The second part of secure teleradiology grid is related to applying appropriate data transmission security protocols and digital signatures in the various nodes of grid. Also human and law aspects of security need to be taken into account because of international nature of teleradiology development. The law should be consistent in different nodes of teleradiology grid.

INTRODUCTION

Why security aspects of teleradiology are so important? With the development of teleradiology images are no longer interpreted at one site (hospital, ambulatory care etc.). They cross institutional and/or national boundaries and are sent to a distant location for interpretation and/or consultation. This fact creates many challenges regarding security issues. We will discuss them in our work.

DOI: 10.4018/978-1-61692-010-4.ch011

In grid technology sharing resources is conditional. Each resource owner makes the resources available subject to constraints on when, where and what can be done. Sharing relationships can vary dynamically over time in terms of resources involved, the nature of access permitted and the participants to whom the access is permitted. Information security in grid can be defined as the preservation of the availability, access to, confidentiality and integrity of information.

Grid are the distributed computer resources cooperating to fulfill the common task. We can consider different types of grid e.g. internal grid of the institution (institutional grid) and grid covering much wider area. The requirements and design of security systems will be different for each type of grid.

The main topic of our work are security aspects of teleradiology grid. Those aspects are related to:

a) centers of archives and applications: which require reliable options for data storage (RAID arrays), backup and access solutions to different media types (CD, DVD, Blu-rays and tape libraries) containing image data,
b) data transmission: types of network connection, bandwidth, topology etc.

We introduce the notion of e-security which is required by teleradiology. The basic features of e-security are confidentiality, integrity, non-repudiation and accountability. The additional features are authorization and certification. They will be discussed in the paper.

Those features can be obtained with the Public Key Infrastructure (PKI) which supplies several tools for achieving them: public key, private key, digital signature, certification centers and public repositories of certificates. PKI is the central security axis around which other elements are located.

The first element are Virtual Private Networks (VPN's) which authorize access of one grid node to another grid node (certificate X.509). VPN is a set of nodes in a public network, such as Internet, which communicate among themselves using encryption technology in order to protect the data against unauthorized access as if they were a private network. VPN is a static configuration. It cannot extend dynamically to encompass other resources and does not provide the remote resource provider of any control of when and whether to share its resources. Therefore VPN function requires extension in the grid context.

There are several hardware and software solutions for VPN implementation. The most commonly used hardware implementation is IPsec and software is OpenVPN. The advantages and disadvantages of each of them will be discussed in the paper.

The second element includes access control (firewalls) to network services and resources used by grid, intrusion detection and prevention systems (IDP) and/or intrusion detection systems (IDS) which support firewalls. Network resources may be for example WWW resources, e-mail, external SQL databases or DICOM modalities such as X-ray, CT, MRI or USG. The main elements of the node in teleradiology are RIS, PACS systems and the main goal is data security in those systems.

Those two elements combined together create secure data transmission system (SDTS) for teleradiology.

Considering data security we have to take also human and law aspects into account. The present state of law regarding teleradiology in Poland will be presented. It can be stated that law is lagging behind the technology development. We will try to explain how digital signature law is influencing security of teleradiology systems and especially how too high number of different electronic signature standards can complicate the implementation of distributed systems.

The conclusions and recommendations aiming at rising the security level of teleradiology grids will be presented.

SECURITY ASPECTS OF CENTERS OF ARCHIVES AND APPLICATIONS

The centers of archives and applications require reliable options for data storage (RAID arrays), backup and access solutions to different media types (CD, DVD, Blu-rays and tape libraries) containing image data. Teleradiology commonly benefits from the development of an increasing media space or faster transfer rate, so it is very important to know pros and cons of near-(on) line storage, backup options, disk arrays and connections interfaces between them and types

Table 1. Near-(on)line storage media

Type of optical storage	Max. size	Typical. transfer rate	Advantages	Disadvantages
CD	~700 MB	52x 9MB/s	low cost	disc surface easy to damage, improper storing conditions could reduce lifespan to 2-3 years
DVD	4.7 GB (SS) 8.5 GB (DL)	16x 21MB/s	low cost, high capacity	disc surface easy to damage, improper storing conditions could reduce lifespan to 2-3 years
DVD-RAM	4.7 GB (SS) 9.4 GB (DS)	2x-3x 2-4MB/s	long life (30 years), optimal for archive storage of image studies	higher price than normal DVDs, drive incompatibilities
MO Discs	600MB-9.1GB	3-6 MB/s	long life technology, ISO approved	high cost, slow transfer rate
Blu-rays (BD)	25-50 GB	8x 36 MB/s	huge capacity	high price, new devices to read/write

of network storage infrastructure, which are later described in this chapter.

Near (On)Line Storage

Near-(on)line storage media are listed in Table 1.

Backup Options Tape Libraries

In order to store in safe place the huge amount of medical images and records the typical backup solution is to use tape libraries with an option of the automatic process of loading tapes from their slots into the drives. There are several different tape formats like DLT, LTO, AIT and at the present time the single tape capacity grows fast reaching up to 800 GB (and 1-2 TB in next years) with up to ~80 MB/s transfer rate. Building a multi-unit tape library could provide hundreds of terabytes for storing medical images for a long time.

Alternative way is to use optical jukeboxes, which could have 500-700 available slots of BD (Blu-ray Discs) with capacity around 30 TB of data. An additional way of ensuring top-ranked backup security is to transfer multiple copies of data to different physical locations, i.e. other city, or even better, another region of country, where the probability of catastrophic disasters like floods, fires, earthquakes is considerably lower. Hard disks could be damaged during planned migration, transport and storing mirror copies of data in the nearest building (i.e. destroying both two towers of World Trade Center) (Fratt, 2008, BRIT). The method of transferring copies to different physical locations requires suitable WAN network infrastructure, but there is a significant progress in the transfer rate and it should be very reliable way of keeping data secure.

Disk Arrays and Connection Interfaces

Understanding RAID (Redundant Array of Inexpensive Disks) levels is the necessary key to implement the right storage security. Typical recommendation should be at least RAID 5 (Striped set with distributed parity or interleave parity, only one of minimum 3 drives array could fail) or RAID 6 (Striped set with dual distributed parity, even with two failed drives of min. 4 drives the array continues to operate normally) per storage server or device (see Table 2).

The optimum choice of hard disk interface type is present dilemma for PACS administrators.

Table 2. The comparison of RAID 5 and RAID 6 disk arrays

Type of disk array	RAID 5	RAID 6
advantages	- higher transfer rates than RAID 6 - more disk space than RAID 6	- the safest solution for critical application data - sustain 2 drives failures in the same time
disadvantages	- two simultaneous drives failures could destroy data	- slower performance than RAID 5 - not supported on older controllers

Newest Serial ATA (SATA) devices could have a volume of 5 to 10 times greater than traditional SCSI interface. On the other side evolution of SCSI interface SAS (Serial Attached SCSI) drives gives enterprise quality, fast speed and near SATA capacity (ex. 1.5 TB) and lower costs than Ultra-SCSI drives, which have lower capacity (around 300GB), but one main advantage, commonly used in database servers - very fast access and rotational speed up to 15000 rpm (15K). The variety of these hard disk types may be chosen for different usage from ultrafast application servers (storage less important than speed UltraSCSI disks recommended) to 10 TB NAS with 12 devices of cheap, fast SATA/SAS ones.

Types of Network Storage Infrastructure

DAS (Direct Attached Storage, Figure 1): That's a typical conventional solution not very suitable for professional medical imaging archive. A server with an option of attaching through SCSI adaptors 4-12 hard disk devices allows capacity about 3TB, but this scenario doesn't scale very well and any failure of server components could cause a long break in accessing the storage data.

NAS (Network Attached Storage, Figure 2): Main advantage of this type of storage is relatively inexpensive scalability and easy deployment in existed network architecture. In addition using DFS feature (Distributed File System) in Microsoft Windows Server's environment several NAS devices could be connected in one logical virtual device increasing storage space available for servers. But there are some drawbacks of NAS - sharing the same network can cause slowing down the transfer rate due to increased network traffic.

SAN (Storage Area Network, Figure 3): In comparison to NAS, SAN also uses network to communicate between storage devices, but has dedicated fiber channel (FC) infrastructure which provides very high performance, good scalability

Figure 1. Direct Attached Storage (DAS) schema

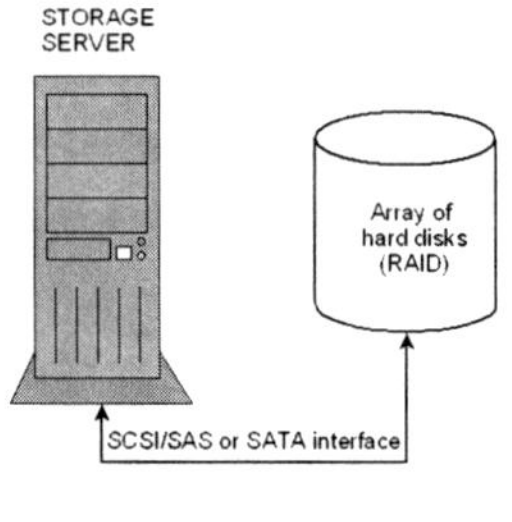

Figure 2. Example of Network Attached Storage (NAS) infrastructure

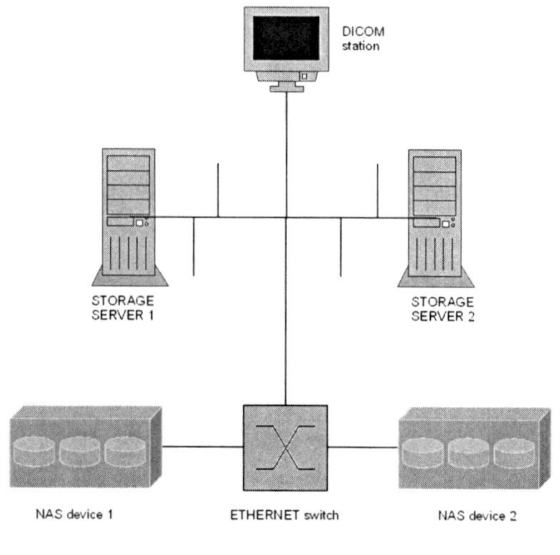

Figure 3. Storage Area Network (SAN)

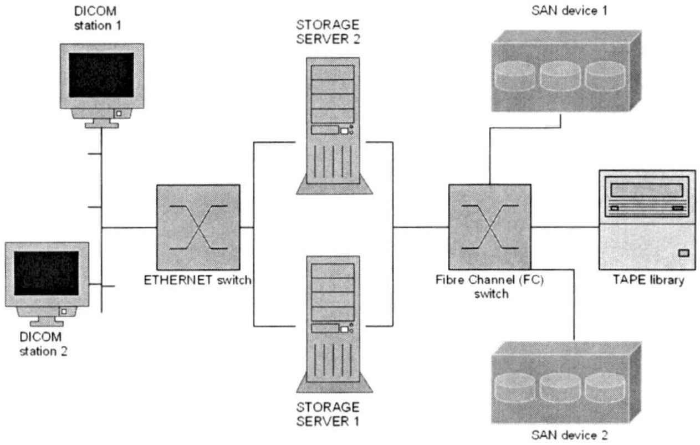

and reliability but generates higher costs than DAS or NAS. This is most often used solution in PACS environment because of possibilities like central server management and big variety of redundancy options.

Grid Storage (Figure 4): For last several years the idea of creating large pools of servers called "grid servers" has been very up to date and could be very promising solution for security and still growing need (exponentially) for increasing volume. If one of them acts as a an interface between grid and PACS server and other ones operate like independent network storage servers, then the interface server through defined policy of HSM (hierarchical storage manager) software manages the copies of files, distributing each copy to a different grid server. Any failure of a single grid server will not destroy data in the grid because of existent other copies that could be retrieved from another grid server (Dryer, 2006).

CAS (Content Addressable Storage, also known as FCS Fixed Content Storage): is a different approach to take advantage of a grid storage, but using a different manner of managing data. Every object (i.e. medical image) placed on grid servers must have its own unique identifier and

Figure 4. Grid Storage diagram

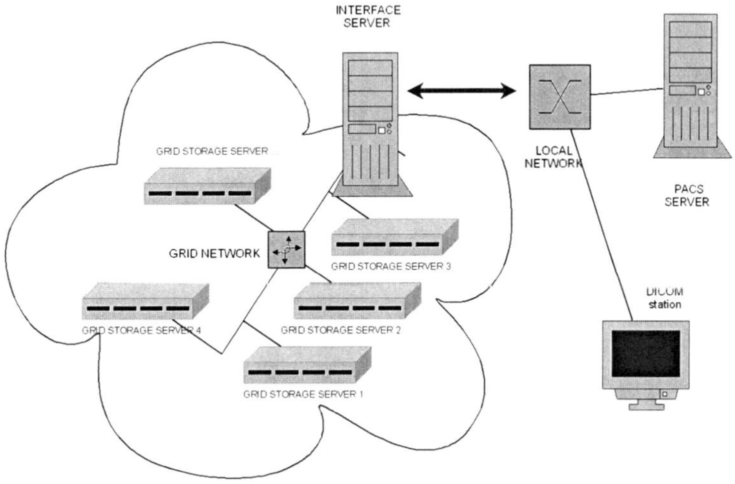

token based on value generated from the data file (typical algorithm is MD5 message digest ver. 5) both to ensure highest security. These objects can be grouped logically together (by the content or any other metadata for example any DICOM fields) and another possibility is to create any number of copies of objects for securing medical data. If an outside application requests object from CAS database, the requested file will be fetched, and then after comparing the actual identifier with its original value stored in database, that object will be transferred to corresponding client's application. Radiological images are the best example of fixed content file, which should be stored for years in unaltered state, written once read many (WORM strategy) and that kind of data could be transferred to requesting physician very fast (Dryer, 2006).

SECURITY ASPECTS OF DATA TRANSMISSION

The aspects related to data transmission include types of network connection, bandwidth and security.

Types of local (wired) network connection speed (bandwidth) are:

a) 100 Mbit/s (Fast Ethernet): commonly used infrastructure, but for improved performance large PACS networks should be upgraded to currently most used Gigabit Ethernet.
b) 1 Gbit/s (Gigabit Ethernet, 1000BASE-T): all modern devices have this standard already built-in, so whenever possible it should be applied to achieve maximal user comfort in downloading image studies. It is optimal and inexpensive choice suitable for medical applications and devices.

Remote use of radiology requires special type of network connection and depends mainly on wireless infrastructure or telecom and cable internet service providers. Teleradiology for a mobile radiologists has different requirements than regional hospital that requires some image interpretations from higher-reference medical center. Both have to transfer data through established connection, but use (A)DSL (Asymmetric Digital Subscriber Line), cable (DOCSIS - Data Over Cable Service Interface Specification standard) or telecom/wireless technology is sufficient only for a mobile radiologist who commonly rather downloads than uploads images. A local hospital is in the opposite situation and should have nearly symmetrical upload channel in comparison to download, which is necessary for fast transfer, life-critical, medical images to the reference medical center. This second scenario involves use of a symmetric, more expensive connection and sometimes this is a basic limitation for successful development of teleradiology.

Teleradiology used in grid systems requires many standard security functions such as: authentication, access control, integrity, privacy and non-repudation. In this chapter we will concentrate mainly on issues related to authentication and access control called in other words authorization.

In grid systems authentication and authorization functions are executed in user context as well in process context. The processes perform computation on behalf of user and resource context used by those processes. According to Foster, Kesselman, Tsudik and Tuecke (1998) we can distinguish following mechanisms of mutual authentication: user-to-resource which means user authentication to resources needed by user, resource-to-user means resource authentication on behalf of a user, process-to-resource means authentication process to resources needed by computing process, process-to-process means mutual authentication between two different processes. Important element is that authentication mechanisms described above are realized on a global level and should cooperate with local access control systems embedded in every node taking part in grid system. Every node in grid provides resources needed to perform computation. Authentication can be done in many ways: using clear text passwords, SSL protocol, Kerberos protocol or other available authentication solutions.

Authentication using clear text passwords is recognized as the weakest solution because it is easy to crack it by specialized tools available on the Internet. Second thing which speaks against clear text password authentication is the lack of security mechanism during passing it to the system by the user.

It is recommended to use authentication mechanisms which eliminate the password. For example they include SSL protocol based on Public Key Infrastructure certificates and using X.509v3 standard. One of the positive aspects of using SSL protocol is that SSL has a proven implementation in a public domain library called SSLeay, which is used in many authentication systems used in the world. And thus SSL is used as a method for authentication and secure communication in many distributed services such as HTTP servers, web browsers, and directory services.

When considering the security architecture of a grid system it is worth to point out what requirements it should meet (Foster, Kesselman, Tsudik and Tuecke, 1998):

1) Single sign-on - The user authenticates only once at the beginning, during starting the work. Any subsequent attempt to authenticate to other nodes, processes or resources is carried out automatically without user intervention.
2) Security of credentials -Access to user credentials such as passwords, private keys is carried out in a secure manner, without any possibility of interception by the other person.
3) Interoperability with local security solutions - Access to resources in the local node is granted on the basis of the local security policy of the node. In such a case it is worth paying attention to the fact how the global authentication method integrates with the local authorization system. One of the solutions is to use intermediate proxy servers between remote users and local resources (e.g. security servers).
4) Uniform structure of the PKI - the common use of uniform PKI standards between the nodes of grid system to express the identity of users. This standard is already mentioned X.509v3 standard which is used by PKI for encoding certificates.
5) Support for multiple technologies - Each node can use different security technologies for doing the same tasks. It is important that it should be based on the same Public Key Infrastructure standards as well as cryptography based on symmetric keys.

As we can see a very important element of the architecture of grid systems is a Public Key Infrastructure. Based on the PKI user authentication is performed between the nodes, ensuring non-repudiation using a digital signature or the integrity of data along with the privacy.

It should be noted here that the digital signature together with uniform standards is a very important element in building the teleradiology grid systems. A digital signature is used for authentication of documents such as electronic patient record (EPR), recommendations for further treatment or research work.

The details on electronic signature will be described in the next chapter.

Grid systems also require efficient and reliable network infrastructure that connects all nodes with each other. In practice, the individual nodes are connected to the Internet, which gives the geographical independence, but also results in that they are vulnerable to security risk associated with various types of malware such as viruses, Trojan horses, back doors or Root Kits. When designing the interfaces between the various nodes of a grid system such items as firewalls must be taken into account to limit access to network resources by

Figure 5. The Virtual Private Network (VPN)

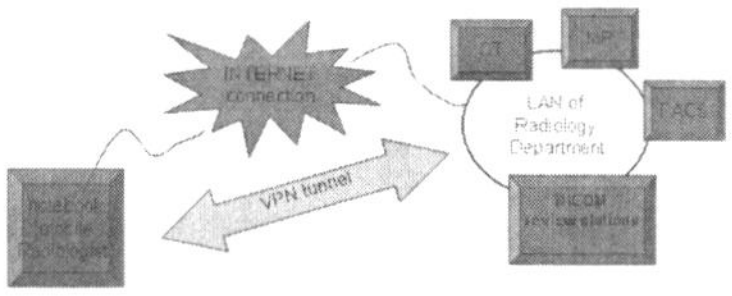

the unauthorized person or the device. When it is impossible to use firewall architecture, instead of restricting, traffic can be monitored by the type of Intrusion Detection Systems (IDS), or by systems Intrusion Detection and Prevention type (IDP), which are able to detect potential security risks and inform the network administrator. In the case of using IDP, it automatically takes action to eliminate the threats detected. These solutions are directly related to each node of the grid system and the resources that are available. Another important aspect is the security of communication between nodes. Maximum security in communication provide Virtual Private Networks solutions which are described next.

VPN (Virtual Private Network, Figure 5): is a way to secure transmission and also to extend local network to any remote device or network through the public internet connection. There are mainly two solutions that are very popular and wide open.

IPsec (Internet Protocol Security): protocol commonly used between network devices likes routers, gateways and firewalls. It typically uses layer 3 (network-protocol) of ISO model, so for applications this protocol is transparent in opposite to SSL/TLS security protocols, which must be integrated at the application level. The main disadvantage is that IPsec require high skills for proper configuration, and often needs expensive packages and hardware to setup connection (Hosner, 2004).

OpenVPN: a software solution (user space) that can be run on variety of operating systems (like Windows, Linux, Macintosh) that uses common used SSL/TLS protocol. Open-source, fast developing, easy to configure is a perfect solution for remote radiologists and teleradiology (Hosner, 2004).

HUMAN AND LAW ASPECTS OF SECURE TELERADIOLOGY

Law regarding secure teleradiology should embrace secure transmission of images and examination results, supervision over the examination (referral, choice and modification of the procedure, conditions of ending the procedure) (Kowski, 2008).

Let us cite the law act regarding teleradiology in Poland (Law Journal, 2006):

"X-ray examinations are performed by radiologists or by physicians being trained in radiology under supervision of radiologist. Electroradiology technicians are entitled to perform themselves only X-ray examination. Other elements of medical procedure must be performed by technicians under radiologists supervision."

This law act implies local supervision of radiologist over technician performing the procedure.

The digital signature law is an important element of teleradiology. In Poland there is the only one acceptable form of digital signature called qualified electronic signature authenticated by the qualified certification centers. Such centers are audited and accredited by the Polish Internal Security Agency. As for today there are three specialized centers in Poland which are enabled to issue qualified electronic signature. Such solution causes many problems. It is based on the fact that every of these three centers applies other format of the digital signature allowed by the law on the digital signature.

The following formats of the digital signature are being used in Poland:

1. CMS (Cryptographic Message Syntax), the format defined by the ETSI standard TS 101 733 and RFC 3125 and RFC 3126.
2. XML-based format, a standard defined by ETSI TS 101 903.
3. PKCS7 binary format which is the precursor of CMS.

A multitude of formats that results in communication and exchange of data among nodes of a grid system becomes complicated due to the fact that each node can use a different standard, and by design it is obvious that grid systems are heterogeneous systems. Therefore at present there is no solution that integrates all available formats of electronic signatures in Poland.

Legal issues in the European context are discussed in the Draft Report on legal framework and related aimed European trends (R-Bay, 2008) from R-Bay project.

General legal issues concern such topics as patient rights, responsibility and liability, professional responsibility, system responsibility.

As regarding system responsibility which is relevant to our work, topics of confidentiality of information, integrity and accessibility can be mentioned (R-Bay, 2008). According to the EU Directive on processing of personal data (95/46/EC REF) medical information is regarded "a special category" i.e. is sensitive.

A system should also ensure the integrity of information and its accessibility in a way that it possible to share the information with other medical personnel, if necessary.

The review of minimum EU requirements for cross-border operation in R-Bay project is based on the questionnaire submitted to project partners. Here are some remarks. The opinion of majority of respondents was that it is necessary to obtain specific consent from the patients both for having radiology images read in another country and for transmission of images.

The interesting question was raised about responsibility for the patient. The majority of opinions was that it should remain at the radiologist at the hospital taking images, not the radiologist interpreting them at a distant location.

Examples from Czech Republic and Estonia (R-Bay, 2008) show that there are different legal problems and some definitions (ex. "health documentation") are not precise. Smaller countries with lack of medical specialists have more flexible law and can have benefits from grid cross-country telemedicine projects.

CONCLUSION

The progress of the last ten years demonstrates a present trend of development in various aspects of the teleradiology. A variety of technological barriers, like connection transfer rate, effectively limited possibilities of using distributed infrastructure for storing image files in the past. Present grid or CAS storage networks solutions in association with today's very high capacity of hard disks and high performance telecommunication connections can guarantee developing secure teleradiological systems. But those elements should not work separately and using them without properly applied security standards and policies would lead to dangerous situations. Any loss, damage and unauthorized access to patient data is unacceptable and can lead to unpleasant consequences.

Another aspect of security in grid systems is a law which should be consistent in the nodes taking part in teleradiology grid. The example of law from Poland (electronic signature) shows that a multitude of standards rather complicates the situation than helps. Therefore during designing of a teleradiology grid the unification of standards which will provide better interconnectivity among nodes should be considered.

Many on-going projects in Europe (eTen Projects), America and Asia in the field of teleradiology grids indicate the importance of security aspects described in our work.

REFERENCES

Dryer, K. J., Hirschorn, D. S., Metha, A., & Thrall, J. H. (2006). *PACS: A Guide to the Digital Revolution*. New York: Springer-Verlag.

eTen projects. (2009). *European Community programme providing funds to help make e-services available throughout the European Union*. Retrieved 28 February, 2009 from http://ec.europa.eu/information_society/activities/eten/opdb/

Foster, I., Kesselman, C., Tsudik, C., & Tuecke, S. (1998). A Security Architecture for Computational Grids. In *5th ACM Conference on Computer and Communication Security*.

Fratt, L. (2008). *Enterprise Long-term Storage: Plan for the Worst, Hope for the Best*. Retrieved 28 February, 2009, from http://www.healthimaging.com/index.php?option=com_articles&view=article&id=15213:enterprise-long-term-storage-plan-for-the-worst-hope-for-the-best.

Hosner, C. (2004). *OpenVPN and SSL VPN Revolution*. SANS Institute, retrieved 28 February, 2009, from http://www.sans.org/reading_room/whitepapers/vpns/openvpn_and_the_ssl_vpn_revolution_1459

Kowski, R. (2008). *Law problems in the development of digital radiology in Poland*. Proceedings of the Conference "Medical Imaging. New trends in technology and law" (In Polish).

Law Journal. (2006). Dz.U. 2006 247 poz.1819, & 60, 4 (In Polish).

R-Bay Project. (2008). *Creating an eMarketplace for the transfer of imaging related eHealth services in Europe*, retrieved 28 February, 2009 from http://www.r-bay.org/twiki/pub/RBay/Deliverables/D4_1_R-Bay_Draft_of_Legal_Framework_v1.pdf

Systems, B. R. I. T. (n.d.). *PACS 101 - things you need to know when embarking on a PACS project*. Retrieved 28 February, 2009, from http://www.brit.com/Product%20Sheet%20PDFs/BRIT%20PACS%20101.pdf

Chapter 12

Tele-Audiology in the United States:

Past, Present, and Future

John Ribera
Utah State University, USA

ABSTRACT

The incorporation of telehealth into the daily clinical practice of audiologists in the United States is in its early stages of development. Some initial research has been conducted in order to validate the use of telehealth technologies in providing hearing and balance evaluation and management services (Krumm, Huffman, Dick, & Klich, 2008; Krumm, Ribera, & Klich, 2007;Krumm, Ribera, & Schmiedge, 2005; Lancaster, Krumm, & Ribera, 2008). More research is needed. This chapter suggests possible applications using existing technology and explores the possibility of virtual audiology clinics nation-wide and internationally.

Whatever the mind of man can conceive and believe, it can achieve—Napoleon Hill

INTRODUCTION

The above quote seems at the root of much of the technological revolution we are experiencing today. This is the stuff of which dreams are made as well as the inspiration for avant-guard thinking such as science-fiction. Who would have imagined 50 years ago that we would someday talk into little plastic boxes without wires and communicate with someone hundreds of miles away? It is thrilling to stand on the threshold of progress with the hopes of adapting modern and future technology to improve the quality of life for countless patients in need of medical evaluation and treatment.

As an audiologist I have given much thought to how technology can be inculcated into healthcare delivery systems for patients with hearing and or balance disorders. Most audiology healthcare providers are located in metropolitan and urban

DOI: 10.4018/978-1-61692-010-4.ch012

areas where population is denser and where there is access to a continuum of healthcare providers and services (ASHA, 2006). However, it is interesting to note that the prevalence of hearing impairment is greater in rural areas (Holt, Hotto, & Cole, 1994). Projections are that audiologists will be in demand for the foreseeable future (Bureau of Labor Statistics, 2008) with an estimated increase of 10% over the next six years. As patients tend to have a longer life expectancy than in the past, there will be an increasing need for audiological services. As universal newborn hearing screening compliance increases there will be additional requirements for pediatric audiologists with specialized training in evaluating and managing children with hearing disorders.

Telehealth/telemedicine seems to possess inherent capabilities of delivering hearing healthcare to remote areas or underserved populations. This chapter will address the history of telemedicine in the United States, recent research in the application of telehealth in audiology, challenges to be overcome, and what the future may hold.

BACKGROUND

Benefits

It seems almost intuitive that there are advantages to providing healthcare at a distance by a) filling a void in healthcare delivery to remote geographic regions, b) expanding access to essential medical services, c) reducing practitioner and/or patient travel time, d) reducing of cost in providing healthcare, d) expanding the dissemination of medical information to patients, e) and enhanced interaction (counseling and consultations) among healthcare providers and between clinicians and patients, to mention only a few.

Another possible benefit from telehealth technology is in support of the international movement to "go green" meaning to be more environmentally friendly and responsible about the carbon footprint we are leaving and to be more conscious of how we manage natural resources. Going green through telehealth seems to be a natural outcome. Use of existing and future technology will allow providers to reduce the amount of paper used, as well as the need for travel resulting in less consumption of fossil fuels. This might be a welcome by-product of adopting telehealth in general and tele-audiology specifically.

Telehealth delivery in audiology is truly in its infancy. There has been reticence on the part of audiologists to adopt this expansion of their scope of practice. There are several possible reasons for a delay in incorporating telehealth as part of the delivery model used by audiologists a) unfamiliarity with the technology, b) lack of confidence in outcomes, c) initial upfront cost for equipment and connectivity, d) training, e) licensure issues, f) reimbursement issues, g) paucity of validation studies, h) lack of standardization, i) safety and security issues, and j) patient acceptance/satisfaction. The challenge for pioneers in this area is to overcome the inertia and develop this delivery system more widely. There is need for more data to validate telehealth technology in audiology. The author invites colleagues from around the world to begin investigating how telehealth can be integrated into the audiologist's practice.

The Alaska Federal Healthcare Access Network (AFHCAN) has been providing audiological services via store and forward digital scans and high resolution images with ear, nose, throat (ENT) specialty physicians. This has resulted in a) reducing patient travel from rural villages, b) reducing wait time, c) reducing ENT patient backlog, and d) a savings of over $100,000 in travel costs per annum (Hofstetter, Kokesh, & Ferguson, 2008).

The American Speech Language and Hearing Association (ASHA) has developed several documents relating to the use of telehealth in speech-language pathology and audiology (ASHA, 2005a, 2005b, & 2005c). The American Academy of Audiology (AAA) has organized a Telehealth Task Force to consider the application of telehealth in the practice of audiology. A group of experienced audiologists with a vision of how this delivery system could be more fully used has been recently asked by AAA to establish guidelines for the use of telehealth in the practice of audiology. Several of the task force members have been involved in telehealth research related to audiology. Recently a resolution was passed by AAA to the effect that a) diagnostic and rehabilitative audiology telehealth or telemedicine services should always be provided by, or supervised by, a qualified audiologist, b) telehealth or telemedicine services should be primarily provided to individuals who have limited access to audiologists in their communities (e.g., homebound), and c) that audiology telehealth or telemedicine services should be validated before implementation to assure confidentiality and accuracy as well as to evaluate feasibility, particularly with difficult to test populations (newborns, infants, individuals with developmental disabilities) for which little or no validation of telehealth or telemedicine services currently exists"(AAA, 2008).

Research

Most of the hearing and balance related research in telehealth within the United States has been conducted at East Carolina University (North Carolina), Kent State University (Ohio), Minot State University (North Dakota), Tripler Army Medical Center (Hawaii), University of Hawaii, (Hawaii), and Utah State University (Utah). A review of the literature on telehealth and audiology can be broken down into categories such as a) overviews of telehealth applications in audiology (Givens, 2003; Ribera & Krumm, 2002), b) auditory brainstem response and otoacoustic emissions (Krumm, Huffman, Dick, & Klich, 2008; Krumm, Ribera, & Klich, 2007; Krumm, Ribera & Schmeidge, 2005; Towers, Pisa & Froelich, 2005), c) speech in noise testing (Ribera, 2005), d) counseling (Andersson, Stromgren, Strom, & Lyttkens, 2002; Kaldo-Sandstrom, Larsen, Andersson, 2004; Laplante-Leveque, Pichora-Fuller & Gagne, 2006), e) professional issues (Denton & Gladstone, 2005), f) audiometrics (Choi, & Oh, 2007; Elangovan, 2005; Lancaster, Krumm, & Ribera, 2008), g) vestibular testing (Yates, & Campbell, 2005), h) training, (Dansie, & Muñoz, 2008; Givens, Blanarovich, Murphy, Simmons, Blach, & Elangovan, 2003; Yates & Campbell, 2005), and i) video otoscopy (Hofstetter, Kokesh, & Ferguson, 2008). Pilot data at Utah State University suggest that programming of hearing aids and mapping of cochlear implants can also be accomplished using a telemedicine approach.

Delivery Models

The question should be asked "Which delivery model(s) might work best for audiology?" This can be answered by determining what the objectives are for providing audiological services via telehealth.

The traditional model of synchronous telehealth is one where a facilitator provides the face-to-face services while the audiologist supervises at a distance. A facilitator may be a nurse or other trained support staff, located at a remote site, and who is trained to assist the audiologist in such tasks as intake history, otoscopy (visual inspection of ear canal and tympanic membrane), patient instruction for each test, placement of earphones, and audiometric testing (air and bone conduction as well as speech tests). A clinic protocol is implemented under the supervision of an audiologist via web camera allowing him/her to visually observe how the tests are being administered. The advantage is that the audiologist can be reassured that the testing protocol is followed correctly and the data are reliable. The disadvantage is that the audiologist is spending time observing and less able to engage in other simultaneous activities at the local (hub) site.

The key to the successful use of a facilitator lies in the level and quality of training. If a "hub and spoke" model is used, training may be conducted simultaneously at several remote sites (the spokes) and broadcast from a central location (the hub) via videoconferencing. The audiologist must have confidence in the skill and knowledge of each remote site facilitator. There might also need to be some face-to-face training to ensure facilitator competency. In the final analysis, it is the healthcare provider (in this case the audiologist) who is ultimately responsible for the evaluation, care and treatment of the patient seen via a tele-audiology delivery system.

What is involved in being a facilitator? How much training is necessary? What is the best way to train a facilitator? These and other questions would need to be addressed during the initial stages of system development. There is evidence that training of a facilitator can be conducted via teleconferencing and results in skill and knowledge acquisition similar to that provided face-to-face (Dansie, & Muñoz, 2008).

Remote computing is an approach that allows the audiologist at the hub to assume control of a computer-based audiometer or other test equipment at the remote site where the patient is located. The role of the facilitator is simplified in this approach. He or she is responsible for all the hands-on tasks that cannot be performed by the audiologist, such as otoscopy, insertion of probe for immittance testing, and placement of earphones, bone oscillator, or electrodes. PC-based audiometers are becoming more and more available. With the right set up of computer application sharing and teleconferencing software an audiologist can take over the commands of a remote audiometer and conduct a comprehensive audiometric test battery and communicate directly with the patient (Krumm, Ribera, & Klich, 2007). This then becomes a virtual audiometer.

Store and forward is a relatively easy asynchronous approach, provided time is not an issue or there is no need for immediate referral. How would this be set up? Data could be collected and sent via regular mail, or transferred by electronic media such as email or by Internet using a web camera and displaying the data for the audiologist to see and interpret. For instance, a tracing of a tympanogram or the photo from a video otoscope could be viewed and interpreted by an audiologist. This would, of course, require good resolution for the audiologist to be able to read the tracing and data. Another approach that might be considered is to have the facilitator do the testing and record the results for the audiologist to review at a later time. This could include a video stream of the test to ensure proper technique was used.

What we do not know at this time is how well tele-audiology will be tolerated by patients with hearing or balance disorders. There may be cultural issues with which to deal. We need studies that evaluate a patient's perception of being treated at a distance and confiding in someone who is not in the same room. Does the patient feel he is receiving the same quality of medical attention via telehealth as he would face-to-face? We just do not know at this point.

Telehealth Technology

There is a continuum of technologies that can be incorporated into a tele-audiology practice. The technology set-up can be very simple such as plain old telephone systems (POTS), or more advanced such as facsimile (fax), email, video conferencing, and video streaming. When using tele-videoconferencing as a mode of hearing healthcare service delivery, it is preferable to have a camera with pan, tilt, and zoom capability. There also exists technology that allows the viewer to track a voice or face. This is a handy feature when there are multiple participants in a broadcast/teleconference. One application of such technology might be the use of tele-audiology in group counseling at one or more remote sites. Audiologists could use this service delivery approach after patients have been fitted with hearing aids. Several post fitting broadcasts would allow the audiologist to ascertain that new hearing aid users receive instruction in communication strategies, and hearing aid maintenance. In addition, the hearing healthcare provider could reiterate information that was presented during the initial hearing aid fitting, but which may have been forgotten or misunderstood. In this type of setting, patients would be free to ask questions of the audiologist or to interact with other hearing aid users either on site or located at other participating sites.

Where feasible, more than one camera might be preferable. For example, if a traditional (synchronous) model of delivery is being used, one camera could focus on the patient and the second could track the actions of the facilitator. Another consideration is the resolution of the video. The higher the resolution is the more expensive the camera. The question that needs to be asked is "What is the purpose of the video?" If it is to verify the correct placement of an insert phone into a new born infant's ear, then high resolution would be the system of choice. If the purpose is merely to see if the facilitator has correctly placed supra aural headphones on the ears of an adult, then a camera with low to mid resolution would suffice.

More and more audiometers are being developed and manufactured that are personal computer (PC)-based. This makes it relatively straightforward to use application sharing software between sites. Much of the research in tele-audiology that has been conducted has relied on computer-based applications. For example, a PC-based audiometer is located at a remote test site and is connected to the Internet. The computer at the remote site has not only the software to run the test equipment, but also video conferencing software with camera and audio capability. The audiologist at the hub (central location) located at a distance from the test site is also connected to the Internet and has compatible video conferencing software with application sharing capability. Once connected, the two sites enable real time interaction. Once control of the remote computer has been relinquished to the audiologist, he/she may begin to control the computer and audiometric test equipment at the remote site.

Telephone consults are probably the most basic and frequently used mode of telehealth. Video phones can provide some information that might be of value to the audiologist. While the video quality is not high definition at this time, the quality and resolution continues to improve with new developments in technology. The use of facsimile (fax) is another approach to hearing healthcare delivery and although the resolution is not as good as the original document being scanned, it does allow for the transmission of valuable information to the audiologist, such as an audiogram from a previous test at another clinic.

Connectivity can present challenges for all end users. There are some limitations with regard to bandwidth. Much depends on how the information is being sent whether by dial-up, DSL, or wide band. Usually the complaint from the end user is there is not enough bandwidth, particularly when using audio and video features simultaneously. There are also network issues such as what type of network to use e.g., local area networks (LAN), wide area networks (WAN), virtual private networks (VPN), or grid clusters. There are security issues such as how to get through fire walls. It is always best to ensure that data are encrypted in order to preclude unauthorized access to sensitive (personal medical) data. Grid technology addresses security issues and should make the transmission of sensitive data safe from outside intrusion.

Challenges to Overcome

There are several issues that have proven challenging to the incorporation of tele-audiology into every clinical practice. Progress has been slow in the area of reimbursement for services delivered via telehealth. Providers need to understand that insurance companies (payors) are not going to reimburse for services unless they are convinced that the services/procedures via telehealth are as valid as those provided face-to-face. This is where validation studies by researchers at universities and other laboratories can make a difference. Insurance companies want data to justify paying a claim for an audiological or other hearing/balance-related procedure.

A second challenging issue is that of licensure. Currently there is no legislation to allow the provision of audiological services across state borders in the United States. There is, however, a model that seems to be working for nursing. Twenty-three states have entered into a Nurse Licensure Compact (Nurse Licensure Compact, 2008) that allows practitioners to provide information to patients living in participating states without needing to be licensed in that state. This is similar in concept to the use of a driver's license issued in the state of California that allows a driver to operate a vehicle in any of the other 49 states, provided he or she abides by the local state laws.

A third issue deals with the cost of tele-audiology. No research to date has been published on the cost benefit for tele-audiology. This is not to suggest that there is no benefit. There is anecdotal information that suggests that without telehealth we face a) an increase in patients who cannot be treated because of distance from the healthcare provider, or b) loss of valuable time of the audiologist spent in travel and related costs when visiting outlying (remote) areas, resulting in periodic or no service.

FUTURE RESEARCH DIRECTIONS

Audiologists may want to begin to do some creative thinking in what the future might hold in terms of providing hearing healthcare in the future. One might take a conservative and simple approach. This approach would include more research, as well as actual implementation of a tele-audiology starting within one or two states. The objective would be to see what works best by starting small and building upon success. A simple approach in telehealth usually means less initial expense; however, it behooves all hearing healthcare providers to make their services available to as many people as possible.

While there is evidence that audiometric testing can be accomplished via telehealth, there is now a need for pioneers in the field to begin putting this evidence to work by incorporating this technology into clinical practice. An audiological test battery might include any or all of the following: air conduction, bone conduction, speech audiometry, electrophysiological tests (auditory brain stem response), and otoacoustic emissions. Further research is needed in immittance testing (middle ear analysis), psychoacoustic tests for tinnitus evaluation, cortical responses, hearing aid adjustments, electroacoustic analysis, as well as cochlear implant mapping. The day may come when a small box is connected to a patient's PC that can be controlled by an audiologist located at a considerable distance to facilitate making adjustments to a cochlear implant or hearing aid in real-time. The possibilities are limitless.

Global Virtual Clinic

In an ideal model there could be a world-wide virtual clinic. Imagine the day when a French-speaking patient goes on line and needs medical intervention for tinnitus (ringing in his ears). Several audiologists, otologists, nurses (who might be from different countries) have previously joined a virtual medical group (team) and agree to be on call for a specified number of hours each week. This could be an application of grid technology on a medical cluster. A call comes into a central clearing house that forwards the question or complaint to the provider (in this case a nurse) who is next in the queue. The nurse responds either by phone or by email to the inquiring patient. This immediate feedback helps to determine the nature and extent of the complaint. An online medical intake history can be filled out by the patient. The nurse makes a referral to the on-call audiologist based on the patient's input or questions. The audiologist can easily gain access to the patient's online responses and determine if he should have audiometric testing or be referred directly to a physician in his immediate area/region for a diagnostic evaluation. If a referral were needed, then the on-call provider could place a referral request into a queue. The next available otologist would respond to the referral and through further interaction with the patient determine the necessity and immediacy of a face-to-face consult.

Given the information provided above, a patient could then be referred to a local clinic (one in his close proximity). If that clinic has limited services a facilitator or nurse could assist in the evaluation, while the physician or audiologist conducts the evaluation at a distance. The clinic would be equipped with a system that is PC-based and connected to the Internet. The audiologist could gain access to the software running the PC and control all the test parameters. At the conclusion of the testing he/she could explain the results to the patient face-to-face using a camera and monitor.

There are several advantages for such a virtual clinic. First, there is a large pool of hearing-related healthcare providers. Second, is the ready and easy access to professionals anytime day or night. Third, is the convenience for the clinician to provide at least initial counseling and triage (screening). Fourth, there is no travel cost or time involved in the initial encounter. This could ensure timely diagnosis and treatment.

There are also disadvantages with this novel idea such as reimbursement issues. How would the hearing team members used in the scenario above be recompensed for their time and expertise? This might not be an issue among European countries where the Euro is the common currency. It could become quite a challenge, however, to bill for services if other currencies were involved. Also, to be evaluated by an international team may result in communication challenges (language differences). What would be the language for the encounter or for reports? Maybe the pool could be restricted to those who were fluent in one or more specific languages. For instance all French-speaking countries could be on the same grid/network or medical team. Third, different protocols or philosophies exist on how to evaluate and treat (manage) a patient. This is not a new challenge. There are areas of healthcare in the United States where there is no consensus on how to treat a certain condition. For example, the issue often arises as to whether or not children with recurring otitis media should have pressure equalization tubes (grommets) inserted. These differences would need to be addressed. Fourth, is the issue of the initial cost, depending on the sophistication of the system to be used.

These and other issues are not insurmountable, but they need to be addressed if tele-audiology is going to be considered as one of many possible approaches to world-wide healthcare. Tele-audiology is like a tool belt. It is only one tool among many and has a specific range of capabilities or applications. There is no one tool or test or therapy that fits the needs of every patient. It is up to the skilled professional to determine what the best use is and when is the best time to employ tele-audiology in providing hearing healthcare services.

CONCLUSION

Audiology is an allied healthcare profession in the United States and encompasses evaluation and treatment of hearing and balance related disorders. While delivery of these services may be different from state to state, the need continues to exist for healthcare providers to service not only those individuals in metropolitan areas, but also those in more remote areas. Although there has been a paucity of research in the area of telehealth and audiology compared to other disciplines, evidence suggests that the field of hearing and balance disorders, no matter who provides the services, is poised to begin embracing telehealth/telemedicine. It will take a few brave professionals to take the initial step and begin developing and implementing delivery models that are compatible with acceptable clinic protocols.

We must learn to crawl before we walk and to walk before we run. This is natural progression for the human race; so it is with telehealth and audiology. There is an ongoing technical revolution with no end in sight. That is both the good news and the bad news. The good news is new technology expands our current capabilities; the negative side of this is the technology changes rapidly, making incorporation of new technology challenging for the healthcare provider. Tele-audiology is really a multidisciplinary issue, where program and systems developers, technicians, healthcare providers, professional organizations, healthcare administrators, insurance payors, and legal counselors, need to jointly examine relevant issues. Each discipline can offer a unique perspective that will enrich the outcome and should ensure consensus.

Grid technology in audiology will undoubtedly start out small and evolve. Maybe it will begin in just one state; then adjoining states might enter into a compact, permitting telehealth patient encounters across state lines. The eventual goal would be to have a virtual clinic with a full spectrum of services that could be delivered via telehealth nation-wide and a protected database with restricted access to qualified grid users. Once the systems, protocols, licensure, reimbursement and connectivity issues are resolved at that level, then a progressive, systematic and responsible approach to international interaction would be a natural next step. This, of course, would be the ideal progression; however, a more likely scenario would follow a parallel evolution model. In this model, there might be simultaneous inter and intra-state development of tele-audiology applications.

As further research data become available we may be able to more clearly see how tele-audiology fits into the healthcare delivery model. It may not be feasible or even desirable to use tele-audiology in all situations. Evidence-based research may well suggest that tele-audiology is best suited for initial screening and that diagnostic evaluations are better conducted face-to-face. Another application of telehealth would be grand rounds or continuing education where case studies are available for comment and discussion internationally. This is rather an intriguing notion that would allow interaction among healthcare providers, facilitating dialogue among international healthcare colleagues, and promoting diverse thinking and problem solving.

REFERENCES

American Academy of Audiology. (2008). *AAA Resolution 2008-06. The use of Telehealth/Telemedicine to Provide Audiology Services*. Retrieved November 15, 2008 from http://www.audiology.org/advocacy/publicpolicyresolutions/Documents/TelehealthResolution 200806.pdf

American Speech-Language-Hearing Association. (2005a). *Audiologists Providing Clinical Services via Telepractice: Technical Report* [Technical Report]. Retrieved November 27, 2008, from www.asha.org/Policy

American Speech-Language-Hearing Association. (2005b). *Audiologists Providing Clinical Services via Telepractice: Position Statement* [Position Statement]. Retrieved November 28, from www.asha.org/policy.

American Speech-Language-Hearing Association. (2005c). *Knowledge and Skills Needed by Audiologists Providing Clinical Services via Telepractice* [Knowledge and Skills]. Retrieved November 27, 2008, from www.asha.org/policy

American Speech-Language-Hearing Association. (2006). *2006 Audiology Survey report: Survey methodology, respondent, demographics, and glossary*. Rockville, MD: Author.

Andersson, G., Stromgren, T., Strom, L., & Lyttkens, L. (2002). Randomized Controlled Trial Of Internet-Based Cognitive Behavior Therapy for Distress Associated with Tinnitus. *Psychosomatic Medicine*, *64*, 810–816. doi:10.1097/01.PSY.0000031577.42041.F8

Bureau of Labor Statistics. (2008). *Occupational Outlook Handbook*, 2008-2009 edition. Retrieved November 28, 2008, from: http://www.bls.gov/oco/oco20016.htm

Choi, Park, Oh, Park (2007). PC-based Tele-Audiometry. *Telemedicine and e-Health 13*(5), 501-508.

Dansie, J., & Muñoz, K. (2008). *Providing Training for Otoacoustic Emissions (OAE)*. Salt Lake City, Utah: Hearing Screening Using Telehealth. Intermountain Area Speech and Hearing Convention. [poster session]

Denton, D., & Gladstone, V. (2005). Ethical and Legal Issues Related to Telepractice. *Seminars in Hearing*, *26*(1), 43–52. doi:10.1055/s-2005-863794

Elangovan, S. (2005). Telehearing and the Internet. *Seminars in Hearing*, *26*(1), 19–25. doi:10.1055/s-2005-863791

Givens, G., Blanarovich, A., Murphy, T., Simmons, S., Blach, D., & Elangovan, S. (2003). Internet-based tele-audiometry system for the assessment of hearing: a pilot study. *Telemedicine Journal Electronic Health*, *9*, 375–378. doi:10.1089/153056203772744707

Hofstetter, P., Kokesh, J., & Ferguson, S. (2008). A telehealth model—delivering hearing healthcare to remote sites. *Telemedicine and e-Health, March 1, 2008, 14*(s1), 24-81.

Holt, J., Hotto, S., & Cole, K. (1994). *Demographic aspects of hearing impairment: questions and answers,* (3rd ed.). Retrieved November 25, 2008, from http://gri.gallaudet.edu/demographics/factsheet.html

Kaldo-Sandstrom, V., Larsen, H., & Andersson, G. (2004). Internet-based cognitive-behavioral self-help treatment of tinnitus: clinical effectiveness and predictors of outcome. *American Journal of Audiology*, *13*(2), 185–192. doi:10.1044/1059-0889(2004/023)

Krumm, M., & Huffman, T., Dick, & Klich, R. (2008). Providing infant hearing screening using OAEs and AABR using telehealth technology. *Journal of Telemedicine and Telecare*, *14*(2), 102–104. doi:10.1258/jtt.2007.070612

Krumm, M., Ribera, J., & Klich, R. (2007). Providing basic hearing tests using remote computing technology. *Journal of Telemedicine and Telecare*, *13*, 406–410. doi:10.1258/135763307783064395

Krumm, M., Ribera, J., & Schmiedge, J. (2005). Using a Telehealth Medium for Objective Hearing Testing: Implications for Supporting Rural Universal Newborn Hearing Screening Programs. *Seminars in Hearing*, *26*(1), 3–12. doi:10.1055/s-2005-863789

Lancaster, P., Krumm, K., & Ribera, J. (2008). Remote hearing screenings via telehealth in a rural elementary school. *American Journal of Audiology*, *17*(2), 114–122. doi:10.1044/1059-0889(2008/07-0008)

Laplante-Leveque, A., Pichora-Fuller, M., & Gagne, J. (2006). Providing an internet-based audiological counseling programme to new hearing aid users: A qualitative study. *International Journal of Audiology*, *45*, 697–706. doi:10.1080/14992020600944408

Nurse Licensure Compact Administrators. (2008). *Nurse Licensure Compact*. Retrieved December 1, 2008 from https://www.ncsbn.org/nlc.htm

Retrieved November 30, 2008, from doi:10.1089/tmj.2008.9979.supp

Ribera, J. (2005). Interjudge Reliability and Validation of Telehealth Applications of the Hearing in Noise Test. *Seminars in Hearing*, *26*(1), 13–18. doi:10.1055/s-2005-863790

Ribera, J., & Krumm, M. (2002) Telepractice in Audiology. *Audiology Online* (www.audiology-online.com), Posted April 1, 2002.

Towers, A., Pisa, J., & Froelich, T. (2005). The Reliability of Click-Evoked and Frequency-Specific Auditory Brainstem Response Testing Using Telehealth Technology. *Seminars in Hearing*, *26*(1), 26–34. doi:10.1055/s-2005-863792

Yates, J., & Campbell, K. (2005). Audiovestibular education and services via telemedicine technologies. *Seminars in Hearing*, *26*, 35–42. doi:10.1055/s-2005-863793

KEY TERMS AND DEFINITIONS

Asynchronous Telehealth: Delivery of healthcare or medically related information via electronic media after data have been collected.

Audiology: An allied healthcare profession dealing with the evaluation and treatment of hearing and balance disorders.

PC-Based Audiometer: Software and hardware system that connects to and is controlled through a personal computer.

Remote Computing: Controlling software applications at a remote site from a local computer.

Tele-Audiology: Provision of audiological services via telehealth technology.

Telehealth: Provision of healthcare services via electronic media.

Synchronous Telehealth: Real-time collection or dissemination of medically-related data.

Virtual Clinic: Provision of clinic services via cyberspace.

Chapter 13
Global Health Network Supercourse and Cancer Epidemiology:
Free Cancer Epidemiology Resources on the Internet

Faina Linkov
University of Pittsburgh Cancer Institute, USA

Elizabeth Radke
University of Pittsburgh Graduate School of Public Health, USA

Mita Lovalekar
University of Pittsburgh Graduate School of Public Health, USA

Ronald LaPorte
University of Pittsburgh Graduate School of Public Health, USA

"A teacher effects eternity. One can never tell where his influence stops." - A. Lincoln

CANCER BURDEN IN DEVELOPED AND DEVELOPING COUNTRIES: THE NEED FOR E-HEALTH APPROACHES

Cancer is a potent cause of death in both the developed and the developing world. The number of global cancer deaths is projected to increase 45% from 2007 to 2030 (from 7.9 million to 11.5 million deaths), influenced in part by an increasing and aging global population (WHO 2008). A recent report from WHO also reveals that cancer has emerged as a major public health problem in developing countries, matching its effect in industrialized nations (Sener 2005). Cancer is the second leading cause of death in the U.S. and in many different parts of the world. With significant improvement in treatment and prevention of cardiovascular diseases, cancer has or will soon become the number one killer in many parts of the world. As elderly people are most susceptible to cancer and population aging continues in many countries, cancer will remain a major health problem around the globe (Ma 2006). Although age is the single greatest risk factor for most cancers, preventable causes of cancer including tobacco use, poor diet and lack of exercise, and infectious

DOI: 10.4018/978-1-61692-010-4.ch013

agents contribute significantly to global cancer trends (Sener 2005).

In addition to this cancer epidemic, we are currently witnessing important technological advancements, including rapid development of Internet-based learning technologies. The Internet is rapidly penetrating hospitals, schools, universities, and homes in the US and around the world. It can therefore be harnessed to reduce the global burden of cancer.

For example, of the 190,000 deaths from cervical cancer that occur annually worldwide, the majority take place in developing countries. Recent advances in our understanding of the causes and natural history of cervical neoplasia and, in particular, the establishment of the central role of human papilloma virus (HPV) infection have created opportunities for the primary and secondary prevention of cervical cancer (Rohan 2003). Sadly, despite recent advances in cervical cancer screening and prevention, many women around the world are needlessly dying of this disease. Given that one of the main predictors of nonattendance for Pap smears is lack of knowledge about the purpose and benefits of screening (Eaker 2004), this situation can potentially be at least partly corrected with better integration of prevention education into the curricula of various schools around the world. Obviously, lack of resources to obtain preventive tools such as the HPV vaccine is also an obstacle.

Clearly, cancer is a menace to all countries. The most common cancers (such as lung cancer) are potentially preventable with appropriate sharing and utilization of prevention information. Cancer prevention is likely the only cost-effective means to reduce the cancer burden in both developing and developed countries. Few studies have examined the science of translation and implementation of prevention information (Ma 2006). There have been even fewer scientific studies examining the translation of prevention research into the classroom. In order to improve global cancer education, global cancer educators need access to good educational lectures and existing data in the area of cancer morbidity and mortality. This chapter will concentrate on describing several resources of cancer information available on the Internet: the Supercourse, SEER, CANCERMondiale, and Cancer Atlas.

Using Existing Electronic Resources for Obtaining Data

Cancer prevention is not possible without access to reliable cancer data. Two core statistics are the cancer incidence rate and the cancer mortality rate, which provide estimates of the average risk of acquiring and of dying from the disease, respectively. About 16% of the world's population is covered by registration systems that produce cancer incidence statistics, while mortality data are available for about 29% (Parkin 2006). Despite the fact that only a small proportion of the world's population is covered by registries, these registries are providing unique epidemiologic information on cancer burden in the U.S. and around the world. This chapter will describe three very important sources of cancer data available on the Internet: SEER, CANCERMondiale, and Cancer Atlas

SEER

The Surveillance, Epidemiology, and End Results (SEER) Program of the National Cancer Institute (NCI) (Figure 1) is an authoritative source of information on cancer incidence and survival in the United States. SEER currently collects and publishes cancer incidence and survival data from population-based cancer registries covering approximately 26% of the US population. SEER coverage includes 23 percent of African Americans, 40 percent of Hispanics, 42 percent of American Indians and Alaska Natives, 53 percent of Asians, and 70 percent of Hawaiian/Pacific Islanders. The SEER Program is the only comprehensive source of population-based information in the United

Figure 1. SEER front page

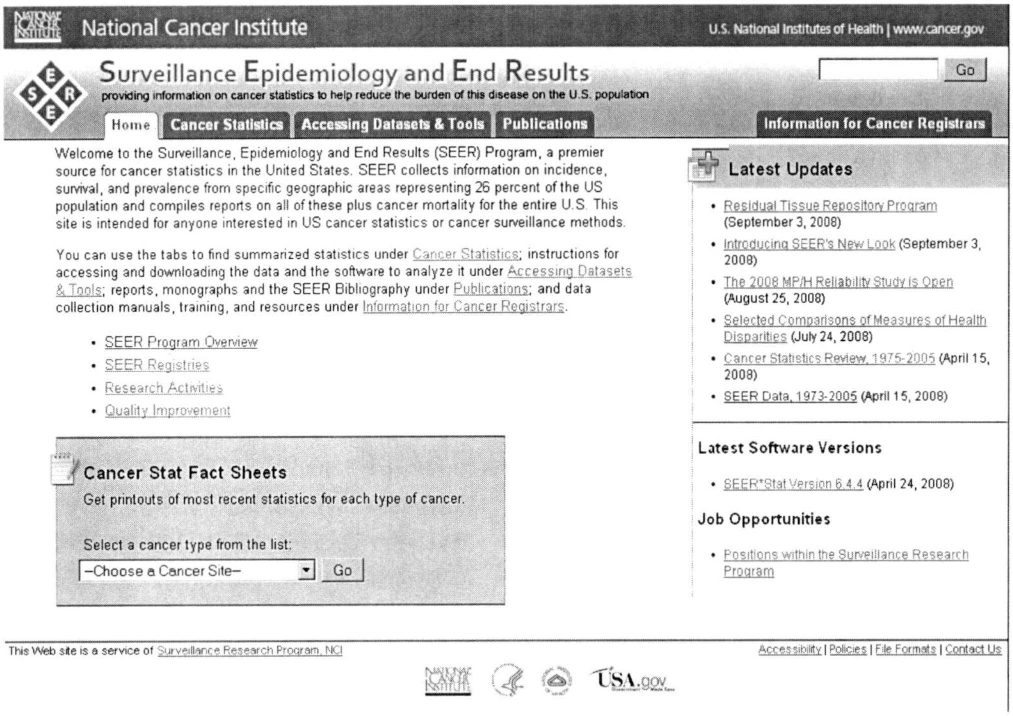

States that includes stage of cancer at the time of diagnosis and patient survival data (SEER 2008).

CANCER*Mondial*

CANCER*Mondial* website (Figure 2) provides access to information on the occurrence of cancer world-wide held by the Descriptive Epidemiology

Figure 2. CANCERMondial front page

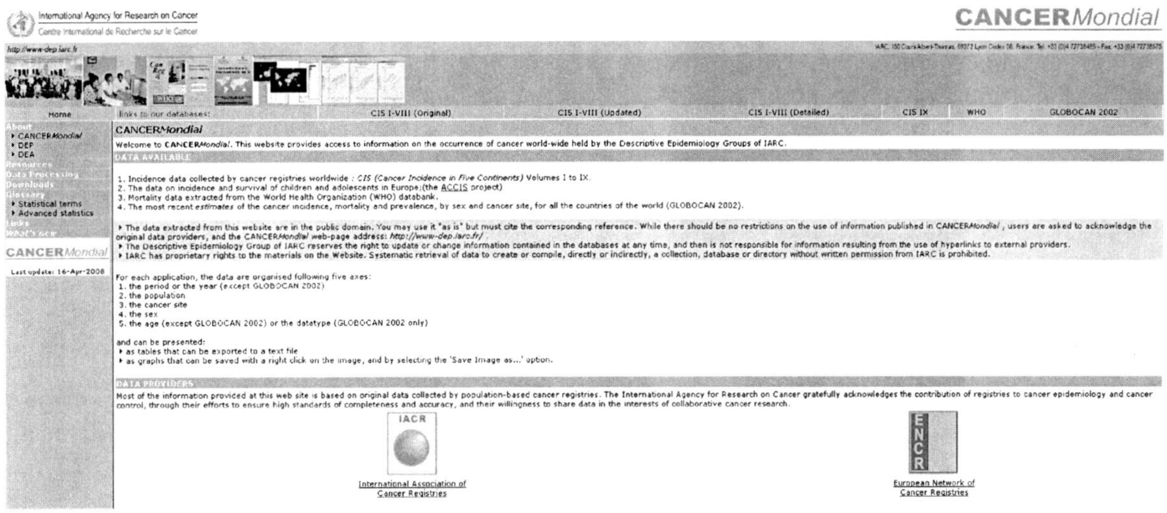

Groups of International Agency for Research on Cancer (IARC). This includes cancer incidence data from registries worldwide. The data extracted from this website are in the public domain. You may use it "as is" but must cite the corresponding reference (IARC 2008), along with the acknowledgement of the original data provider.

For each application, the data are organized following five axes:

1. the period or the year (except GLOBOCAN 2002)
2. the population
3. the cancer site
4. the sex
5. the age (except GLOBOCAN 2002) or the datatype (GLOBOCAN 2002 only) and can be presented:
   as tables that can be exported to a text file
   as graphs that can be saved with a right click on the image, and by selecting the 'Save Image as...' option.

Cancer Atlas

The "Atlas of Cancer Mortality in the United States, 1950-94" (Figure 3) was released in December 1999. Two Web sites are associated with the Atlas. "The Atlas On-Line" is an interactive version of the Atlas, which enables the user to view and print everything in the Atlas. The user can also download the maps and figures appearing in the Atlas, as well as the data used to generate the maps. "Customizable Maps" enables the user to create maps by controlling parameters such as number of ranges, ranging method, and colors. The user can also zoom, pan, and view an individual state, state economic area, or county. This system does not have data for cancer mortality outside the United States. (Devesa 1999)

The **Cancer Mortality Maps & Graph** Web Site provides interactive maps, graphs (which are accessible to the blind and visually-impaired),

Figure 3. Atlas of Cancer Mortality front page from Dan Grauman's Supercourse lecture http://www.pitt.edu/~super1/lecture/lec1241/001.htm

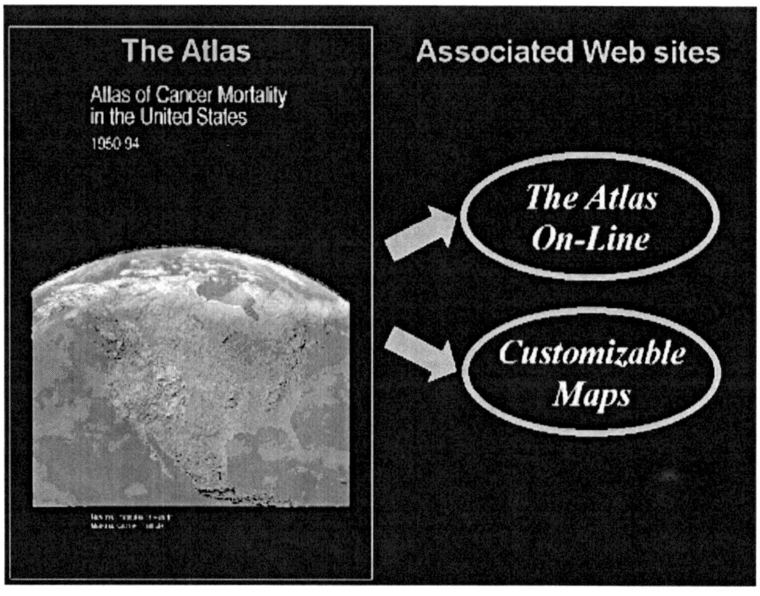

text, tables and figures showing geographic patterns and time trends of cancer death rates for the time period 1950-1994 for more than 40 cancers (NCI 2008)

Databases of Cancer Grants

In addition to cancer surveillance databases, there are systems that assemble cancer research. The International Cancer Research Portfolio contains information about actively funded research from several countries classified by type of cancer, area of research, and funding organization (ICRP 2008). In the United States, the Computer Retrieval of Information on Scientific Projects (CRISP) is a database that includes biomedical research projects and programs supported by the Department of Health and Human Services, including those involving cancer (HHS 2008). These databases and others are necessary for international scientists to obtain information on projects that are already funded in cancer research. This can potentially lead to scientific collaboration and innovation.

All of the previously discussed databases provide important, easily accessible resources in the area of cancer. However, in addition to these types of cancer information, it is important for faculty members around the world to have easy access to theoretical foundations of cancer epidemiology. Outside the US and UK, schools of public health are not easily found and access to inexpensive educational materials in the area of epidemiology is not always good. This is especially problematic for the developing world, where digital divide oftentimes separates haves and have nots. The Global Health Network Supercourse, described in detail in the next part of this chapter, provides a very unique combination of educational materials that in conjunction with freely available statistical information, such as SEER, can become a good source of public health information for scientists and instructors in both developing and developed countries.

Supercourse: The On-Line System for Obtaining PowerPoint Lectures in the Area of Cancer

The Parent Supercourse comprises 4200 PowerPoint lectures on prevention that are housed in a lecture library on the Internet (www.pitt.edu/~super1/). It is an open source system where scientists across the world share their best lectures for free and every lecture is "copy left", instead of copy right, and thus usable by anyone. In the past 10 years the Global Health Network Supercourse built a network of over 50,000 scientists from 174 countries. The Supercourse developers are working on bringing the concept of a Supercourse model to cancer prevention. The Cancer Prevention Supercourse will be used to "Whisk research into the classroom" as we described in the British Medical Journal (LaPorte 2002). Our goal is to research how best to translate cancer prevention science into the classrooms of the world for better prevention of cancer. Our research is national and international, with over 30% of the faculty from developing countries. We are one of the few epidemiology groups concerned about the "unreached" populations around the world.

The problem of research to classroom translation is evident in almost all college classrooms where cancer prevention is taught. Recently we have examined a sample of books used in cancer courses in the Graduate School of Public Health and the Medical School at the University of Pittsburgh. The most recent references in these books for cancer prevention research were 3-10 years old. Clearly, we are not translating the latest research into the classroom in timely manner.

Lectures

The lectures are like any PowerPoint lectures that would be used as building blocks of curricula in various educational institutions. They are designed to help teachers educate students about cancer prevention. This does not necessarily mean that the lectures will produce immediate functional or behavioral changes, but does suggest that changes will likely occur in the future. We are thus researching how to advance knowledge and education by not excluding people from developing countries and the un-reached. Cancer education is viewed as being vitally important in the war against cancer.

This is an innovative concept that can lead to a marked improvement in the translation of knowledge to the classroom in developing countries, in developed countries and your classroom. If we marry cancer prevention with the Internet and make this information accessible, we can have a profound effect on the world through improved communication of cancer prevention information.

Cancer Network

The Supercourse has 329 faculty and researchers interested in cancer research. There are 46 experts from the National Cancer Institute, and many more from other prestigious institutions such as the American Cancer Society (7 members), Dana-Farber Cancer Institute (9 members), Fred Hutchinson Cancer Research Center (20 members) and the Memorial Sloan Kettering Cancer Center (6 members). The Supercourse library has many important lectures in the area of cancer prevention and control (Figure 4). A few examples of valuable contributors are:

- Dr. Dan Grauman from NCI (National Cancer Institute), demonstrating how to use the Cancer Atlas
- Dr. Leeland Hartwell, Nobel Prize Laureate, who recently donated a ground-breaking lecture on yeast and cancer
- Dr. Gilbert Omenn, professor at the University of Michigan and former president of the American Association for Advancement in Science (AAAS), donated several lectures including the one on cancer prevention
- Dr. Baruch Blumberg, whose revolutionary work in the area of Hepatitis B was very important for the prevention of liver cancer.

This vibrant network of cancer professionals is not static, it is continuously evolving and attracting more and more professionals from various disciplines each year.

Target Group: Educators of the World

Using our lectures, educators can teach from elementary school, to graduate school to "leisure learning for retirees". An elementary school teacher will understand most of the cancer prevention lectures, and can modify or customize the lectures

Figure 4. Cancer Network: selected lectures

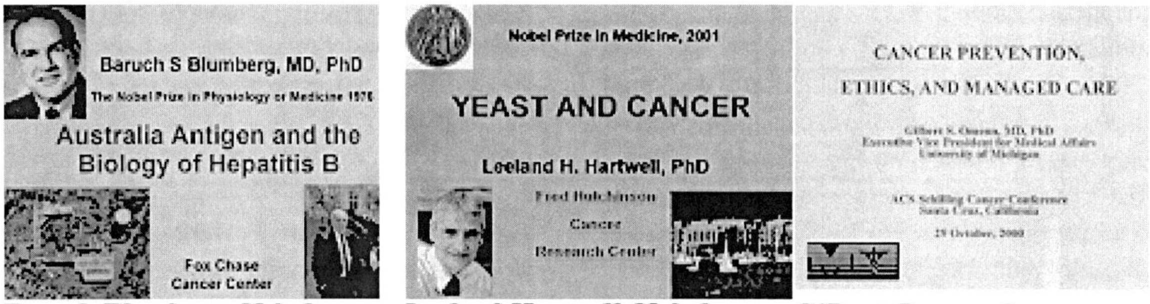

Baruch Blumberg, Nobel Prize Laureate | Leeland Hartwell, Nobel Prize Laureate | Gilbert Omenn, former president of AAAS

for young children. If we can improve teaching in the classroom, we can reach many students today and for generations to come. By networking the experts and targeting the teachers, we have a powerful combination. We have established one of the first mechanisms where we can tap into the collective intelligence of cancer experts, and readily disseminate their knowledge to teachers.

This will also benefit faculty members, students, nurses, doctors, rehabilitation professionals, and all educators. For example, if one needed to present a lecture on breast cancer, there are 15 lectures that have slides on global breast cancer. Typically, it takes, an expert teacher 10-15 hours to prepare a lecture on a new topic. With the Supercourse, one can have an exciting lecture in 1-3 hours. Using this template model, we can prepare better lectures, at 1/5 the time. Much of the preparation time is eliminated. There is no need to "reinvent" the wheel, all we need to do is to share template lectures. This is particularly important for the public health topics that already have large numbers of existing lectures. For example, Supercourse has many lectures on smoking and health, including several lectures dedicated to the work of Sir Richard Doll. For junior faculty members, it does not make sense to reinvent new lectures on smoking and health, if they can have free access to the lecture given by Dr. Doll.

Additionally, there is a need to build more programs for translation of research from labs to practice. Supercourse could become a unique tool for guiding junior faculty members in the development and implementation of anti-smoking research programs and many other important public health efforts. Thus, the SEER, Cancer Atlas and CANCER*Mondial* are systems to evaluate the trends of cancer. The Supercourse is a means to educate about prevention, and if these prevention efforts are successful, one can track these public health changes through the SEER and other programs

Progress Report: Internet and Prevention

The speed at which the information revolution is occurring is remarkable. Since 1975 the speed and memory of computers has increased 1,000,000 fold and prices have plummeted. A $2,000 PC is equivalent to a $10,000,000 supercomputer in 1975. The Economist pointed out that if automobile technology improved as rapidly as IT, a car would speed along at 100,000 miles per hour, get 200,000 miles per gallon of gas, and cost $5.00. Acquisition and dissemination of knowledge in cancer prevention has not been as rapid as IT. However, bringing the Internet into cancer prevention could markedly accelerate the pace of progress in our field by bringing together those involved in cancer prevention, education and other areas of science.

Telepreventive Medicine Concept

Remarkable improvements in cancer prevention have occurred in the US and across the world this century. We argue that the 21st century will be the era of Teleprevention (Eaker 2004). Our scientific approaches have been driven by the new information technologies that have begun to play a major role in cancer prevention. We have coined the word **"telepreventive medicine"**. This new field uses the tools of the Internet to share information with large numbers of healthy people to prevent disease. It is different from telemedicine, which targets expensive telecommunications technologies to a small number of sick people to "cure" disease. We believe that a telepreventive medicine approach will have a much greater effect on improving the health of the world. However, the research field of telepreventive medicine is in its infancy. Teleprevention is rapidly becoming a new field in public health.

Progress Report and Current Status

Cancer prevention is increasingly becoming global. Destruction of the ozone layer might be related to melanomas in Auckland and California; global migrations bring new patterns of cancer, world trade of tobacco impacts cancer risk, and cancer prevention. Despite the globalization of cancer prevention, there has been little globalization of prevention research. We have established the technologies where global education is now possible, and educators can learn from each other.

What will make our research more successful is the building of an International Library of Lectures for Cancer Prevention on the Internet. As part of our parent Supercourse, we have already gathered a large and vibrant group of scientists, and have networked faculty from 174 countries. We already have hundreds of faculty specializing in cancer epidemiology. About 20-30% of our lectures are coming from developing countries, providing a good contrast to major biomedical journals that publish only a very small percentage of materials from the developing world.

As of August 2009, the Supercourse has 177 lectures dedicated to cancer epidemiology. These lectures are available in six different languages. Among the lecture authors, Supercourse has four researchers from the National Cancer Institute who have provided 13 lectures on cancer. Among other notable authors, we have two AES members who have donated four lectures, three NAS members who donated five lectures, two Nobel Prize Laureates who donated two lectures, and three Institute of Medicine members who donated five lectures. Supercourse has a large selection of lectures that have a great relevance to cancer epidemiology and cancer control. These include 38 lectures devoted to smoking control and 253 lectures on environmental health.

Supercourse lectures, which provide great theoretical background on cancer epidemiology and public health research methods in general, become even more valuable when used in conjunction with existing data resources like Cancer*Mondiale*, SEER, and Cancer Atlas. By linking these two areas, theory is supported by practical opportunities to explore the data, evaluate cancer trends, and produce new publications. Collaborative efforts between public health faculty members around the world, supported by collaboration with cancer data promises to be a unique and low cost approach to better cancer research locally and globally.

"If everyone is moving forward together, then success takes care of itself."-Henry Ford

We would like to invite all faculty members around the world to join the Supercourse network. For more information, please e-mail Super1@pitt.edu

REFERENCES

Cancer Mortality Maps & Graphs. (2008). National Cancer Institute. Retrieved from http://www3.cancer.gov/atlasplus/

CANCERMondial. (2008). International Agency for Research on Cancer. Retrieved from http://www-dep.iar.fr/

Computer Retrieval of Information on Scientific Projects. (2008). Department of Health and Human Services. Retrieved from http://crisp.cit.nih.gov/

Devesa, S., Grauman, D. J., Blot, W. J., Pennello, G., & Hoover, R. N. (1999) *Atlas of cancer mortality in the United States: 1950-94*. Washington, DC: US Govt Print Off. NIH 99-4564: 360.

Eaker, S., Adami, H., Granath, F., Wilander, E., & Sparen, P. (2004). A Large Population-Based Randomized Controlled Trial to Increase Attendance at Screening for Cervical Cancer. *Cancer Epidemiology, Biomarkers & Prevention*, *13*, 346–354.

ICRP: A Joint Initiative of International Cancer Research Funding Organizations. (2008). International Cancer Research Portfolio. Retrieved from http://www.cancerportfolio.org/index.jsp

Laporte, R. E. (2002). Whisking research into the classroom. *BMJ (Clinical Research Ed.)*, *324*(7329), 99. doi:10.1136/bmj.324.7329.99

Ma, X., & Yu, H. (2006). Global burden of cancer. *The Yale Journal of Biology and Medicine*, *79*(3-4), 85–94.

Overviewof the SEER Program. (2008). Surveillance Epidemiology and End Results. Retrieved from http://seer.cancer.gov/about

Parkin, D. M., & Fernandez, L. M. (2006). Use of statistics to assess the global burden of breast cancer. *The Breast Journal*, *12*(Suppl 1), S70–S80. doi:10.1111/j.1075-122X.2006.00205.x

Rohan, T. E., Burk, R. D., & Franco, E. L. (2003). Toward a reduction of the global burden of cervical cancer. *American Journal of Obstetrics and Gynecology*, *189*(4Suppl), S37–S39. doi:10.1067/S0002-9378(03)01079-2

Sener, S. F., & Grey, N. (2005). The global burden of cancer. *Journal of Surgical Oncology*, *92*(1), 1–3. doi:10.1002/jso.20335

WHO. (2008). *Are the number of cancer cases increasing or decreasing in the world?* World Health Organization Online Q&A. Retrieved from http://www.who.int/features/qa/15/en/index.html.

Compilation of References

(2005). *Plunkett's Health Care Industry Almanac*. Houston, TX: Plunkett Research, Ltd.

A Simple API for Grid Applications (SAGA). (n.d.). Retrieved from http://saga.cct.lsu.edu/index.php?option=com_content&task=view&id=71&Itemid=158

Aas, I. H. M. (1997). Organizational change: decentralization in hospitals. *The International Journal of Health Planning and Management*, *12*, 103–114. doi:10.1002/(SICI)1099-1751(199704)12:2<103::AID-HPM461>3.0.CO;2-5

Aas, I. H. M. (2001). Telemedical work and co-operation. *Journal of Telemedicine and Telecare*, *7*, 212–218. doi:10.1258/1357633011936426

Aas, I. H. M. (2002). Learning in organizations working with telemedicine. *Journal of Telemedicine and Telecare*, *8*, 107–111. doi:10.1258/1357633021937569

Aas, I. H. M. (2005). Organizational cooperation in teleradiology. *Journal of Telemedicine and Telecare*, *11*, 45–50. doi:10.1258/1357633053430449

Aas, I. H. M. (2006a). Organizational centralization in radiology. *Journal of Telemedicine and Telecare*, *12*, 27–32. doi:10.1258/135763306775321344

Aas, I. H. M. (2006b). Organizational decentralization in radiology. *Journal of Telemedicine and Telecare*, *12*(Suppl. 1), 1–3. doi:10.1258/135763306777978524

Aas, I. H. M. (2007). The organizational challenge for health care from telemedicine and e-health. Oslo, The Work Research Institute. Retrieved November 20, 2008, from http://www.afi.no/stream_file.asp?iEntityId=2088

Abel-Smith, B. (1989). Health economies in developing countries. *The Journal of Tropical Medicine and Hygiene*, *92*, 229–241.

About, E. R. *A*. (2010). Retrieved from http://www.era.pl/en/home/company/ptc

Abrahamian, H., Schueller, A., Mauler, H., Prager, R., & Irsigler, K. (2002). Transfer of knowledge from the specialist to the generalist by videoconferencing: effect on diabetes care. *Journal of Telemedicine and Telecare*, *8*, 350–355. doi:10.1258/135763302320939248

ActiveBPEL. (n.d.). Retrieved from http://www.activevos.com/community-open-source.php

Ad-Dab'bagh, Y., et al. (2005). Native space cortical thickness measurement and the absence of correlation to cerebral volume. In K. Zilles, (ed.), *Proceedings of the 11th Annual Meeting of the Organization for Human Brain Mapping*, Toronto, NeuroImage 2005.

Afford, W. (2003). *Corrosive reform: failing health systems in Eastern Europe, ILO Socio-Economic Security Programme, Geneva 2003*. Accessible at http://www.ilo.org/public/english/bureau/inf/features/03/health.htm

After the outbreak. (2003, April 3rd). *Economist*.

Ahmed, W., Lenz, D., Liu, J., Robinson, P. J., & Ghafoor, A. (2008). XML-Based Data Model and architecture for a knowledge-based grid-enabled problem-solving environment for high-throughput biological imaging. *IEEE Transactions on Information Technology in Biomedicine*, *12*, 226–237. doi:10.1109/TITB.2007.904153

Akhtar, R. (Ed.). (1991). *Health Care Patterns and Planning in Developing Countries* (pp. 1–336). New York: Greenwood Press.

Alberts, D. S., Garstka, J. J., & Stein, F. P. (1999). Network Centric Warfare: Developing and Leveraging Information Superiority. *CCRP Publ.* From: http://www.dodccrp.org/files/Alberts_NCW.pdf

Alberts, D. S., Garstka, J. J., & Stein, F. P. (2000). *Network Centric Wardare: Developing and Leveraging Information Superiority*, (pp 1-284). Washington, DC: CCRP Publication Series. Retrieved from http://www.dodccrp.org/publications/pdf/Alberts_NCW.pdf

Alberts, D. S., Garstka, J. J., Hayes, R. E., & Signori, D. A. (2001). *Understanding Information Age Warfare*. Washington, DC: CCRP Press. Retrieved from http://%20 www.dodccrp.org/ publications/ pdf/ Alberts_UIAW.pdf

Aloisio, G., Barba, M. C., Biasi, E., Cafaro, M., Fiore, S., & Mirto, M. (2005). A web service-based Grid portal for Edgebreaker compression. *Methods of Information in Medicine*, *44*(2), 233–238.

Alonso, J. M., Ferroero, J. M. Jr, Hernánde, Z. V., Moltò, G., Saiz, J., & Trénor, B. (2008). A grid-based approach for the acce;eration of simulation in cardiology. *IEEE Transactions on Information Technology in Biomedicine*, *12*(2), 138–144.

Alonso, J. M., Ferrero, J. M., Hernandez, V., Molto, G., Saiz, J., & Trenor, B. (2008)... *IEEE Transactions on Information Technology in Biomedicine*, *12*(2). doi:10.1109/TITB.2007.907982

Amendolia, R., Estrella, F., Hauer, T., Manset, D., McCabe, D., McClatchey, R., et al. Grid databases for shared image analysis in the mammogrid project. In *Proc. 8th Int. Database Eng. Appl. Symp. (Ideas2004)*, pp. 302–311.

Amendolia, S. R., Estrella, F., Hassan, W., Hauer, T., Manset, D., McClatchey, R., et al. (2004). MammoGrid: A Service Oriented Architecture Based Medical Grid Application. In *Proceedings of the 3rd International Conference on Grid and Cooperative Computing – GCC'04*. Wuhan, China, (LNCS Vol. 3251, pp 939-942). Berlin: Springer-Verlag.

American Academy of Audiology. (2008). *AAA Resolution 2008-06. The use of Telehealth/Telemedicine to Provide Audiology Services*. Retrieved November 15, 2008 from http://www.audiology.org/advocacy/publicpolicyresolutions/Documents/TelehealthResolution 200806.pdf

American Speech-Language-Hearing Association. (2006). *2006 Audiology Survey report: Survey methodology, respondent, demographics, and glossary*. Rockville, MD: Author.

American Speech-Language-Hearing Association. (2005a). *Audiologists Providing Clinical Services via Telepractice: Technical Report* [Technical Report]. Retrieved November 27, 2008, from www.asha.org/Policy

American Speech-Language-Hearing Association. (2005b). *Audiologists Providing Clinical Services via Telepractice: Position Statement* [Position Statement]. Retrieved November 28, from www.asha.org/policy.

American Speech-Language-Hearing Association. (2005c). *Knowledge and Skills Needed by Audiologists Providing Clinical Services via Telepractice* [Knowledge and Skills]. Retrieved November 27, 2008, from www.asha.org/policy

AMGA – the ARDA Metadata Catalogue Project. (n.d.). Retrieved from http://amga.web.cern.ch/amga/

Ammen, E., & Versweyveld, L. (1998). Virtual Medical Worlds Magazine - A Euromed on-line information building block for HPCN related telemedicine. *Future Generation Computer Systems*, *14*(1-2), 131–136. doi:10.1016/S0167-739X(98)00015-6

Andalusi, I., Blanquer, I., Breton, V., Dobrev, A., van Dooselaere, C., & Hernandez, V. (2008). The SHARE road map: healthgrids for biomedical research and healthcare. *Studies in Health Technology and Informatics*, *138*, 238–278.

Anderson, R. J., & Boumbulian, P. J. (1997). Beyond the safety net in Dallas. *Health Affairs*, *16*, 27–29. doi:10.1377/hlthaff.16.4.27

Anderson, P. (2007). What is Web 2.0? Ideas, technologies and implications for education. *JISC Technology and Standards Watch,* (Feb. 2007). Retrieved from http://www.jisc.org.uk/media/documents/techwatch/tsw0701b.pdf

Andersson, G., Stromgren, T., Strom, L., & Lyttkens, L. (2002). Randomized Controlled Trial Of Internet-Based Cognitive Behavior Therapy for Distress Associated with Tinnitus. *Psychosomatic Medicine*, *64*, 810–816. doi:10.1097/01.PSY.0000031577.42041.F8

Andrew, D., Jurik, & Alfred, C.W. (2008). Remote Medical Monitoring. *Computer Magazine,* 96-99.

Andronico, G. Barbera, R. Falzone, A. Lo Re, G., Pulvirenti, A., Rodolico, A. (2005). The GENIUS web portal – an easy way yo access the Grid. *Methods Inf. Med.*

Anirban, G., Anirban, C., Dheepak, R. A., & Shaken, A. (2007). Streamlining drug discovery research by leveraging grid workflow manager. *Infosys Nov. 2007.* Retrieved from http://www.infosys.com/industries/life-sciences/white-papers/streamlining-drug-discovery.pdf

Anjum, A., Bloodsworth, P., Habib, I., Lansdale, T., McClatchey, R., Mehmood, Y. & The neuGRID Consortium. (2009). *Reusable Services from the neuGRID Project for Grid-Based Health Applications.* Accepted as Poster at the International Healthgrid'09 Conference.

Anvari, M. (2007). Impact of information technology on human resources in healthcare. *Healthcare Quarterly, 10,* 84-88. Retrieved November 9, 2008 from <http://www.longwoods.com/product.php?productid=19320&cat=513&page=1>

Apollo Path-PACS. (2008). [Computer software]. Retrieved November 10, 2008, from http://www.apollopacs.com/pathpacs

Application for Medical Diagnostics. (2008). Retrieved from http://www.sblsoftware.com/embedded-medical.aspx

Arbona, A., Benkner, S., Engelbrecht, G., Fingberg, J., Hofmann, M., & Kumpf, K. (2007)... *IEEE Transactions on Nanobioscience*, *6*(2), 136–141.

Arsanjani, A. (2004). *Service-oriented modeling and architecture*. IBM technical article. Retrieved October 20, 2008, from http://www.ibm.com/developerworks/library/ws-soa-design1/

Ash, A. (1997). Telemedicine: Technology and Equipment Enabling New Models of HealthCare Delivery. *Informatics in HealthCare Australia*, *6*(3), 90–96.

ASME. *(Assoc. for the Study of Med. Educ.)*. (2008). Understanding Medical Education Series, description available at http://www.asme.org.uk/pub_ume.htm

Associated Press. (2007). FDA is rejecting more drugs than in the past. Retrieved from http://www.msnbc.msn.com/id/20321830/

Attaran, A. (2004). Where did it go wrong. *Nature*, *430*, 2–3.

Auf der Heide, E. (2006). The importance of evidence-based disaster planning. *Annals of Emergency Medicine*, *1*, 34–49.

Axelsson, R., & Axelsson, S. B. (2006). Integration and collaboration in public health - a conceptual framework. *The International Journal of Health Planning and Management*, *21*, 75–88. doi:10.1002/hpm.826

Ballester, F., Michelozzi, P., & Iñiguez, C. (2003). Weather, climate, and public health. *Journal of Epidemiology and Community Health*, *57*, 759–760.

Balogh A.A., Preul M.C., Laszlo K., Schornak M., Hickman M., Deshmukh P., & Spetzler R.F. (2006). Multilayer image grid reconstruction technology: four-dimensional interactive image reconstruction of microsurgical neuroanatomic dissections. *Neurosurgery, 58*(1 Suppl):ONS157-65. Discussion ONS157–65.

Banta, D. (2003). The development of health technology assessment. *Health Policy (Amsterdam)*, *63*, 121–132. doi:10.1016/S0168-8510(02)00059-3

Barillot, C., Benali, H., Dojat, M., Gaignard, A., Gibaud, B., & Kinkingnéhun, S. (2006). Federating distributed and heterogeneous information sources in neuroimaging: the NeuroBase Project. *Studies in Health Technology and Informatics*, *120*, 3–13.

Barnett, T.P.M., (20040. *The Pentagon's New Map,* (pp. 1-435). New York: G.P. Putnam & Sons.

Bartocci, E., Cacciagrano, D., Cannata, N., Corradini, F., Merelli, E., Milanesi, L., & Romano, P. (2007)... *IEEE Nanobioscience*, *6*(2), 142–148.

Becich, M. J., Gilberston, J. R., Gupta, D., Grzybicki, D. M., & Raab, S. S. (2008). Patient Safety and Healthcare Research: The Critical Role of Path Informatics in Error Reduction and Quality Initiatives. *Clinics in Laboratory Medicine*, *24*(4), 913–943. doi:10.1016/j.cll.2004.05.019

Beckwith, B. A., Mahaadevan, R., Balis, U. J., & Kuo, F. (2006). Development and evaluation of an open source software tool for the identification of pathology reports. *BMC Med Inform Decis. Mak., 6,* 12-22. Retrieved November 10, 2008, from http://www.pubmedcentral.nih.gov/picrender.fcgi?artid=1421388&blobtype=pdf

Bee, P. E., Bower, P., Lovell, K., Gilbody, S., Richards, D., Gask, L., & Roach, P. (2008). Psychotherapy mediated by remote communication technologies: a meta-analytic review. *BMC Psychiatry*, *8*, 60. doi:10.1186/1471-244X-8-60

Begent, R. (2008). *Developing standards for recording, sharing and integrating data from Antibody Society*. San Diego, CA: The Antibody Society.[Web Site]. Retrieved November 10, 2008, from http://www.antibodysociety.org/data/GIAATE_by_prof_Begent_09March2008.pdf

Beier, K. P., Freer, J., Griffiths, J. M., Levine, H., Sauter, J., & Treloar, D. (2001). The VIBE of the burning agent: simulation and modeling of burns and their treatment using agent-based programming, virtual reality, and human patient simulation. In Westwood, J. D. (Eds.), *Medicine Meets Virtual Reality 2001* (pp. 551–560). Amsterdam: IOS Press.

Beitiger, J., Johnson, W., Bivens, H., Humphreys, S., & Rhea, R. (2000). Constructing the ASCI Grid. *Proc. 9th IEEE Symposium on High Performance Distributed Computing*.

Bello, I. S., Arogundade, F. A., Sanusi, A. A., Ezeoma, I. T., Abioye-Kuteyi, E. A., & Akinsola, A. (2004). Knowledge and utilization of Information Technology among health care professionals and students in Ile-Ife, Nigeria: a case study of a university teaching hospital. *I. Med. Internet Res.*, *6*(4), e45.

Beowulf.org. *The Beowulf Cluster Site*. (2009). Retrieved from http://www.beowulf.org/

Berman, J. J., & Moore, G. W. (2006). *LDIP (Laboratory digital image project): RDF data specifications: the simple alternative to complex data standards.* Association for Pathology Informatics. Retrieved November 10, 2008, http://www.pathologyinformatics.org/Resources/jjb_gwm.pdf

Bescos, C., Schmitt, D., Kaas, J., Garcia-Barbero, M., & Kentchev, P. (2005). Interoperability and HealthGrid. *Methods of Information in Medicine*, *44*(2), 190–192.

Beynon, M. D., Kurc, T., Catalyurek, U., Chang, C., Sussman, A., & Saltz, J. (2001). Distributed processing of very large datasets with DataCutter. *Parallel Computing*, *27*(11), 1457–1478. doi:10.1016/S0167-8191(01)00099-0

Bidgood, W. D., Horii, S. C., Prior, F. W., & Van Syckle, D. E. (1997). Understanding and using DICOM, the data interchange standard for biomedical imaging. *Journal of the American Medical Informatics Association, 4*, 199–212.

Biggs, S. (1997). Interprofessional collaboration: Problems and prospects. In Ovretveit, J., Mathias, P., & Thomson, T. (Eds.), *Interprofessional working for health and social care* (pp. 186–200). Houndsmills, UK: MacMillan Press Ltd.

Binder, B., Hofman-Wellenhof, R., & Salmhofer, W. (1511-1514). Okcu, A., Kerl, H. & Soyer, H.P. (2007). Teledermatological monitoring of leg ulcers in cooperation with home care nurses. *Archives of Dermatology*, 143.

Biomoby Consortium. (2008). Interoperability with Moby 1.0 – it's better than sharing your toothbrush. *Briefings in Bioinformatics*, *9*(3), 220–231.

Blignaut, P. J. (1999). Software for primary healthcare in a developing country. Background and problem statement. *Computers in Nursing*, *17*(6), 291–296.

Blum, A., Hofman-Wellenhof, R., Luedtke, H., Ellwanger, U., Steins, A., & Roehm, S. (2004). Value of the clinical history for different users of dermoscopy compared with results of digital image analysis. *European Academy of Dermatology and Venerology*, *18*, 665–669. doi:10.1111/j.1468-3083.2004.01044.x

Boakai, M. Fofana. (2008). The African e-Health program. *All Africa's Boakai Fofana blogs on a Rockefeller Foundation conference on how to use information technology to improve access to health care*, Italy.

Bologna Declaration. (1999). Retrieved from http://www.bologna-bergen2005.no/Docs/00-Main_doc/990719BOLOGNA_DECLARATION.PDF

Bosch-Sijtsema, P. (n.d.). *Virtual organisations and knowledge development: A Case of Expectations*. University of Groningen, Groningen, The Netherlands. Retrieved from http://www.uni-hildesheim.de/~chlehn/isko2001/abstracts/bosch_petra.html

Bouchama, A. (2005). The 2003 European heat wave. *Int. Care Med.*, *30*(1), 1–3.

Boyd, C., Williams, W., Skinner, D., & Wilson, S. (2005). *A comparison of approaches to assessing network-centric warfare (NCW) concept implementation, Systems Engineering/Test and Evaluation Conference (SETE) 2005*. Retrieved from http://www.concepts.aero/ documents/SETE-2005- NPI.pdf#search=%22Boyd%20C%20Williams%20 W%20 Skinner%20D%20Wilson%20S%20a%20comparison%20of%20approaches%22

Boyd, J. R. COL. USAF. (1987). *Patterns of Conflict*. unpubl Briefing (accessible as "Essence of Winning and Losing", http://www.d-n-i.net).

Bradford, Z. B., & Brown, F. J. (2008). *America's Army: A Model for Interagency Effectiveness*, (pp. XIV + 1-250). Westport, CN: Praeger Security International.

Braverman, A. M. (2004). Father of the Grid. *University of Chicago Magazine 96*(4). Retrieved from http://magazine.uchicago.edu/0404/features/index.shtml

Brennan, R. J., & Nandy, R. (2001). Complex humanitarian emergencies: a major global challenge. *Emerg. Med.*, *13*(2), 147–156.

Breton, V., Blanquer, I., Hernandez, V., Legré, Y., & Solomonidés, T. (2006). Proposing a roadmap for HealthGRIDs. *Studies in Health Technology and Informatics*, *120*, 319–329.

Brown, F. J. (2002). Imperatives for tomorrow. *Military Review*, (September-October): 81–91.

Brown, M. S., Goldin, J. G., Rogers, S., Kim, H. J., Suh, R. D., & McNitt-Gray, M. F. (1999). Computer-aided lung nodule detection in CT: results of large-scale observer test. *Academic Radiology*, *12*, 681–686. doi:10.1016/j.acra.2005.02.041

Brown, H. G., Poole, M. S., & Walsum, K. V. (2002). Trust, trait theory, and collaboration in telemedicine: a circumplex perspective. In *Proc 36th Hawaii International Conference on System Sciences (HICSS'03)*. Washington DC: IEEE Computer Society.

Buneman, P., Khanna, S., & Tan, W. C. (2001). A Characterization of Data Provenance. In *ICDT, 2001* (pp. 316–330). Why and Where.

Burduli, A., Sheklashvili, G., & Kldiashvili, E. (2008). The application of medical databases for elearning. *Ukr Z Telemed Med Telemat*, *6*, 275–277.

Bureau of Labor Statistics. (2008). *Occupational Outlook Handbook*, 2008-2009 edition. Retrieved November 28, 2008, from: http://www.bls.gov/oco/oco20016.htm

Burke, L., & Weill, B. (2000). *Information Technology for the Health Professionals*. Upper Saddle River, NJ: Prentice-Hall Inc.

Buunk, B. P. Jonge. de J., Ybema, J.F, & Wolff, de C.J. (1998). Psychosocial aspects of occupational stress. In P. J. D. Drenth, H. Thierry, & C.J. de Wolff (eds.), *Handbook of work and organizational psychology. Volume 2: Work Psychology*, (2nd ed., pp. 145-182). East Sussex, UK: Psychology Press Ltd.

Buxton, P. J. (1999). Teleradiology – practical aspects and lessons learnt. *European Journal of Radiology*, *32*, 116–118. doi:10.1016/S0720-048X(99)00136-9

Byrne, J. P. (2006). *Daily Life During the Black Death* (pp. 1–344). Westport, CT: Greenwood Press.

caBIG, caTissue. (2006). Retrieved from https://cabig.nci.nih.gov/tools/catissuecore; https://cabig.nci.nih.gov/workspaces/Architecture/caGrid; http://gforge.nci.nih.gov/projects/cacorecvs/

caBIG. (2005). *Compatibility Guidelines Revision 2*. Retrieved November 10, 2008, from http://cabig.nci.nih.gov/guidelines_documentation/caBIGCompatGuideRev2_final.pdf

caBIG. (2008). *GRID & metadata with ISO 11179*. [Web Site]. Retrieved November 10, 2008, from https://cabig.nci.nih.gov/

California HealthCare Foundation. (November 2005). *National Consumer Health Privacy Survey 2005*. CHCF Org. Available at: http://www.chcf.org/topics/view.cfm?itemID=115694

Callen, J. L., Buyankhishig, B., & McIntosdh, J. H. (2007). Clinical information sources used by hospital doctors in Mongolia. *International Journal of Medical Informatics*, (Jul): 21.

Camarasu, S., Benoit-Cattin, H., Montagnat, J., & Racoceanu, D. (2008). Content-based medical image indexing and retrieval on Grids, First International Symposium on ICT for Health, Ateneo de Manila University, Manila, Philippines. *Philippine J Info Tech. 1*, 46.

Cambazoglu, B., Sertel, O., & Kong, J. (2007). Efficient processing of pathological images using the grid: Computer-aided prognosis of neuroblastoma. In *Proc. Challenges of Large Applications in Distributed Environments,* CLADE'07, June 25, 2007, (pp. 35-41), Monterey, California.

CAMT -computer aided medical transcription. (2008). [Web Site]. Retrieved November 10, 2008, from http://www.escription.com/products/index.htmlhttp://www.nuance.com/dictaphone/products/powerscribe/pathology/

Cancer Mortality Maps & Graphs. (2008). National Cancer Institute. Retrieved from http://www3.cancer.gov/atlasplus/

CANCERMondial. (2008). International Agency for Research on Cancer. Retrieved from http://www-dep.iar.fr/

Careau, E., Vincent, C., & Noreau, L. (2008). Assessing interprofessional teamwork in a videoconference-based telerehabilitation setting. *Journal of Telemedicine and Telecare*, *14*, 427–434. doi:10.1258/jtt.2008.080415

Cascio, W. F. (1999). Virtual workplaces: Implications for organizational behaviour. In C.L. Cooper & D.M. Rousseau (eds.), *Trends in organizational behaviour. Volume 6. The virtual organization*. (pp. 1-14). Chichester, UK: John Wiley & Sons Ltd.

Cavalier, J. C., & Klein, J. D. (1998). Effects of cooperative versus individual learning and orienting activities during computer-based instruction. *ETR&D*, *46*(1), 5–17.

Cebrowski, A. K., & Garstka, J. J. (1998). Network-centric warfare: its origin and future. *US Nav. Inst. Proc. 1*, (pp. 28-35). Retrieved from http://www.usni.org/magazines/proceedings/ archive/month.asp?ID=205

CERNER. (2008). *CoPATHplus solution*. [Computer Software]. Retrieved November 10, 2008, from http://www.cerner.com/public/Cerner_3.asp?id=30881

Chang, W. (2008). *Network-centric Service Oriented Enterprise* (pp. 1–540). Dordrecht, The Netherlands: Springer.

Chanlat, J.-F. (1997). Conflict and politics. In Sorge, A., & Warner, M. (Eds.), *The IEBM Handbook of Organizational Behaviour* (pp. 472–480). London: International Thomson Business Press.

Chen, L., Evans, T., Anand, S., Boufford, J.I., & Brown, H., Chowdhury, et al. (2004). Human resources for health: overcoming the crisis. *Lancet*, *364*, 1984–1990.

Chen, F., Romano, N. C., Nunamaker, J. F., & Briggs, R. O. (2002). A collaborative project management architecture. In *Proc 36th Hawaii International Conference on System Sciences (HICSS'04)*. Washington, DC: IEEE Computer Society.

Chisholm, R. F. (Ed.). (1998). *Developing network organizations: Learning from practice and theory*. Reading, MA: Addison-Wesley.

Choi, Park, Oh, Park (2007). PC-based Tele-Audiometry. *Telemedicine and e-Health 13*(5), 501-508.

Chowdhry, B. S., Rajput, A. Q. K., & Chowdhry, N. P. (2007). *Major challenges and opportunities in the practice of research and development in the area of bioinformatics. In 5th annual international conference, "Role of medical universities in promotion of research", at Liaqat University of Medical & Health Sciences, Jamshoro, PK* (p. 70).

Chowdhry, N. P., Ansari, A. W., Memon, A. A., & Fatima, M. (2008). Bioinformatics awareness system for skin diseases using stem cells therapy in the perspective of e-Health. In *Handbook of communications in Computer and information Sc* (pp. 261–267). Berlin: Springer Verlag.

Chowdhry, N. P., Ansari, A. W., & Baloch, A. K. (2008). Diagnostic image archive system for rapid web based access to the consultant through metropolitan area networks. In *proc. of the Med-e-Tel, the international educational and networking forum for E-Health, Telemedicine and Health ICT, Luxembourg,* (Vol. 1, pp. 300-306).

Claus, B. L., & Johnson, S. R. (2008). Grid computing in large pharmaceutical molecule modeling. *Drug Discov. Today 13*(13-14), S 78-83, Collins, F.S. & McKusick, V.A. (2001). Implications of the Human Genome Project for Medical Science. *Journal of the American Medical Association*, *285*, 540–544.

Cluster Computing Info Centre. (2010). Retrieved from http://www.gridbus.org/~raj/cluster/

Cohen, S. G., & Mankin, D. (1999). Collaboration in the virtual organization. In C.L. Cooper & D.M. Rousseau (Eds.), *Trends in organizational behaviour. Volume 6. The virtual organization* (pp. 105-120). Chichester, UK: John Wiley & Sons Ltd.

Collins, F. S., Morgan, M., & Patrinos, A. (2003). The human genome project: Lessons from large-scale biology. *Science*, *300*, 286–290. doi:10.1126/science.1084564

Computer Retrieval of Information on Scientific Projects. (2008). Department of Health and Human Services. Retrieved from http://crisp.cit.nih.gov/

Cooper, C., & Block, R. (2006). *Disaster: Hurricane Katrina and the Failure of Homeland Security* (pp. 3–333). New York: Times Books/Henry Holt and Company.

Coulter, A., & Ham, C. (2002). *The global challenge of health care rationing* (pp. 1–267). Buckingham, UK: Open University Press.

Coveney, P. V., & Fowler, P. W. (2005). Modelling biological complexity: a physical scientist's perspective. *J.R. Soc. Interface*, *2*(4), 267–280.

Crook, G., Gibson, C. J., Adam, C., Levesque, L., O'Reilly-Brunelle, B., & Hwee, J. (2009). Chapter 7: Towards an Electronic Health Record. In CHIMA (Ed.), *Fundamentals of Health Information Management*. Ottawa: CHA Press.

Cuevas, de C., Arredondo, T., Cabrera M.F., Sulzenbacher, H. & Meise, U. (2006). Randomized clinical trial of telepsychiatry through videoconference versus face-to-face conventional psychiatric treatment. *Telemedicine and e-Health, 12*, 341-350.

Curran, V. R., Sharpe, D., Forristall, J., & Flynn, K. (2008). Student satisfaction and perceptions of small group process in case-based interprofessional learning. *Medizinische Technik*, *30*(4), 431–433.

Da Silveira, M., & Guelfi, N. (2009). The Concept of a Platform for Remote Monitoring Patient's Health State. In Jordanova, M., & Lievens, F. (Eds.), *Global Telemedicine and eHealth Updates: Knowledge Resources* (*Vol. 2*, pp. 278–282). Luxembourg: Luxexpo.

Dansie, J., & Muñoz, K. (2008). *Providing Training for Otoacoustic Emissions (OAE)*. Salt Lake City, Utah: Hearing Screening Using Telehealth. Intermountain Area Speech and Hearing Convention. [poster session]

Davis, D. (1998). Continuing medical education: Global health, global learning. *BMJ (Clinical Research Ed.)*, *316*(7128), 385–389.

Day, B., Mckay, R. B., Ishman, M., & Chung, E. (2004). The new normal: lessons learned from SARS for corporations operating in emerging markets. *Management Decision*, *42*(6), 794–806.

Day, Y. F., Dagtas, S., Iino, M., Khokhar, A., & Ghafoor, A. (1995). Object-oriented conceptual modeling of video data. In *Proc. 11th Int. Conf. Data Eng.* (pp. 401-408).

Deapen, D. (2006). Cancer surveillance and information: balancing public health with privacy and confidentiality concerns (United States). *Cancer Causes & Control*, *17*, 663–637. doi:10.1007/s10552-006-0002-1

Denton, D., & Gladstone, V. (2005). Ethical and Legal Issues Related to Telepractice. *Seminars in Hearing*, *26*(1), 43–52. doi:10.1055/s-2005-863794

Detmer, D. (2000). Information technology for quality health care: a summary of United Kingdom and United States experiences. *Quality in Health Care*, *9*, 181–189. doi:10.1136/qhc.9.3.181

Detmer, D. (2001). Transforming health care in the internet era. *World Hospitals and Health Services*, *37*, 2.

Detmer, D. E. (2000). Information technology for quality health care: a summary of United Kingdom and United States experiences. *Quality in Health Care*, *9*, 181–189. doi:10.1136/qhc.9.3.181

Devesa, S., Grauman, D. J., Blot, W. J., Pennello, G., & Hoover, R. N. (1999) *Atlas of cancer mortality in the United States: 1950-94*. Washington, DC: US Govt Print Off. NIH 99-4564: 360.

Devitt, N., & Murphy, J. (2004). A survey of the information management and technology training needs of doctors in an acute NHS trust in the United Kingdom. *Health Information and Libraries Journal*, *21*(3), 164–172.

Dhar, V., & Olson, M. H. (1989). Assumptions underlying systems that support work group collaboration. In Olson, M. H. (Ed.), *Technological support for work group collaboration* (pp. 33–50). Hillsdale, NJ: Lawrence Erlbaum Associates Publishers.

Diamond, C., Goldstein, M., Lansky, D., & Verhulst, S. (2008). An architecture for privacy in a networked health information environment. *Cambridge Quarterly of Healthcare Ethics*, *17*, 429–440. doi:10.1017/S0963180108080559

Dianic, A. (2006). The need for scalability in network-centric warfare – it's all in the semanitcs. *SEC BSSD Bulletin January*, 1-11. Retrieved from http://www.pdf-search-online.com/dianic-pdf-40.html

Dick, R. S., Steen, E. B., & Detmer, D. E. (1997). *The Computer-Based Patient Record: An Essential Technology for Health Care*. Washington, DC: National Academy Press.

Digital Library. (2010). *Wikipedia*. Retrieved from http://en.wikipedia.org/wiki/Digital_library

DIR2007. (2007). *DIR 2007/47/EC - Nueva directiva sobre equipos médicos*. [Web Site]. http://en.wikipedia.org/wiki/Medical_device

Dirnhofer, R., Jackowski, Ch., Vock, P., Potter, K., & Thali, M. J. (2006). VIRTOPSY: Minimally Invasive, Imaging-guided Virtual Autopsy. *Radiographics, 26*(5), 1305-1356. Retrieved November 10, 2008, from http://radiographics.rsnajnls.org/cgi/content/figsonly/26/5/1305

Dixon, N. M., Allen, N., Burgess, T., Kilner, P., & Dchweitzer, S. (2005). *Company Command: Unleashing the Power of the Army Profession* (pp. 1–198). NY: West Point.

Dixon, R., & Stahl, J. (2008). Virtual visits in a general medicine practice: A pilot study. *Telemedicine and e-Health, 14*(6), 525-530.

Drews, J. (2000). Drug discovery: a historical perspective. *Science*, *287*(5460), 1960–1964.

Dryer, K. J., Hirschorn, D. S., Metha, A., & Thrall, J. H. (2006). *PACS: A Guide to the Digital Revolution*. New York: Springer-Verlag.

Eaker, S., Adami, H., Granath, F., Wilander, E., & Sparen, P. (2004). A Large Population-Based Randomized Controlled Trial to Increase Attendance at Screening for Cervical Cancer. *Cancer Epidemiology, Biomarkers & Prevention*, *13*, 346–354.

Eddrippulige, S., Marasinghe, R. B., Smith, A. C., Fujisawa, Y., Herath, W. B., & Jiffry, M. T. (2007). Medical students' knowledge and perception of e-health: results of a study in Sri Lanka. *Medinfo*, *12*(Pt.2), 1406–1409.

EDRM. (2008). *The Electronic Discovery Reference Model.* [Web Site]. Retrieved November 10, 2008, from http://www.edrm.net/

EGEE. *Enabling the Grid for E-sciencE, 2007 Conference, Live Demo Competition.* (2007). Retrieved October 20, 2008, from http://indico.cern.ch/contributionDisplay.py?contribId=174&sessionId=23&confId=18714.

Ekeland, A. G. (1999). Teleradiologi - virkemiddel for solidarisk helsepolitikk? *Tidsskrift for Den Norske Laegeforening*, *119*, 4345–4347.

EKOS Research Associates. (2007, August). (Submitted to). Electronic Health Information and Privacy Survey [Canada Health Infoway, Health Canada, and the Office of the Privacy Commissioner of Canada, Ottawa.]. *What Canadians Think.*

Elangovan, S. (2005). Telehearing and the Internet. *Seminars in Hearing*, *26*(1), 19–25. doi:10.1055/s-2005-863791

Electronic Health Record Meets Digital Library. (n.d). Retrieved from http://www.pubmedcentral.nih.gov/articlerender.fcgi?artid=79039

El-Ghazali, T., & Albert, Y. Zomaya. (2008). *Grid Computing for bioinformatics and computational biology*. Chichester, UK: Wiley InterScience.

Embedded System. (n.d.). *Wikipedia*. Retrieved from http://en.wikipedia.org/wiki/Embedded_system

English, T. (1997). Personal paper: medicine in the 1990s needs a team approach. *British Medical Journal*, *314*, 661.

ESRI. (n.d.). Retrieved from http://www.esri.com/library/brochures/pdfs/gis-for-defense

eTen projects. (2009). *European Community programme providing funds to help make e-services available throughout the European Union*. Retrieved 28 February, 2009 from http://ec.europa.eu/information_society/activities/eten/opdb/

EUCOM. (2009). *Teams of Leaders Coaching Guide 1.0*. Stuttgart, Germany: US Army European Command.

European Commission. (2007). *From Bergen to London*. Retrieved from http://ec.europa.eu/education/policies/educ/bologna/report06.pdf

European Institute of Medicine. (2003). *Health is Wealth: Strategic Vision for European Healthcare at the Beginning of the 21st Century*. Salzburg, Austria: European Academy of Arts and Sciences.

European Institute of Telesurgery. (n.d.). Retrieved from http://www.eits.fr/

European Policy Center. (2008, 1st November). *European Health Policy in an International Perspective Report*. Retrieved from http://www.epc.eu/en/er.asp?AI=439&LV=293&PG=ER/EN/detail&TYP=ER&see=y&t=2

Evans, G. (1993). Health and security in the global village. *World Health Forum*, *14*, 133–135.

Evans, W. E., & McLeod, H. L. (2003). Pharmacogenomics – drug disposition, drug targets, and side effects. *The New England Journal of Medicine*, *348*(6), 538–549. Retrieved from http://content.nejm.org/cgi/content/full/348/6/538.

EXOCOM Group. Business Strategy and Consulting IT Division for Office of Health and the Information Highway, Health Canada. (2001). *Privacy Technology Review*. Retrieved November 14, 2008 from http://www.hc-sc.gc.ca/hcs-sss/pubs/ehealth-esante/2001-priv-tech/index-eng.php#anne

Farag, A. A., El-Baz, A., Gimelfarb, G., El-Ghar, M. A., & Eldiasty, T. (2005). Quantitative nodule detection in low dose chest CT scans: new template modeling and evaluation for CAD system design. *Med Image Comput Assist Interv*, *8*(pt1), 720–728. doi:10.1007/11566465_89

FDA (US Food and Drug Administration). (2004). *Innovation or Stagnation. White Paper.* Washington, DC: Author.

Fernandez, I. (2002). Barcelona 2002: law, ethics, and human rights. Global battle cry: health is a right, not a commodity. *Canadian HIV/AIDS Policy & Law Review*, *7*, 80–84.

Ferrer-Roca, O., Figueredo, A., Franco, K., & Diaz-Cardama, A. (2005). Telemedicine Intelligent Learning. Ontology for Agent Technology. *Trans. on Adv. Res*, *1*(2), 46-54. Retrieved November 10, 2008, from http://internetjournals.net/journals/tar/2005/TARVol1Num2.pdf

Ferrer-Roca, O., Marcano, F., & Quintana, J. J. (2008). Small Size Virtual Slides in Pathology. *Virchows Arch*, *452* (suppl 1), s9-s10. Retrieved November 10, 2008, from http://www.springerlink.com/content/e672131738 6258u3/?p=1eff7f89dee44ce085fc696b4faf4e69&pi=0

Finch, T., May, C., Mair, F., Mort, M., & Gask, L. (2003). Integrating service development with evaluation in telehealthcare: an ethnographic study. *British Medical Journal*, *327*, 1205–1209. doi:10.1136/bmj.327.7425.1205

FMRIB Software Library. (n.d.). Retrieved from http://www.fmrib.ox.ac.uk

Fogg, B. J. (2003). *Persuasive Technology: Using Computers to Change What We Think and Do* (pp. 1–282). San Francisco: Morgan Kaufman.

Fortin, J.-P., Gagnon, M.-P., Cloutier, A., & Labbé, F. (2002). Evaluation of a telemedicine demonstration project in the Magdalene Islands. *Journal of Telemedicine and Telecare*, *9*, 89–94. doi:10.1258/135763303321327948

Fost, I., & Kesselman, C. (1999). *The Grid: Blueprint for a future computing infrastructure*. San Francisco: Morgan Kaufmann Publishers, Inc.

Foster, I., Kesselman, C., & Tuecke, S. (2001). The Anatomy of the Grid. *International Journal of High Performance Computing Applications*, *15*(3). doi:10.1177/109434200101500302

Foster, I. (2002). *What is the grid? A three point checklist. Argonne National Library & University of Chicago*. Retrieved November 10, 2008, from http://www-fp.mcs.anl.gov/~foster/Articles/WhatIsTheGrid.pdf

Foster, I., & Kesselman, C. (2003). *The Grid 2: Blueprint for a new Computing Infrastructure,* (The Elsevier Series in Grid Computing, pp. 1-748). San Francisco, CA: Morgan Kaufman.

Foster, I., Kesselman, C., Tsudik, C., & Tuecke, S. (1998). A Security Architecture for Computational Grids. In *5th ACM Conference on Computer and Communication Security*.

Fratt, L. (2008). *Enterprise Long-term Storage: Plan for the Worst, Hope for the Best*. Retrieved 28 February, 2009, from http://www.healthimaging.com/index.php?option=com_articles&view=article&id=15213:enterprise-long-term-storage-plan-for-the-worst-hope-for-the-best.

Frelick, K. M., & Jovellano, J. (2009). Chapter 13: Legal Aspects of Health Information Management. In CHIMA (Ed.), *Fundamentals of Health Information Management*. Ottawa: CHA Press.

Frenk, J., Sepulveda, J., Gomez-Dantes, O., McGuinness, M. J., & Knaul, F. (1997). The future of world health: the new world order and international health. *BMJ (Clinical Research Ed.)*, *314*, 1404–1407. Retrieved from http://www.ncbi.nlm.nih.gov/pmc/articles/PMC2126640/pdf/9161318.pdf.

Freund, J., Comaniciu, D., Ioannis, Y., Liu, P., McClatchey, R., & Morley-Fletcher, E. (2006). Health-e-child: an integrated biomedical platform for grid-based paediatric applications. *Studies in Health Technology and Informatics*, *120*, 259–270.

Frost & Sullivan Country Industry Forecast – European Union Healthcare Industry. (2004, May 11). Retrieved from http://www.news-medical.net/print_article.asp?id=1405

Gabbay, J., & Walley, T. (2006). Introducing new health interventions. *British Medical Journal*, *332*, 64–65. doi:10.1136/bmj.332.7533.64

Galperin, M. Y. (2005). The molecular biology database collection: 2005 update. *Nucleic Acids Research*, *33*, D5–D24.

Galperin, M. Y. (2008). Genomes of model organisms: know thy tools. *Environ. Biol.*, *10*(6), 1383–1391.

Ganguly, P., & Ray, P. (1998). *Telemedicine over Enterprise-wide Networks: A Case Study.* IEEE Global Telecommunications Conference (GLOBECOM98), Sydney, November. Retrieved from http://www.apuhc.org/pradeep

GAO. (2004). *Emerging Infectious Diseases: Review of State and Federal Disease Surveillance Efforts* (GAO 04-877, I-IV, pp. 1-64). Washington, DC: Government Accounting Office.

Garcia-Rojo, M. (1998). *Management and automation in pathology laboratories*. Retrieved November 10, 2008, from http://www.mcmaster.ca/inabis98/rojo/rojo0500/two.html

Garrett, L. (1994). *The Coming Plague: Newly Emerging Diseases in the World out Of Balance* (pp. 3–750). New York: Penguin.

Garstka, J. J. (2000). Network Centric Warfare: an overview of emerging theory. *Phalanx*, *4*, 28–33.

Garstka, J. J. (2004, 28th January). Implementation of network centric warfare. *Force Transformation Trends*. Retrieved from http://www.oft.osd.mil

Gentili, A., Chung, C., & Hughes, T. (2008). Use of the MIRC DICOM Service for Clinical Trials to Automatically Create Teaching File Cases from PACS. *Radiographics 27*, 269-275. Retrieved November 10, 2008, from http://radiographics.rsnajnls.org/cgi/content/full/27/1/269

Germain, C., Breton, V., Clarysse, P., Gaudeau, Y., & Glatard, T., Jeannot, et al. (2005). Grid-enabling medical image analysis. *Journal of Clinical Monitoring and Computing*, *19*(4–5), 339–349. doi:10.1007/s10877-005-0679-9

Gerrard, L., Grant, A. M., & Maclean, J. R. (1999). Factors that may influence the implementation of nurse-centred telemedicine services. *Journal of Telemedicine and Telecare*, *5*, 231–236. doi:10.1258/1357633991933765

Giger, M. L., Doi, K., MacMahon, H., Metz, C. E., & Yin, F. F. (1990). Pulmonary nodules: computer-aided detection in digital chest images. *Radiographics*, *10*, 41–51.

Gilelet, F., Fichera, R., Schreck, G., Yates, S., & Wenninger, S. (2004). *Grid gets big, but the term is confusing*. Retrieved from http://www.egenera.com/reg/pdf/forrester_grid.pdf

Gils, van M.R. (1984). Interorganizational relations and networks. In P.J.D. Drenth, H. Thierry, P.J. Willems & C.J. de Wolff de (Eds.), *Handbook of work and organizational psychology*, (Vol. 2, pp. 1073-1100). Chichester, UK: John Wiley & Sons Ltd.

Giménez, J. A., Alvarez, R., & Alfaro, J. (2007). *El control interno y externo de la calidad de las técnicas inmunohistoquímicas en relación con la Norma UNE-EN ISO 15189:2003*. Paper presented at the meeting of the XXIII Congreso de la Sociedad Española de Anatomía Patológica, Palacio de Congresos de Tarragona, may 2007. Retrieved November 10, 2008, from http://www.seapcongresos.com/2007/clubes/gestion/gimenez.htm

Givens, G., Blanarovich, A., Murphy, T., Simmons, S., Blach, D., & Elangovan, S. (2003). Internet-based tele-audiometry system for the assessment of hearing: a pilot study. *Telemedicine Journal Electronic Health*, *9*, 375–378. doi:10.1089/153056203772744707

Glaser, J., Henley, D. E., Downing, G., & Brinner, K. M. (2008). Advancing personalized health care through health information technology: An update from the American Health Information Community's Personalized Health Care Workgroup. *Journal of the American Medical Informatics Association*, *15*(4), 391–396. doi:10.1197/jamia.M2718

Glatard, T., Emsellem, D., & Montagnat, J. (2006). Generic web service wrapper for efficient embedding of legacy codes in service-based workflows (workshop). In *Proceedings of the Grid-Enabling Legacy Applications and Supporting End Users Workshop (GELA'06)*, (pp. 44--53), Paris, France, June 2006.

Glatard, T., Montagnat, J., Pennec, X., Emsellem, D., & Lingrand, D. (2006). *MOTEUR: a data-intensive service-based workflow manager.* Research Report I3S, number I3S/RR-2006-07-FR, (pp. 37), Sophia Antipolis, France, Mar 2006. *glite, A lightweight middleware for grid computing*. (2008). Retrieved October 20, 2008, from http://glite.web.cern.ch/glite/

Goble, C. (2001). The low down on e-science and grids for biology. *Comparative and Functional Genomics*, *2*, 365–370. doi:10.1002/cfg.115

Godman, M. (2008). But is it unique to nanotechnology? Reframing nanoethics. *Science and Engineering Ethics*, *14*, 391–403. doi:10.1007/s11948-008-9052-y

Gokhale, A. A. (1995). Collaborative learning enhances critical thinking. *J. Technological Education*, *7*(1), 22–30.

Gonzalez, M., Quesada, G., Urrutia, I., & Gavidia, J. (2006). Conceptual design of an e-health strategy for the Spanish health care system. *International Journal of Health Care Quality Assurance*, *19*(2), 146–157. doi:10.1108/09526860610651681

Goodfellow, T., Bali, R. G., Wickramasinghe, N., & Naguib, R. N. G. (2008). From data to decisions: introducing knowledge management to effect superior operations in a radiology department. *Int J Biomedical Engineering and Technology*, *1*, 259–272. doi:10.1504/IJBET.2008.016960

Gortiz, L.G., Karnabatidis, D., Siabatidis, D. & Nikifordis, G. (2006). Clinical-oriented collaboration over the Web during interventional radiology procedures. *Telemedicine and e-Health, 12*, 448-456.

Görtler, J., Berghoff, M., Kayser, G., & Kayser, K. (2006). Grid technology in tissue-based diagnosis: fundamentals and potential developments. *Diagnostic Pathology, 1*, 23. August 24, 2006, from: http://www.diagnosticpathology.org/content/1/1/23

Gray, C. S. (2006). Clausewitz, history, and the future strategic world. In Murray, W., & Sinnreich, R. H. (Eds.), *The Past as Prologue: the Importance of History to the Military Profession* (pp. 111–132). Cambridge, UK: Cambridge University Press.

Greenhalgh, T., Glenn, R., Bate, P., Macfarlane, F., & Kyriakidou, O. (2004). Diffusion of innovations in service organisations: systematic review and recommendations. *The Milbank Quarterly*, *82*, 581–629. doi:10.1111/j.0887-378X.2004.00325.x

Gregg, W., & Moscovice, I. (2003). The evolution of rural health networks: implications for health care managers. *Health Care Management Review*, *28*, 161–178.

Grifftihs, J.-M., Sauter, J., Parunak, H. V. D., Wolf, E., & von Lubitz, D. K. J. E. (2000). Models, models everywhere: brain injury, datapocalypse, and the art of computing. In C. Webb (Ed.), *Proc. NIH Pulse Workshop*, NIH, Leesburg, VA, June 29-30.

Grimshaw, D., Willmott, H., & Rubery, J. (2005). Inter-organizational networks: Trust, power, and the employment relationship. In Marchington, M., Grimshaw, D., & Rubery, J. (Eds.), *Fragmenting work: blurring organizational boundaries and disordering hierarchies* (pp. 34–61). Oxford, UK: Oxford University Press.

Gurcan, M. N., Sahiner, B., Petrick, N., Chan, H. P., Kazerooni, E. A., Cascade, P. N., & Hadjiiski, L. (2002). Lung nodule detection on thoracic computed tomography images: preliminary evaluation of a computer-aided diagnosis system. *Medical Physics*, *29*, 2552–2558. doi:10.1118/1.1515762

Hagedoorn, J., & Duysters, J. (2002). Learning in dynamic inter-firm networks: The efficacy of multiple contacts. *Organization Studies*, *23*, 525–548. doi:10.1177/0170840602234002

Haine, J.-Y. (2005). Military matters: ESDP transformed? *NATO Review*, Summer. Retrieved from http://www.nato.int/docu/review/2005/issue2/english/military.html

Haroske, G., Meyer, W., Kunze, D., & Boeking, A. (1998). Quality control measures for dna image cytometry in a telepathology network. *Advances in Clinical Pathology*, *2*(2), 143–145.

Haroske, G., Meyer, W., Oberholzer, M., Bocking, A., & Kunze, K. D. (2000). Competence on demand in DNA image cytometry. *Pathology, Research and Practice*, *196*(5), 285–291.

Harris, M. A., Levy, A. R., & Teschke, K. E. (2008). Personal privacy and public health: Potential impacts of privacy legislation on health research in Canada. *Canadian Journal of Public Health*, *99*(4), 293–296.

Harrison, R., Clayton, W., & Wallace, P. (1996). Can telemedicine be used to improve communication between primary and secondary care? *British Medical Journal*, *313*, 1377–1380.

Haythorntwaite, C. *(2005). Knowledge flow in interdisciplinary teams. In* Proc 38th Hawaii International Conference on System Sciences (HICSS'05). *Washington DC: IEEE Computer Society.*

Health and Medicine Digital Library – Online Medical Library – Academic Info. (2010). Retrieved from http://www.academicinfo.net/medlibrary.html

Health, A. (n.d.). *Add Health research on genetic influence in social networks is featured in HarvardScience*. Retrieved from http://www.cpc.unc.edu/projects/addhealth/news/add-health-research-on-genetic-influence-in-social-networks-is-featured-in-harvardscience

Health-e-Child. *The EU FP6 Information Societies Technology Project*. (2008). Retrieved October 20, 2008, from http://www.health-e-child.org/

HealthGrid. (2004). *HealthGrid white paper*. Retrieved November 10, 2008, from http://initiative.healthgrid.org/the-initiative/healthgrids-concept/white-paper.html

Hebert, M.A., Jansen, j.J., Brant, R., & Hailey, D. & Pol, van M. (2004). Successes and challenges in a filed-based, multi-method study of home telehealth. *Journal of Telemedicine and Telecare*, *10*(suppl. 1), 41–44. doi:10.1258/1357633042614348

Hernandez, V., & Blanquer, I. (2005). The grid as a healthcare provision tool. *Methods of Information in Medicine*, *44*(2), 144–148.

Hernandez, V., Blanquer, I., Solomonides, T., Breton, V., & Legre, Y. (Eds.). (2006). *Challenges and Opportunities of HealthGrids: Proceedings of Healthgrid 2006,* (pp. 407.). Washington, DC: IOS Press, Washington, DC.

Hertog, den F., & Tolner, T. (1997). Groups and teams. In A. Sorge & M. Warner M (Eds.), *The IEBM Handbook of organizational behaviour*, (pp. 492-501). London: International Thomson Business Press.

Hjelm, M. (2001). Telemedicine and in-patient. *Hospitals International*, *37*, 2.

Hjelm, N. M., Wootton, R., & Staines, D. (2003). Social capital, gold for telemedicine? *World Hospitals and Health Services*, *39*(3), 11–12, 42, 44.

Hofstetter, P., Kokesh, J., & Ferguson, S. (2008). A telehealth model—delivering hearing healthcare to remote sites. *Telemedicine and e-Health, March 1, 2008, 14*(s1), 24-81.

Holger, K., & Andreas, W. (2006). *Protocols and Architectures for Wireless Sensor Networks*. Chicester, UK: Wiley & Sons.

Holt, J., Hotto, S., & Cole, K. (1994). *Demographic aspects of hearing impairment: questions and answers*, (3rd ed.). Retrieved November 25, 2008, from http://gri.gallaudet.edu/demographics/ factsheet.html

Hosner, C. (2004). *OpenVPN and SSL VPN Revolution*. SANS Institute, retrieved 28 February, 2009, from http://www.sans.org/reading_room/whitepapers/vpns/openvpn_and_the_ssl_vpn_revolution_1459

Hristovski, D., Friedman, C., Rindflesch, T., & Peterlin, B. (2006). Exploiting Semantic Relations for Literature-Based Discovery. *AMIA ... Annual Symposium Proceedings / AMIA Symposium. AMIA Symposium, 2006*, 349–353.

Hubbard, T. (2002). Biological information: making it accessible and integrated (and trying to make sense of it). *Bioinform., 18*(Suppl. 2), S140.

Humayun, A., Fatima, N., Naqqash, S., Hussain, S., Rasheed, A., Imtiaz, H., & Imam, S. Z. (2008). Patients' perception of actual practice of informed consent, privacy and confidentiality in general medical outpatient departments of two tertiary care hospitals of Lahore. *BMC Medical Ethics, 9*(14), 1–8.

Husain, O. A., & Watts, K. C. (1987). Preparatory methods for DNA hydrolysis, cytochemistry, immunocytochemistry and ploidy analysis. Their application to automated and routine diagnostic cytopathology. *Analytical and Quantitative Cytology and Histology, 9*(3), 218–224.

Ichikawa, K. date, S., Kaishima, T., & Shimojo, S. (2005). A framework supporting the development of a Grid portal for analysis based on ROI. *Methods of Information in Medicine, 44*(2), 265–269.

ICRP: A Joint Initiative of International Cancer Research Funding Organizations. (2008). International Cancer Research Portfolio. Retrieved from http://www.cancerportfolio.org/index.jsp

IEC60601. (2006). *IEC 60601-1:2006 - Seguridad en los equipos electromédicos incluyendo los PESS o subsistemas electrónicos programables*. Retrieved November 10, 2008, from http://www.tecnologias-sanitarias.com/electromedicina/en60601-1.htm, http://www.tecnologias-sanitarias.com/electromedicina/IEC60601-1_ed3-info.pdf

IHS. (2008). *ISO Information/Image technology collection*. [Web Site]. Retrieved November 10, 2008, from http://engineers.ihs.com/collections/iso/information-image-9.htm

ISO Information/ Image technology collection. (2008). Retrieved November 10, 2008, from http://engineers.ihs.com/collections/iso/information-image-9.htm

ISO11073. (2008). *ISO/IEEE 11073 – Plug & Play Standard*. Retrieved November 10, 2008, from http://www.ieee1073.org/

ISO11179. (2004). *ISO* 11179 - Metadata Standard. Retrieved November 10, 2008, from http://dublincore.org/documents/1999/07/02/dces/, http://www.ukoln.ac.uk/metadata/newsagent/metadata/, http://hpcrd.lbl.gov/SDM/XMDR/overview.html, http://xmdr.org/

ISO13250. (2003). *ISO 13250 - Topic maps*. Retrieved November 10, 2008, from http://www.isotopicmaps.org/sam/sam-xtm/

ISO13485. (2003). ISO 13485:2003. Medical devices -- Quality management Systems. Retrieved November 10, 2008, from http://www.tecnologias-sanitarias.com/calidad/iso13485-2003/

ISO14971. (2007). ISO 14971:2007 Medical devices -- Application of risk management to medical devices. Retrieved November 10, 2008, from http://www.tecnologias-sanitarias.com/iso14971/index.htm

ISO17025. (2005). *ISO 17025:2005. General requirements for the competence of testing and calibration laboratories*. Retrieved November 10, 2008, from http://www.aiha.org/1documents/lab/lqapnews03-0406.pdf

Jafari, R. (2006). *Medical Embedded Systems*. Doctoral Dissertation, University of California, Los Angles, CA. Retrieved from http://www.utdallas.edu/~rjafari/publications/JAFARI_Dissertation.pdf

Jannett, P., Yeo, M., Pauls, M., & Graham, J. (2003). Organizational readiness for telemedicine: implications for success and failure. *Journal of Telemedicine and Telecare*, *9*(2), 27–30. doi:10.1258/135763303322596183

Jannett, P., & Jackson, A., & Ho, K., & Healy, T., & Kazanjian, A., & Wollard, R., & Haydt, S., & Bates, J. (2005). The essence of telehealth readiness in rural communities: an organizational perspective. *Journal of Telemedicine and eHealth, 11*, 137-145.

Jessen, W. (2007, December 4). Social Networks and Health. Posted to *Highlight HEALTH: Discover the Science of Health*. Retrieved from http://www.highlighthealth.com/highlight-health-web-site/social-networks-and-health-the-research-and-the-reviews/

Jianggan, L. (2008). An Australian quest for e-Health. *Future Gov, free weekly newsletter.*

Johansson, F. (2006). *The Medici Effect* (pp. 1–206). Boston: Harvard Business School Press.

Jonas, K. W. (2005). *Network-centric operations: European capabilities*, Report A1899. Assembly of WEU, Interparliamentary European Security and Defense Assembly

Josef, J., Ernest, M., & Fellenstein, C. (2004). Evolution of Grid Computing architecture and Grid adoption models. *IBM Systems Journal*, *43*(4), 624–645. doi:10.1147/sj.434.0624

Kaelber, D. C., Jha, A. K., Johnston, D., Middleton, B., & Bates, D. W. (2008). A research agenda for personal health records (PHRs). *Journal of the American Medical Informatics Association*, *15*, 729–736. doi:10.1197/jamia.M2547

Kalawsky, R.S., Nee, S.P., Homes, I. & Coveney, P.V. (2005). A grid-enabled lightwiright computational steering client: a .NET PDA implementation. *Philos. Trans. A. math. Phys. Eng. Sci., 363*(1833), 1885-94.

Kalawsky, R.S., O'Brien, J., & Coveney, P.V. (2005). Improving scientists' interaction with complex computational-visualization environments based on a distributed grid infrastructure. *Philos. Trans. A. Math. Phys. Eng. Sci, 363*(1833), 1867-84.

Kaldo-Sandstrom, V., Larsen, H., & Andersson, G. (2004). Internet-based cognitive-behavioral self-help treatment of tinnitus: clinical effectiveness and predictors of outcome. *American Journal of Audiology*, *13*(2), 185–192. doi:10.1044/1059-0889(2004/023)

Kamel Boulos, M. N., Hetherington, L., & Wheeler, S. (2007). Second Life: an overview of the potential of 3-D virtual worlds in medical and health education. *Health Information and Libraries Journal*, *24*(4), 233–245.

Kamel Boulos, M. N., & Wheeler, S. (2007). The emerging Web 2.0 social software: an enabling suite of sociable technologies in health and health care education. *Health Information and Libraries Journal*, *24*(1), 2–23.

Karasavvas, K. A., Baldock, R., & Bureger, A. (2004). Bioinformatics integration and agent technology. *Biomed. Inform.*, *37*(3), 205–219.

Kayser, G., Radziszowski, D., Bzdyl, P., Sommer, R., & Kayser, K. (2006). Theory and implementation of an electronic, automated measurement system for images obtained from immunohistochemically stained slides. *Analytical and Quantitative Cytology and Histology*, *28*(1), 27–38.

Kayser, K., Molnar, B., & Weinstein, R. S. (2006). *Virtual Microscopy*. Berlin: VSV Interdisciplinary Medical Publishing.

Kayser, K., Görtler, J., Goldmann, T., Vollmer, E., & Hufnagl, P. & Kayser G. (2008). Image standards in tissue-based diagnosis (diagnostic surgical pathology). *Diagnostic Pathology, 3*, 17. Retrieved from http://www.diagnosticpathology.org/content/3/1/17

Kersten, H. B., Thompson, E. D., & Frohna, J. G. (2008). The use of evidence-based medicine in pediatrics: past, present, and future. *Current Opinion in Pediatrics*, *20*(3), 326–331.

Ketelaar, P. (2008). Best practices of mobile e-Health in the Netherlands: The lessons learned. In *proc. of the Med-e-Tel, the international educational and networking forum for E-Health, Telemedicine and Health ICT, Luxembourg*, (pp. 1818 9334, 228-229).

Kincade, K. (1999). Wireless hits the ground running. *Telemedicine and Telehealth Networks*, *5*(6), 14–18.

Kobb, R., & Lane, R., & Stallings, D. (2008). E-learning and telehealth: Measuring your success. *Telemedicine and e-Health, 14*(6), 576-579.

Kola, I., & Landis, J. (2004). Can the pharmaceutical industry reduce attrition rates? *Nature Reviews. Drug Discovery*, *3*(8), 711–715.

Konieczny, E. (2010). *Embedded Medical Innovations*. Retrieved from http://www.embeddedintel.com/technology_applications.php?article=1065

Kopper, K. (2005). *The LINUX ENTERPRISE CLUSTER*. San Francisco, CA: No Starch Press. Retrieved from http://books.google.com/books?id=wiCGoCq8n4oC&dq=cluster%2Bcomputing&printsec=frontcover&source=bl&ots=NoUyFCqT3s&sig=Rx054L-cBDPbybnU0ClS2_zAZ0&hl=en&ei=bb7PSaK1FaectAOMm8ygAw&sa=X&oi=book_result&resnum=8&ct=result#PPP1,M1

Kowski, R. (2008). *Law problems in the development of digital radiology in Poland*. Proceedings of the Conference "Medical Imaging. New trends in technology and law" (In Polish).

Krauter, K., Buyya, R., & Maheswaran, M. (2002). A taxonomy and survey of grid resource management systems for distributed computing. *Software, Practice & Experience*, *32*, 135–164. doi:10.1002/spe.432

Krumm, M., & Huffman, T., Dick, & Klich, R. (2008). Providing infant hearing screening using OAEs and AABR using telehealth technology. *Journal of Telemedicine and Telecare*, *14*(2), 102–104. doi:10.1258/jtt.2007.070612

Krumm, M., Ribera, J., & Klich, R. (2007). Providing basic hearing tests using remote computing technology. *Journal of Telemedicine and Telecare*, *13*, 406–410. doi:10.1258/135763307783064395

Krumm, M., Ribera, J., & Schmiedge, J. (2005). Using a Telehealth Medium for Objective Hearing Testing: Implications for Supporting Rural Universal Newborn Hearing Screening Programs. *Seminars in Hearing*, *26*(1), 3–12. doi:10.1055/s-2005-863789

KUB. *Virtual Organisation*. (n.d.). Retrieved from http://www.strategyforbusiness.co.uk/html/virtual_organisation.html

Kulkarni, R., & Nathanson, L. A. (2005). Medical Informatics in medicine. *E-Medicine*. Retrieved from http://www.emedicine.com/emerg/topic879.htm

Kumar, V. S., Rutt, B., Kurc, T., Catalyurek, U. V., Pan, T. C., & Chow, S. (2008). Large-Scale Biomedical Image Analysis in Grid Environments. *IEEE Transactions on Information Technology in Biomedicine*, *12*(2), 154–161. doi:10.1109/TITB.2007.908466

Kun, L. (2001)... *Computer Methods and Programs in Biomedicine*, *64*(3), 155–167.

Kyle, R., & Murray, B. (Eds.). (2008). *Clinical Simulation: Operations, Engineering, and Management* (pp. 1–821). Amsterdam: Elsevier Press.

Kyprianou, M. (2005). Healthcare: Is Europe getting better? *The new European Healthcare Agenda – The European Voice conference*. Retrieved from http://www.noticias.info/asp/aspcommunicados.asp?nid=45584

Lacher, D., Nelson, E., Bylsma, W., & Spena, R. (2000). Computer use needs of internists: a survey of members of the American College of Physicians-American Society of Internal medicine. *In Proc. AMIA Symp.*, *2000*, 453–456.

Lagadec, E. (2007). *Unconventional Crises, Unconventional Responses: Reforming Leadership in the Age of Catastrophic Crises and Hypercomplexity* (pp. 1–68). Baltimore, MD: Johns Hopkins University Press.

Lam, D., & MacKenzie, C. (2005). Human and organizational factors affecting telemedicine utilization within U.S. military forces in Europe. *Telemedicine Journal and e-Health*, *11*, 70–78. doi:10.1089/tmj.2005.11.70

Lancaster, P., Krumm, K., & Ribera, J. (2008). Remote hearing screenings via telehealth in a rural elementary school. *American Journal of Audiology*, *17*(2), 114–122. doi:10.1044/1059-0889(2008/07-0008)

Lane, K. (2006). Telemedicine news. *Telemedicine and e-Health, 12*(5), 507-511.

Laplante-Leveque, A., Pichora-Fuller, M., & Gagne, J. (2006). Providing an internet-based audiological counseling programme to new hearing aid users: A qualitative study. *International Journal of Audiology*, *45*, 697–706. doi:10.1080/14992020600944408

Laporte, R. E. (2002). Whisking research into the classroom. *BMJ (Clinical Research Ed.)*, *324*(7329), 99. doi:10.1136/bmj.324.7329.99

Lareng, L. (2002). Telemedicine in Europe. *European Journal of Internal Medicine*, *13*, 1–13. doi:10.1016/S0953-6205(01)00188-1

Latifi, R., & Muja, S., & Bekhteshi, F., & Merrell, R. (2006). The role of telemedicine and information technology in the redevelopment of medical systems: The case of Kosova. *Telemedicine and e-Health, 12*(3), 332-340.

Lavoie, A. (2006, January 26th). The genes in your congeniality: Researchers identify genetic influence in social networks. *Harvard Science.* Retrieved from http://www.harvardscience.harvard.edu/culture-society/articles/the-genes-your-congeniality

Law Journal. (2006). Dz.U. 2006 247 poz.1819, & 60, 4 (In Polish).

Lee, J. W., & McKibbin, W. J. (2003). Globalization and disease: the case of SARS. *Asian Economic Papers*, *3*(1), 113–131. doi:.doi:10.1162/1535351041747932

Lee, M. Y., Albright, S. A., Alkasab, T., Damassa, D. A., Wang, P. J., & Eaton, E. K. (2003). Tufts Health Sciences Database: lessons, issues, and opportunities. *Academic Medicine*, *78*, 254–264.

Lee, H. W., Park, Y. R., Sim, J., Park, R. W., Kim, W. H., & Kim, J. H. (2006). The Tissue Microarray Object Model A Data Model for Storage, Analysis, and Exchange of Tissue Microarray Experimental Data. *Archives of Pathology & Laboratory Medicine*, *130*, 1004–1013.

Leeder, S., Raymond, S., & Greenberg, H. (2007). The need for leadership in global health. *The Medical Journal of Australia*, *187*(9), 532–535.

Lerch, J. P., & Evans, A. C. (2005). Cortical thickness analysis examined through power analysis and a population simulation. *NeuroImage*, *24*, 163–173. doi:10.1016/j.neuroimage.2004.07.045

Lewis, W. W. (2006). *The Power of Productivity: Wealth, Poverty, and the Threat to Global Stability* (pp. 1–339). Chicago: Chicago University Press.

Li, M., & Easrman, C. J. (2003). Working with funding agencies in the delivery of healthcare in the Asia Pacific region. *MJA*, *178*, 13–16.

Librarian, D. *a librarian's choice of the best of the Web, Health & Medicine*. (2009). Retrieved from http://www.digital-librarian.com/health.html

Liebman, M. N. (2000). Bioinformatics. In *proc. of the 23 Annual EMBS International Conference, Istanbul, Turkey*, (pp.7211-7215).

Lindberg, I., Öhrling, K., & Christenson, K. (2007). Midwives' experience of using videoconferencing to support parents who were discharged early after childbirth. *Journal of Telemedicine and Telecare*, *13*, 202–205. doi:10.1258/135763307780908102

Lindsay, M. A. (2005). Finding new drug targets in the 21st century. *Drug Discovery Today*, *10*(23-24), 1683–1687.

Lingrand, D., Montagnat, J., & Glatard, T. (2008). Estimating the execution context for refining submission strategies on production grids (workshop). In *Proceedings of the Assessing Models of Networks and Distributed Computing Platforms (ASSESS / ModernBio) (CCgrid'08),* (pp. 753 – 758).

Lipnack, J., Stamps, J., Prevou, M., Hannah, M., (in press). *Teams of Leaders Handbook,* (pp. 1-175). Fort Leavenworth, KS: Battle Command Knowledge System Combined Arms Center – Knowledge.

Littler, D., Leverick, F., & Wilson, D. (1998). Collaboration in new technology based product markets. *International Journal of Technology Management*, *15*(1-2), 139–159.

Liu, B. J., Zhou, M. Z., & Documet, J. (2005). Utilizing data grid architecture for the backup and recovery of clinical image data. *Computerized Medical Imaging and Graphics*, *29*(2–3), 95–102.

Liu, K., Mitchell, K. J., Chapman, W. W., & Crowley, R. S. (2005). Automatic clinical annotation in tissue bank specimen. Automating Tissue Bank Annotation from Pathology Reports – Comparison to a Gold Standard Expert Annotation Set. *AMIA ... Annual Symposium Proceedings / AMIA Symposium. AMIA Symposium*, *2005*, 460–464.

Liu, M., Cao, J., Gang, G., Li-Jun, C., & Li, X. (2005). A distributed power efficient data gathering and aggregation protocol for wireless sensor networks, parallel and distributed processing and applications. *international symposium,* (3758, 743-756).

Löhr, H., & Ramasamy, H. Sadeghi, A-R., Schulz, S., Schunter, M. & Stüble, C. (2006). *Enhancing Grid Security Using Trusted Virtualization.* Paper accepted for 1st Benelux Workshop on Information and System Security, November 8-9, Antwerpen, Belgium. Retrieved from https://www.cosic.esat.kuleuven.be/wissec2006/papers/12.pdf

LONI Software Tools. (n.d.). Retrieved from http://www.loni.ucla.edu/Software/

Lou, Y. (2001). Small group and individual learning with technology. *Review of Educational Research*, *71*(3), 449–521.

Lure Wasko, M., & Sara, F. (2000). "it's what one does": why people help others in electronic communities of practice. *The Journal of Strategic Information Systems*, *9*(1-3), 155–173.

Ma, X., & Yu, H. (2006). Global burden of cancer. *The Yale Journal of Biology and Medicine*, *79*(3-4), 85–94.

MacKenzie, C. M., et al. (2006, 2 August). *Reference Model for Service Oriented Architecture 1.0, OASIS Committee Specification 1.*

Manset, D., McClatchey, R., Oquendo, F., & Verjus, H. (2005). A Model-driven Approach for Grid Services Engineering. In *Proceedings of the 2005 International Conference on Software Engineering and their Applications - ICSSEA'05, (France), ICSSEA 2005.* (Vol 1. pp 135-142).

Manset, D., Pourraz, F., Tsymbal, A., Revillard, J., Skaburskas, K., McClatchey, R., et al. (in press). Gridifying Biomedical Applications: Experiences of the Health-e-Child Project. In *Handbook of Research on Computational Grid Technologies for Life Sciences, Biomedicine and Healthcare.* Hershey, PA: Information Science Reference.

Manset, D., Verjus, H., & McClatchey, R. (2007). *Managing Separation of Concerns in Grid Applications Through Architectural Model Transformations,* (LNCS Vol. 4758, pp. 308-310). Berlin: Springer-Verlag.

Maresko, D. (n.d.). Development, relief aid, and creating peace: humanitarian aid in Liberia's war of the 1990s. *OJPCR (The Online Journal of Peace and Conflict Resolution* *6*(1), 94-120.

Mars, M., & Dlova, N. (2008). Teledermatology by videoconference: experience of a pilot project. *South African Family Practice*, *50*, 70–70d.

Martin, R., & Hoover, J. N. (2008). Guide to cloud computing. *Information Week, June 21*. Retrieved from http://www.informationweek.com/news/services/hosted_apps/show Article. jhtml?articleID=208700713

May, C., Harrison, R., Finch, T., MacFarlane, A., Mair, F., & Wallace, P. (2003). Understanding the normalization of telemedicine services through qualitative evaluation. *Journal of the American Medical Informatics Association*, *10*, 596–604. doi:10.1197/jamia.M1145

Mazziotta, J. C., Toga, A. W., Evans, A. C., Fox, P., & Lancaster, J. L. (1985). A Probabilistic Atlas of the Human Brain: Theory and Rationale for its development. *NeuroImage*, *2*(3), 89–10.

McClatchey, R., Manset, D., & Solomonides, T. (2006). Lessons learned from MammoGrid for integrated biomedical solutions. In *19th IEEE Int. Symposium on Computer-Based Medical Systems, CBMS 2006*.

McEntire, D. A. (1999). Issues in disaster relief: progress, perpetual problems and prospective solutions. *Intl. J. Disaster Prevention and Management*, *8*(5), 351–361.

Meingast, M., Roosta, T., & Sastry, S. (2006). Security and privacy issues with health care information technology. In *Proceedings of the 28th IEEE EMBS Annual International Conference,* New York, August 30- September 3, (pp. 5453-5458).

Merell, R., & Doarn, C. (2008). Is it time for a telemedicine breakthrough? *Telemedicine and e-Health, 14*(6), 505-506.

Michelon, T., Magne, P., & Simon-Delavell, F. (2005). Lessons of the 2003 Heat-Wave in France and action taken to limit the effects of future heat waves. In Kirch, W., Bertollini, R., & Menne, B. (Eds.), *Extreme Weather Events and Public Health Responses* (pp. 131–140). Berlin: Springer.

Miles, S., Groth, P., Branco, M. &, Moreau, L. (2005). *The requirements of recording and using provenance in e-Science experiments*. Technical Report, Electronics and Computer Science, University of Southampton, UK.

Modal, I., Jabarin, M., Kurs, R., Barak, P., Hanan, I. & Kitain, L. (2006). Cost effectiveness, safety, and satisfaction with video telepsychiatry versus face-to-face care in ambulatory settings. *Telemedicine and e-Health, 12*, 515-520.

Mohammad, I., & Imad, M. (2004). *Handbook of Sensor Networks: Compact Wireless and Wired Sensing Systems*. Boca Raton, FL: CRC Press.

Mohrman, S. A., Cohen, S. G., & Mohrman, A. M. (Eds.). (1995). *Designing team-based organizations: New forms for knowledge work*. San Francisco: Jossey-Bass Publishers.

Monnier, J., Knapp, R. G., & Frueh, B. C. (2003). Recent advances in telepscyhiatry: An updated review. *Psychiatric Services (Washington, D.C.)*, *54*, 1604–1609. doi:10.1176/appi.ps.54.12.1604

Montagnat, J., Breton, V., & Magnin, I. E. (2003). Using grid technologies to face medical image analysis challenges. In *Proceedings of BioGrid 2003: 3rd Int. Symp. Cluster Comput. Grid (CCGrid 2003)*, (pp. 588–593).

Moore, D., Green, J., Jay, S., Leist, J., & Maitland, F. (1994). Creating a new paradigm for CME: Seizing opportunities within the health care revolution. *The Journal of Continuing Education in the Health Professions*, *14*, 4–31. doi:10.1002/chp.4750140102

Moore, G. W., & Berman, J. J. (1994). Performance analysis of manual and automated systemized nomenclature of medicine (SNOMED) coding. *American Journal of Clinical Pathology*, *101*(3), 253–256.

Moura, A., & Del Giglio, A. (2000). Education via internet. *Revista da Associação Médica Brasileira*, *46*(1), 47–51.

Moura, S. L., Coutinho, F. J., Siqueira, S. W., & Melo, R. N. (2005). Integrating Repositories of Learning Objects Using Web-Services and Ontologies. *IJWSP, 1*(1-2), 57-72. Retrieved November 10, 2008, from http://nwesp.org/ijwsp/2005/vol1/6.pdf

MRIcro, Brain Extraction Tool (BET). (n.d.). Retrieved from http://www.sph.sc.edu/comd/rorden/mricro.html

Muller, H., Michoux, N., Bandon, D., & Geissbuler, A. (2004). A review of content-based image retrieval systems in medical applications-clinical benefits and future directions. *International Journal of Medical Informatics*, *73*, 1–23. doi:10.1016/j.ijmedinf.2003.11.024

Myers, K. M., Valentine, J. M., & Melzer, S. M. (2007). Feasibility, acceptability, and sustainability of telepsychiatry for children and adolescents. *Psychatric Services*, *58*, 1493–1496. doi:10.1176/appi.ps.58.11.1493

Nannings, B., & Abu-Hanna, A. (2006). Decision support telemedicine systems: A conceptual model and reusable templates. *Telemedicine and e-Health, 12*(6), 644-654.

Nash, D. B., & Quigley, G. D. (2008). Looking forward to the end of autonomy. *Headache*, *48*(5), 719–726.

National Center for Health Statistics. *Health Expenditures*. (2002). Hyatsville, MD: CDC/NCHS. Retrieved from http://www.cdc.gov/nchs/fastats/hexpense.htm

National Coalition on Healthcare. (2004). *Building a Better Health: Specifications for Reform*. Washington, DC: Author.

NATO. (2005). *NATO Network Enabled Capability; Feasibility Study*. Brussels: NATO Consultation, Command and Control Agency.

Neerincx, P. B. T., & Leunissen, J. A. M. (2005). Evolution of web services in bioinformatics. *Briefings in Bioinf.*, *6*(2), 178–188.

Networking, S. (n.d.). *Wikipedia*. Retrieved from http://en.wikipedia.org/wiki/Social_network

NeuGrid Project. (2008). Retrieved October 20, 2008, from http://www.neugrid.eu/.

NIEeS GridInfo. *Virtuial Organisation*. (2006, March 12). Retrieved from http://gridinfo.niees.ac.uk/index.php/Virtual_Organisation

Nikula, R. E. (1999). Organisational learning within health care organisations. *International Journal of Medical Informatics*, *56*, 61–66. doi:10.1016/S1386-5056(99)00039-8

Nilsen, L. L., & Moen, A. (2008). Teleconsultation – a collaborative work and opportunities for learning across organizational boundaries. *Journal of Telemedicine and Telecare*, *14*, 377–380. doi:10.1258/jtt.2008.007012

Nirupama, B., & Sanjay, J. (2005). *Wireless Sensor Network A Systems Perspective*. Boston: Artech House.

Noji, E. K. (2005). Disasters: introduction and state of the art. *Epidemiologic Reviews*, *27*(1), 3–8.

Nordhaug, O. (Ed.). (1993). *Human capital in organizations. Competence, training, and learning*. Oslo, Norway: Scandinavian University Press.

Nurse Licensure Compact Administrators. (2008). *Nurse Licensure Compact*. Retrieved December1, 2008 from https://www.ncsbn.org/nlc.htm

O'Reilly, R., Bishop, J., Maddox, K., Hutchinson, L., Fisman, M., & Takhar, J. (2007). Is telepsychiatry equivalent to face-to-face psychiatry? Results from a randomized controlled equivalence trial. *Psychatric Services*, *58*, 836–843. doi:10.1176/appi.ps.58.6.836

Oberholzer, M., Christen, H., Haroske, G., Helfrich, M., Oberli, H., & Jundt, G. (2003). Modern telepathology: a distributed system with open standards. *Current Problems in Dermatology*, *32*, 102–114. doi:10.1159/000067381

OBO. (2008). *The Open Biomedical Ontologies*. [Web Site]. Retrieved November 10, 2008, from http://obofoundry.org/.

OECD (Organization for Economic Co-operation and Development). (2004). *OECD Health Data 2004,* CD-ROM, (also downloadable at www.oecd.org/health/healthdata).

Office of the Information and Privacy Commissioner. (2002). *Privacy Review: Chatham- Kent IT Transition Pilot Project*, (pp. 1-32). Toronto: Ontario. Available at http://www.ipc.on.ca/images/Resources/up-042202.pdf

Ogasawara, K., Endoch, A., & Sakurai, T. (2001). What do radiographers think about teleradiology in Japan. *Journal of Telemedicine and Telecare*, *7*, 161–166. doi:10.1258/1357633011936327

Olive, M., Rahmouni, H., Solomonides, T., Solomonides, T., Breton, V., & Legré, Y. (2008). SHARE, from vision to road map: technical steps. *Studies in Health Technology and Informatics*, *129*(Pt.2), 1149–1153.

Olive, M., Rahmouni, H., & Solomonides, T. (2007). From HealthGRID to SHARE: a selective review of projects. *Studies in Health Technology and Informatics*, *126*, 306–313.

Olive, M., Rahmouni, H., & Solomonides, T. (2008). *SHARE the journey: a European Healthgrid Roadmap, EU Commission: Information Society and Media*. Retrieved from http://ec.europa.eu/information_society/activities/health/docs/publications/200810share-roadmap.pdf

Oliveira, I. C., Oliveiura, J. L., Lopéz-Alonso, V., Martin-Sanchez, F., Maojo, V., & Sousa Pereira, A. (2005). Grid requirements for the integration of biomedical information resources for health applications. *Methods of Information in Medicine*, *44*(2), 161–167.

Onen, C. L. (2004). Medicine in resource-poor settings: time for a paradigm shift? *Clinical Medicine (London, England)*, *4*, 355–360.

ORACLE. (2007). *DICOM XML-Schemes*.[Web Site]. Retrieved November 10, 2008, from http://download.oracle.com/docs/cd/B28359_01/appdev.111/b28416/ap_schemas.htm

Oster, S., Langella, S., Hastings, S., Ervin, D., Madduri, R., & Phillips, J. (2008). caHrid 1.0: an enterprise grid infrastructure for biomedical research. *Journal of the American Medical Informatics Association*, *15*(2), 138–149.

Oster, S., Langella, S., Hastings, S., Ervin, D., Madduri, R., Kurc, T., et al. (2007). caGrid 1.0: A Grid Enterprise Architecture for Cancer Research. *AMIA Annu Symp Proc. 2007*, (pp. 573-577). Retrieved November 10, 2008, from http://bmi.osu.edu/resources/publications/cagrid-amia-2007.pdf

Osterholm, M., & Branswell, H. (2005). *Emerging pandemic: costs and consequences of an avian influenza outbreak, Global health Initiative/Woodrow Wilson International Center for Scholars*. Retrieved from http://www.wilsoncenter.org/index.cfm?event_id=142787&fuseaction=topics.event_summary&topic_id=116811

Overviewof the SEER Program. (2008). Surveillance Epidemiology and End Results. Retrieved from http://seer.cancer.gov/about

Ovretveit, J. (Ed.). (1993). *Coordinating community care. Multidisciplinary teams and care management*. Buckingham, UK: Open University Press.

Ovretveit, J. (1996). Five ways to describe a multidisciplinary team. *Journal of Interprofessional Care*, *10*, 163–171. doi:10.3109/13561829609034099

Ovretveit, J. (1997). Planning and managing interprofessional working and teams. In Ovretveit, J., Mathias, P., & Thomson, T. (Eds.), *Interprofessional working for health and social care* (pp. 34–52). London: Macmillan Press Ltd.

Pak, H. (2007). Telethinking. *Telemedicine and e-Health*, *13*(5), 483-486.

Pal, S. K., & Mittal, B. (2004). Fight against cancer in countries with limited resources: the post genomic era scenario. *Asian Pacific Journal of Cancer Prevention*, *5*, 328–333.

Pallikonda, M., Radhakrishan, S. & Subbaraj, P., (2008). *Remote monitoring of post operative patients using wireless sensor networks*, (9) 247-257.

Pan, T. C., Gurcan, M. N., Langella, S. A., Oster, S. W., Hastings, S. L., & Sharma, A. (2007). GridCAD: Grid-based computer-aided detection system. *Radiographics*, *27*(3). doi:10.1148/rg.273065153

PandemicFlu.gov. (n.d.). Retrieved from http://www.pandemicflu.gov/global/index.html

Papazoglou, M. P. (2003). Service-oriented computing: concepts, characteristics and directions. In *Proceedings of the 4th International Conference on Web Information Systems Engineering, WISE 2003, Roma, Italy*.

Parashar, M., & Browne, J. C. (2005). Conceptual and implementation models for the grid. *Proceedings of the IEEE*, *93*(3), 653–668. doi:10.1109/JPROC.2004.842780

Parkin, D. M., & Fernandez, L. M. (2006). Use of statistics to assess the global burden of breast cancer. *The Breast Journal*, *12*(Suppl 1), S70–S80. doi:10.1111/j.1075-122X.2006.00205.x

Paul, D. L. (2005). Collaborative activities in virtual settings: Case studies of telemedicine. In *Proc 38th Hawaii International Conference on System Sciences (HICSS'04)*. Washington, DC: IEEE Computer Society.

Pearson, S., Balis, U. J., Fuller, J., Kowalski, B., Locke, A. P., & Tillman, D. (2006). AUTO8-A Managing and Validating Laboratory Information Systems: Approved guideline. *CLSI (NCCLS). Documents. International Chamber of Commerce*, *26*(36).

Pedersen, C. A., & Gumper, K. F. (2008). ASHP National Survey on Informatics: Assessment of the adoption and use of pharmacy informatics in U.S. hospitals-2007. *American Journal of Health-System Pharmacy*, *65*(23), 2244–2264. doi:10.2146/ajhp080488

Peldschus, K., Herzog, P., Wood, S. A., Cheema, J. I., Costello, P., & Schoepf, U. J. (2005). Computer-aided diagnosis as a second reader: spectrum of findings in CT studies of the chest interpreted as normal. *Chest*, *128*, 1517–1523. doi:10.1378/chest.128.3.1517

Peltier, S., & Ellisman, M. (2003). The Grid, blueprint for a new computing infrastructure. in *The Biomedical Informatics Research Network*, (2nd ed.). Amsterdam, The Netherlands: Elsevier. Retrieved from http://www.nbirn.net

Pérez del Rey, D., Crespo, J., Pérez, L. J., Dorado, J., Bueno, G., & Feliu, V. (2005). Biomedical Image Processing Integration through INBIOMED: A Web Services-Based Platform. *Lecture Notes in Computer Science, (. LNBI*, *3745*, 34–43.

Perry, M. (2006). *Humanitarian relief challenges in the wake of South East Asian tsunami disaster*. Department of Management Working Paper Series, Monash University, Austalia. Retrieved from http://www.buseco.monash.edu.au/mgt/research/working-papers/2006/wp16-06.pdf

PI. (2008). *Pathology Informatics*. [Web Site]. Retrieved November 10, 2008, from http://www.pathologyinformatics.org/

Pileggi, S. F., Palau, C.E. & Esteve, M. (n.d.). *Integrating wireless sensor networks with Grid Computing and RFID technology for products monitoring into airports*.

Plaszczak, P., & Wellner, R. (Eds.). (2006). *Grid computing: The savvy manager's guide*. San Francisco: Morgan Kaufman Publishers.

Pollock, J. T., & Hodgson, R. (2004). *Adaptive Information: Improving Business Through Semantic Interoperability, Grid Computing, and Enterprise Integration, (Wiley Series in System Engineering Management)*. Chichester, UK: John Wiley & Sons, Inc.

Polska Telefonia Cyfro Has HSDPA Across Entire 3G Network. (2006, October 30th). Retrieved from http://www.3g.co.uk/PR/October2006/3834.htm

Porter, R. (1997). *The Greatest Benefit to Mankind: A Medical History of Humanity* (pp. 3–831). New York: Norton.

Porter, R. (2006). *The Cambridge History of Medicine* (pp. 1–408). New York: Cambridge University Press.

Powell, W. W. (1990). Neither market nor hierarchy: network forms of organization. *Research in Organizational Behavior*, *12*, 295–336.

Price, H. (2007). Delivering Tele-Health in kent England, Best practices of European E-Health Expertise, proc. of the Med-e-Tel, the international event and conference for E-Health. In *Telemedicine and Health ICT,* Luxembourg, (pp. 1818-9334, 291).

Purdy, J. (2000, July). An Intimate Invasion [Electronic Version]. *USA Weekend Magazine*. Retrieved November 3, 2008 from http://www.usaweekend.com/00_issues/000702/000702privacy.html

Puskeppeleit, M. (2008). Improving telemedicine onboard Norwegian ships and drilling platforms – A study of intersectorial co-operation in maritime medicine. [Göteborg: Nordic School of Public Health.]. *MPH*, *2008*, 13.

Quin, L., Shuo, L., Yuan, H., et al. (2008). *Securing tele-Health applications in a web-based e-Health portal,* (pp. 3-9).

Radetzky, U., Leser, U., Schultze-Rauschenbach, S. C., Zimmermann, J., Lüssem, J., Bode, T., & Cremers, A. B. (2006). Adapters, shims, and glue – services interoperability for in silico experiments. *Bioinform., 22*(9), 1137–1143.

Rajeev, S., Ananda, A., & Mun, C. C., Wei, T, O., (2006). *Mobile, wireless, and sensor networks: Technology, Applications, and Future Directions.*

R-Bay Project. (2008). *Creating an eMarketplace for the transfer of imaging related eHealth services in Europe,* retrieved 28 February, 2009 from http://www.r-bay.org/twiki/pub/RBay/Deliverables/D4_1_R-Bay_Draft_of_Legal_Framework_v1.pdf

Redfern, S., & Naughton, N. (2002). Collaborative virtual virtual environments to support communication and community in internet-based distance education. *Journal of Information Technology Education, 1*(3), 202–211.

Ribera, J. (2005). Interjudge Reliability and Validation of Telehealth Applications of the Hearing in Noise Test. *Seminars in Hearing, 26*(1), 13–18. doi:10.1055/s-2005-863790

Ribera, J., & Krumm, M. (2002) Telepractice in Audiology. *Audiology Online* (www.audiologyonline.com), Posted April 1, 2002.

Rice, R. E., Grant, A. E., Schmitz, J., & Torobin, J. (1990). Individual and network influences on the adoption and perceived outcomes of electronic messaging. *Social Networks, 12*, 27–55. doi:10.1016/0378-8733(90)90021-Z

Richards, C. (2004). *Certain to Win: the Strategy of John Boyd Applied to Business* (pp. 1–187). St. Paul, MN: Xlibris.

Richards, C. (2008). Operations other than war: what they are, and why. *Intl. J. Risk Assessment and Management, 9*(4), 376–393.

Richardson, R. (2008). E-Health Networks, International Telemedicine and E-Health initiatives. In *proc. of the Med-e-Tel, the international educational and networking forum for E-Health, Telemedicine and Health ICT,* (pp. 224).

Ricks, T. E. (2007). *Fiasco: the American Military Adventure in Iraq* (pp. 3–492). New York: Penguin.

Rifkin, J. (1998). *The Biotech Century: Harnessing the Gene and Remaking the World* (pp. 1–271). New York: Tarcher.

Rifkin, J. (2001). *The Age of Access* (pp. 3–312). New York: Tarcher/Putnam.

Rifkin, J. (2005). *The European Dream: How Europe's Vision of the Future Is Quietly Eclipsing the American Dream,* (pp. 1-434). New York: Tarcher (Penguin).

Rindfleisch, T. C. (1997). Privacy, information technology, and health care. *Communications of the ACM, 40*(8), 92–100. doi:10.1145/257874.257896

Riva, G. (2000). From telehealth to e-health: Internet and distributed virtual reality in health care. *Journal of CyberPsychology & Behavior, 3*(6), 989–998. doi:10.1089/109493100452255

Riva, G. (2002). The emergence of e-health: using virtual reality and the internet for providing advanced healthcare services. *International Journal of Healthcare Technology and Management, 4*(1/2), 15–40. doi:10.1504/IJHTM.2002.001127

Rogers, E. M. *(2003).* Diffusion of innovations, (5th, Ed.). *New York: Free Press.*

Rohan, T. E., Burk, R. D., & Franco, E. L. (2003). Toward a reduction of the global burden of cervical cancer. *American Journal of Obstetrics and Gynecology, 189*(4Suppl), S37–S39. doi:10.1067/S0002-9378(03)01079-2

Role Based Access Control (RBAC). (n.d.). Retrieved from http://en.wikipedia.org/wiki/RBAC

Rosenbaum, S., MacTaggart, P., & Borzi, P. C. (2006). Medicaid and health information: Current and emerging legal issues. *Health Care Financing Review, 28*(2), 21–30.

Rosenthal, U., Boin, A. R., & Comfort, L. K. (1993). *Managing Crises: Threats, Dilemmas, Opportunities* (pp. 5–354). Springfield, IL: Charles C. Thomas.

Roure, D., Jennings, N. R., & Shadbolt, N. R. (2005). The semantic grid: past, present and future. *Proceedings of the IEEE*, *93*(3), 669–681. doi:10.1109/JPROC.2004.842781

Roure, D. D., Jennings, N. R., & Shadbolt, N. R. (2005). The semantic grid: Past, present, and future. *Proceedings of the IEEE*, *93*, 669–681. doi:10.1109/JPROC.2004.842781

Rubin, C. (Ed.). (2007). *Emergency Management: The American Experience 1900-2005* (pp. 1–274). Fairfax, VA: PERI.

Ruch, P., Tbahriti, I., Gobeill, J., Baud, R., Lovis, C., & Geissbühler, A. (2006). *Automatic Assignment of SNOMED Categories: Preliminary and Qualitative Evaluations*. Paper presented at the meeting of the Semantic mining conference on SNOMED CT. Retrieved November 10, 2008, from http://www.hiww.org/smcs2006/proceedings/5RuchSMCS2006final.pdf

Ruckhaus, E., Ruiz, E., & Vidal, M.-E. (2008). Query Evaluation and optimization in the Semantic Web. *TPLP*, *8*(3), 393–409.

Ruiz, J. G., Mintzer, M. J., & Leipzig, R. M. (2006). The Impact of E-Learning in Medical Education. *Academic Medicine*, *81*(3), 207–212.

Sadiq, S.K., Mezzeo, M.D., Zasada, S.J., Manos, S., Stoica, I., Gale, C.V. et al. (2008). Patient-specific simulation as a basis for clinical decision-making. *Philos. Transact. A. Med. Phys. Eng. Sci. 366*(1878), 3199-219.

Salmoni, A. J., & Gonzales, M. L. (2008). Online collaborative learning: quantifying how people learn together online. *Medizinische Technik*, *30*(7), 710–716.

Saltz, J., hastings, S., Langella, S., Oster, S., Kurc, T., & payne, P. et al. (2008). The roadmap for caGrid, an enterprise Grid architecture for biomedical research. *Studies in Health Technology and Informatics*, *138*, 224–237.

Saltz, J., Oster, S., Hastings, S., Langella, S., Kurc, T., & Sanchez, W. (2006)... *Bioinformatics (Oxford, England)*, *22*(15), 1910–1916. doi:10.1093/bioinformatics/btl272

Sams-Dodd, F. (2005). Target-based drug discovery: is something wrong? *Drug Discovery Today*, *10*(2), 139–147.

Sandkuhl, K., & Fuchs-Kittowski, F. (1999). Telecooperation in decentralized organizations: conclusions based on empirical research. *Behaviour & Information Technology*, *18*, 339–347. doi:10.1080/014492999118922

Scheffler, R. M., Liu, J. X., Kinfu, J., & Dal Poz, M. L. (2008). Forecasting the global shortage of physicians: an economic- and needs-based approach. *Bull. World health Organ*, Geneva. Retrieved from http://www.scielosp.org/pdf/bwho/v86n7/a11v86n7.pdf

Schilling, M. A. (2005). *Strategic management of technological innovation*. New York: McGraw-Hill Irwin.

Schmitt, F. C. (2007). Image Biobanking: Biomaterial to personalized cancer diagnosis and treatment. In Ferrer-Roca, O. (Ed.), *Quality control in Telemedicine: Biobanking* (pp. 68–72). Tenerife, Spain: Ediciones Catai.

Schrader, T., & Kldiashvili, E. (2008). Virtual health care center in Georgia. *Diagnostic Pathology*, *3*(suppl 1), S4. .doi:10.1186/1746-1596-3-S1-S4

Schrader, T., Niepage, S., Leuthold, T., Saeger, K., Schluns, K., Hufnagl, P., et al. (2006). The diagnostic path, a useful visualisation tool in virtual microscopy. *Diagnostic Pathology*. doi:10.1186/1746-1596-1-40, 08 November 2006, 1:40, from: http://www.diagnosticpathology.org/content/1/1/40

Scotch, M., Yip, K. Y., & Cheung, K. H. (2008). *Development of Grid-like Applications for public health using Web 2.0 mashup techniques*. Journal American Medical Informatics Association.

SEAP. (2000). *Catalogo de técnicas y procedimientos*. [Web Site]. Retrieved November 10, 2008, from http://www.conganat.org/seap/informacion/catalogo.htm

SEAP. (2003). CECP - Programa de control externo de calidad en patología. *Rev. Española Patología, 36*(3), 347-349. Retrieved November 10, 2008, from http://www.conganat.org/seap/cecp/index.htm

Seely Brown, J. & Duguid, P. (1991). Organizational learning and communities of practice: toward a unified view of working, learning, and innovation. *Organization Science 2*(1 -Special Issue: Papers in honor of (and by) James G. March), 40-57.

Seers, K. (2007). Evaluating complex interventions. *Worldwide Evid. Based Nurs., 4*(2), 67–68.

Sener, S. F., & Grey, N. (2005). The global burden of cancer. *Journal of Surgical Oncology, 92*(1), 1–3. doi:10.1002/jso.20335

Senge, P. M., Kleiner, A., Roberts, C., Ross, R. B., & Smith, B. J. (Eds.). (1994). *The fifth discipline fieldbook. Strategies and tools for building a learning organization.* New York: Doubleday.

Shannon, G., Nesbitt, T., Bakalar, R., Kratochwill, E., Kvedar, J., & Vargas, L. (2002). Organizational models of telemedicine and regional telemedicine networks. *Telemedicine Journal and e-Health, 8*, 61–70. doi:10.1089/15305620252933400

Shefter, S. M. (2006). Workflow technology: the new frontier. How to overcome the barriers and join the future. *Lippincott's Case Management, 11*(1), 25–34.

Shershneva, M., & Olson, C. A. (2005). Education through telemedicine networks: setting quality standards. *Journal of Telemedicine and Telecare, 11*, 127–134. doi:10.1258/1357633053688732

Shostak, S. (1999). *Evolution of Sameness and Difference: Perspectives on the Human Genome Project* (pp. 3–342). Boca Raton, FL: CRC Press.

Shulman, A. D. (1996). Putting group information technology in its place: Communication and good work group performance. In Clegg, S. R., Hardy, C., & Nord, W. R. (Eds.), *Handbook of Organization studies* (pp. 357–374). London: Sage Publications.

Silenas, R., Waller, S. G., D'Amore, A. R., & Carlton, P. K. (2008). US Armed Forces medical operations other than war. *Int. J. Risk Assessment and Management, 9*(4), 367–375.

Singh, A., Chen, C., Liu, W., Mitchell, W., & Schmidt, B. (2008). A Hybrid Computational grid architecture for comparative Genomics. *IEEE Transactions on Information Technology in Biomedicine, 12*, 218–225. doi:10.1109/TITB.2007.908462

Sjøvold, E. (Ed.). (2006). *Teamet. Utvikling, effektivitet og endring i grupper* [The team. Development, efficiency and change in groups]. Oslo, Norway: Universitetsforlaget.

Skaburskas, K., Estrella, F., Shade, J., Manset, D., Revillard, J., Rios, A., et al. (2007). Health-e-Child: A Grid Platform for European Paediatrics. In *Proceedings of the 2007 Computing in High Energy and Nuclear Physics International Conference - CHEP07, (USA), 2007 Publication in Journal of Physics: Conference Series.*

Sloot, P., Tirado-Ramos, A., Altintas, I., Bubak, M., & Boucher, C. (2006). From molecule to man: Decision support in individualized E-Health. *Computer, 39*(11), 40–46. doi:10.1109/MC.2006.380

Sloot, P., Coveney, P., Bubak, M.T., Vandamme, A.M., & Nuallain, O, B., van de Vijver, D. & Boucher, C. (2008). Multi-science decision support for HIV drug resistance treatment. *Stud. Health Inform., 138*, 188–198.

Sluimer, J. D., Vrenken, H., Blankenstein, M. A., Fox, N. C., Scheltens, P., Barkhof, F., & van der Flier, W. M. (n.d.). *Whole-brain atrophy rate in Alzheimer disease - Identifying fast progressors. SOAP Attachment.* (n.d). Retrieved from http://www.w3.org/TR/SOAP-attachments

SNCFP. (2005). Catalogo nacional de calificación profesional. Familia profesional de sanidad. *Anatomía patológica y citología. BOE 238 5.* Retrieved November 10, 2008, from http://www.mepsyd.es/educa/incual/pdf/2/SAN_125_(5).pdf

Snow, C. C., Lipnack, J., & Stamps, J. (1999). The virtual organization: Promises and payoffs, large and small. In C.L. Cooper, D.M. Rousseau, (Eds.), *Trends in organizational behaviour, Volume 6, The virtual organization* (pp. 15-30). Chichester, UK: John Wiley & Sons Ltd.

Solomonides, A., McClatchey, R., Odeh, M., Brady, M., Mulet-Parada, M., Schottlander, D., & Amendolia, S. (2003). Mammogrid and ediamond: Grids applications in mammogram analysis. In *Proc. International Association for Development of the Information Society International Conference, IADIS Int. Conf.: e-Soc.*, (pp. 1032–1033).

Souvik, R., & Zhang, Z. (2004). An efficient anonymity protocol for Grid Computing. In *Proc. of the 5th IEEE/ACM, international workshop on Grid Computing,* (pp. 200-207). Washington, DC: IEEE computer society.

Srinivasan, P., Libbus, B., & Kumar, A. (2004). Mining MEDLINE: Postulating a Beneficial Role for Curcumin Longa in Retinal Diseases. In Hirschman, L., & Pustejovsky, J. (Eds.), *HLT-NAACL 2004 Workshop: BioLINK 2004, Linking Biological Literature, Ontologies and Databases* (pp. 33–40). Boston: Association for Computational Linguistics.

SRP. (2008). *Speach recognition in pathology*. [Computer software]. Retrieved November 10, 2008, from http://www.escription.com/products/index.html, http://www.nuance.com/dictaphone/products/powerscribe/pathology/

Stead, W. W. (1998). The networked health enterprise: A vision for 2008. *Journal of the American Medical Informatics Association, 5*, 412–415.

Structural Image Evaluation using Normalisation of Atrophy (SIENA). (n.d.). Retrieved from http://www.fmrib.ox.ac.uk/fsl/siena/index.html.

Sucurello, F. (2008). A Tele-homecare System for patients with chronic diseases. In *Proc. of the Med-e-Tel, the international trade event and conference for E-Health, Telemedicine and Health ICT*, Luxembourg (1818-9334, pp. 41-42).

Summers, R. M., Jerebko, A. K., Franaszek, M., Malley, J. D., & Johnson, C. D. (2002). Colonic polyps: complementary role of computer-aided detection in CT colonography. *Radiology, 225*, 391–399. doi:10.1148/radiol.2252011619

Swedlow, J. R., Goldberg, I., Brauner, E., & Sorger, P. K. (2003). Informatics and quantitative analysis in biological imaging. *Science, 300*, 100–102. doi:10.1126/science.1082602

Systems, B. R. I. T. (n.d.). *PACS 101 - things you need to know when embarking on a PACS project.* Retrieved 28 February, 2009, from http://www.brit.com/Product%20Sheet%20PDFs/BRIT%20PACS%20101.pdf

Taylor, H. (2007). Lack of trust in both FDA and pharmaceutical companies makes drug safety a concern. *Healthcare News* 7(6), April 25. Retrieved from http://www.harrisinteractive.com/news/newsletters/healthnews/HI_HealthCareNews_2007_v07_i06.pdf

Taylor-Gooby, P. (2006). Trust, risk, and healthcare reform. *Health Risk & Society, 8*(2), 97–103.

Temal, L., Dojat, M., Kassel, G., & Gibaud, B. (2008). Towards an ontology for sharing medical images and regions of interest in neuroimaging. *Journal of Biomedical Informatics, 41*(5), 766–778. doi:10.1016/j.jbi.2008.03.002

Thali, M. J. (2006). Virtopsy: Virtual Autopsy. In Ferrer-Roca, O. (Ed.), *Personalizad virtual medicine: p-health* (pp. 159–162). Tenerife, Spain: Ediciones Catai.

The distributed computing. (n.d.). Retrieved January 9, 2009, from Wikipedia: http://en.wikipedia.org/

The Economist. (2003, April 10). Epidemics and economies.

The Globus Alliance. (n.d.). Retrieved from http://www.globus.org/

The Healthgrid White Paper. (2005)... *Stud. Technol. Inform., 112*, 249–321.

The Information Societies Technology Project: Health-e-Child EU Contract IST-2004-027749 Description of Work

The Mind and the Body are the Same Thing. (2010). Retrieved from http://mentalhealth.about.com/gi/o.htm?zi=1/XJ&zTi=1&sdn=mentalhealth&cdn=health&tm=15&gps=37_59_882_523&f=00&su=p284.9.336.ip_p736.8.336.ip_&tt=2&bt=1&bts=1&zu=http%3A//serendip.brynmawr.edu/exhibitions/Mind/Descartes.html

The University of Washington School of Public Health's Center for Public Health Informatics. (n.d.). Retrieved on October 14, 2008 from http://www.cphi.washington.edu/research.html.

Tierney, K. J. (2006). Testimony on needed emergency management reforms. *J. Homeland Security and Disaster Management 4*(3), Article 15.

Tobias, J., Chilukuri, R., Komatsoulis, G. A., Mohanty, S., Sioutos, N., Warzel, D. B., et al. (2006). The CAP cancer protocols - a case study of caCORE based data standards implementation to integrate with the Cancer Biomedical Informatics GRID. *BMC Med Inform Decis Mak, 6,* 25-44. Retrieved November 10, 2008, from http://www.biomedcentral.com/1472-6947/6/25

Toffler, A., & Toffler, H. (2007). *Revolutionary Wealth: How it will be created and how it will change our lives*. New York: Doubleday Business.

Towers, A., Pisa, J., & Froelich, T. (2005). The Reliability of Click-Evoked and Frequency-Specific Auditory Brainstem Response Testing Using Telehealth Technology. *Seminars in Hearing*, *26*(1), 26–34. doi:10.1055/s-2005-863792

Tweed, T., & Miguet, S. (2003). Medical image database on the grid: Strategies for data distribution. In *Proc. HealthGrid 2003 Workshop*, (pp. 152–162).

UMLS. (2008). *UMLS Semantic Network*. [Web Site]. Retrieved November 10, 2008, from http://semanticnetwork.nlm.nih.gov/

US Mission to the UN Release 65. (2002). USAI leads public and private partners to improve health and save lives through food fortification, USUN, New York, May 8, 2002.

Vahid, F., & Givargis, T. (2002). *Embedded System Design, A Unified Hardware/Software Approach*. Chichester, UK: John Wiley & Sons. Retrieved from http://esd.cs.ucr.edu/

Vallat, B. (2007). Avian influenza epizootie: where do we stand in 2007. *CSIRO Snowdon Lecture*, 11 July 2007 (chapter 2). Retrieved from http://www.csiro.au/files/files/pqlo.pdf

Van Rooyen, M. J., Hansch, S., Curtis, D., & Burnham, G. (2001). Emerging issues and future needs in humanitarian assistance. *Prehospital and Disaster Medicine*, *16*(4), 216–222.

Virolab. (2006). Retrieved from http://www.virolab.org:8080/virolab/ and

VLA. (2006). *Virtual lab automation*. [Computer software]. Retrieved November 10, 2008, from http://www.vmware.com/pdf/virtual_lab_automation_whitepaper.pdf

Vladzymyrskyy, A. V., et al. (2008). Clinical efficiency of telemedicine in trauma and orthopedics. In *proc. of the Med-e-Tel, the international educational and networking forum for E-Health, Telemedicine and Health ICT*, Luxembourg, (pp. 224).

von Lubitz, D. K. J. E. (2008). Medical readiness for operations other than war: Boyd's OODA Loop and training using advanced distributed simulation technology. *Intl J. Risk Assessment and Management*, *9*(4), 409–432.

von Lubitz, D. K. J. E., & Beakley, J. (in press). "Teams of Leaders" concept in homleland security and disaster management operations. *Int l.J. Homeland Security and Disaster Management.*

von Lubitz, D. K. J. E., & Patricelli, F. (2006). Network-centric Healthcare Operations; Data Warehousing and the Associated Telecommunication Platforms. *Intl. J.Services and Standards*, *3*(1), 97–119.

von Lubitz, D. K. J. E., & Patricelli, F. (2008). Telecommunications infrastructure for worldwide network-centric healthcare operations and the associated information system. *Intl. J. Business and Systems Research*, *2*(1), 34–51.

von Lubitz, D. K. J. E., & Wickramasinghe, N. (2006a). Healthcare and technology: the doctrine of network-centric healthcare. *International Journal of Electronic Healthcare*, *4*, 322–344.

von Lubitz, D. K. J. E., & Wickramasinghe, N. (2006b). Networkcentric healthcare and bioinformatics: unified operations within three domains of knowledge. *Expert Systems with Applications*, *30*, 11–23.

von Lubitz, D. K. J. E., & Wickramasinghe, N. (2006c). Dynamic Leadership In Unstable And Unpredictable Environments. *Intl. J. Innovation Learning*, *4*, 339–350.

von Lubitz, D. K. J. E., & Wickramasinghe, N. (2006d). Networkcentric healthcare: outline of entry portal concept. *Intl. J. Electronic Business Management*, *4*(1), 16–28.

von Lubitz, D. K. J. E., & Wickramasinghe, N. (2006e). Creating germane knowledge in dynamic environments. *Int. J. Innovation and Learning*, *3*(3), 326–347.

von Lubitz, D. K. J. E., Wickramasinghe, N., & Yanovsky, G. (2006). Networkcentric healthcare operations: the telecommunications structure. *Int. J. Networking and Virtual Org.*, *3*(1), 60–85.

von Lubitz, D., & Patricelli, F. (2007). Network-centric healthcare operations: data warehousing and the associated telecommunications platforms. *International Journal of Services and Standards*, *3*(1), 97–119. doi:10.1504/IJSS.2007.011830

von Lubitz, D. K. J. E., Levine, H., & Wolf, E. (2002). The Goose, the Gander, or the Strasbourg Paté for All: Medical Education, World, and the Internet. In Chin, W., Patricelli, F., & Milutinovic, V. (Eds.), *Electronic Business and Education: Recent Advances in Internet Infrastructures* (pp. 189–210). Boston: Academic Publishers.

von Lubitz D. & Wickramasinghe N. (2006). Network-centric healthcare: applying the tools, techniques and strategies of knowledge management to healthcare. *International Journal of Management*, 60-85.

von Lubitz, D. K. J. E., Beakley, J., & Patricelli, F. (2008a). "All hazards approach" to network-centric disaster management: the role of information and knowledge management, and Boyd's OODA Loop in disaster leadership. *The Journal of Disaster Study, Policy and Management,* May 13. doi:10.1111/j.0361-3666.2008.01060.x, available at http://www.blackwell-synergy.com/toc/disa/0/0

von Lubitz, D. K. J. E., Beakley, J., & Patricelli, F. (2008b). Disaster Management: The Structure, Function, and Significance of Network-Centric Operations. *Journal of Homeland Security and Emergency Management, 1/1*(5). Available at: http://www.bepress.com/jhsem/vol5/iss1/1

von Lubitz, D. K. J. E., Beier, K. P., & Freer, J. Griffiths, J.M., Levine, H., Sauter, J., et al. (2001). *IMERSEME in VIBEs: Interactive/Immersive Medical Education/Research Simulation and Modeling Environment (IIMERSME) and Virtual Interactive Burn Environment (VIBE) as a "New Generation" approach to global bio-medical education, training, and research.* Proc ITEC 2001, Lille (France), April 24-26, 2001.

von Lubitz, D. K. J. E., Carrasco, B., Fausone, C. A., Gabbrielli, F., Kirk, J., Lary, M. J., et al. (2005). Bioterrorism, medical readiness, and distributed simulation training of first responders. In J. Johnson, M. Cwiek, G. Ludlow, (eds.), *Community and Response to Terrorism (Vol. II): A Community of Organizations: Responsibilities and Collaboration Among All Sectors of Society,* (pp. 267-312). Westport, CT: Praeger/Greenwood Publ. Group.

Voss, H. (2009). *Telepsykiatri i Danmark – hvad ved vi fra udlandet? Udenlandske erfaringer med anvendelse af videokonference i psykiatrien. DSI projekt nr. 2654.* København, Denmark: Dansk Sundhedsinstitut.

Vuonovirta, T., Timonen, M., Keinänen-Kiukaaniemi, S., Timonen, O., Ylitalo, K., Kantse, O., & Taanila, A. (2009). The attitudes of multiprofessional teams to telehealth adoption in northern Finland health centres. *Journal of Telemedicine and Telecare*, *15*, 290–296. doi:10.1258/jtt.2009.090108

Wagner, E. H. (2000). The role of patient care teams in chronic disease management. *British Medical Journal*, *320*, 569–572. doi:10.1136/bmj.320.7234.569

Walther, J. B., Bunz, U., & Bazarova, N. N. *(2005). The rules of virtual groups. In* Proc 38th Hawaii International Conference on System Sciences (HICSS'04). *Washington, DC: IEEE Computer Society.*

Wang, S., Armstrong, M. P., & Bennett, D. A. (2002). Conceptual basics of middleware design to support Grid Computing of geographic information. In *Proc. of International Conference on Geographic Information Science*, September, 25 - 28, Boulder, CO, (pp. 197-200).

Ward, R., Stevens, C., Brentnall, P., & Briddon, J. (2008). The attitudes of healthc care staff to information technology: a comprehensive review of the research literature. *Health Info Libr.*, *25*(2), 81–97.

Ward, R., & Wamsley, G. (2007). From a painful past to an uncertain future. In Rubin, C. (Ed.), *Emergency Management: The American Experience 1900-2005* (pp. 207–242). Fairfax, VA: PERI.

Web Service Description Language (WSDL). (n.d.). Retrieved from http://www.w3.org/TR/2007/REC-wsdl20-primer-20070626/

Web Services Business Process Execution Language (WSBPEL). (n.d.). Retrieved from http://www.oasis-open.org/committees/tc_home.php?wg_abbrev=wsbpel

Wegener, D., Sengstag, T., Sfakianakis, S., Ruping, S., & Assi, A. (2007, December 10-13). GridR: An R-Based Grid-Enabled Tool for Data Analysis in ACGT Clinico-Genomics Trials. In *IEEE International Conference on e-Science and Grid Computing,* (pp. 228 - 235).

Weinstein, R. S., Dunn, B. E., & Graham, A. R. (1997). Telepathology networks as models of telemedical services by cybercorps. *Nature Medicine*, *1*, 235–241.

Weiss, T. (2001, November 29). Grid computing to aid breast cancer research. *CNN news*. Retrieved October 3, 2008 from http://archives.cnn.com/2001/TECH/industry/11/29/grid.cancer.research.idg/

Welch, G., Sonnenwald, D. H., Fichs, H., Cairns, B., Mayer-Patel, K., & Söderholm, H. M. (2009). 3D medical collaboration technology to enhance emergency healthcare. *Journal of Biomedical Discovery and Collaboration*, *4*(4).

Welsh, T., & Pringle, M. (2001). Social capital. *British Medical Journal*, *323*, 177–178. doi:10.1136/bmj.323.7306.177

Werner, P. (2004). Willingness to use telemedicine for psychiatric care. *Telemedicine and e-Health, 10*, 286-293.

Whitten, P., & Kuwahara, E. (2004). A multi-phase telepsychiatry programme in Michigan: organizational factors affecting utilization and user perceptions. *Journal of Telemedicine and Telecare*, *10*, 254–261. doi:10.1258/1357633042026378

WHO. (1946). *Constitution of the World Health Organization.* Retrieved from http://www.who.int/gb/bd/PDF/bd46/e-46_p2.pdfhttp://www.who.int/gb/bd/PDF/bd46/e-bd46_p2.pdf

WHO. (2008). *Are the number of cancer cases increasing or decreasing in the world?* World Health Organization Online Q&A. Retrieved from http://www.who.int/features/qa/15/en/index.html.

Wickramasinghe, N., & Schaffer, J. L. (2006). Creating knowledge-driven healthcare processes with the Intelligence Continuum. *International Journal of Electronic Healthcare*, *2*(2), 164–174.

Wickramasinghe, N., & von Lubitz, D. K. J. E. (2007). *Knowledge-Based Enterprise: Theories and Fundamentals* (pp. 1–380). Hershey, PA: IDEA Group Publishing.

Wiecha, J., & Barrie, N. (2002). Collaborative online learning: a new approach to distance CME. *Academic Medicine*, *77*(9), 928–929.

Wiese, C.R. (2006). Organizing Homeland Security after Katrina: is adaptive management what's missing. *Publ. Adm. Rev. May-June 2006*, 302-318.

Wiljer, D., Urowitz, S., Apatu, E., DeLenardo, C., Eysenbach, G., & Harth, T. (2008). Patient accessible electronic health records: Exploring recommendations for successful implementation strategies. *Journal of Medical Internet Research*, *10*(4), e34. doi:10.2196/jmir.1061

Williams, K. A., Sullivan, F., Suner, S., Shapiro, M., Kobayashi, L., Woolard, B., & Hill, W. (2008). Rhode Island disaster initiative. *Intl. J. Risk Assessment and Management*, *9*(4), 394–408.

Wilson, C. (2004). *CRS Report for Congress, 2004, Network Centric Warfare: Background and Oversight Issues for Congress* (pp. 1–35). Washington, DC: Congressional Research Service and The Library of Congress.

WIPO. (2008). *World Intellectual property organization: WO/2001/098774. Systems for automated and remote histological analysis and new drug assessment.* [Web Site]. Retrieved November 10, 2008, from http://www.wipo.int/pctdb/en/wo.jsp?gIA=IL2001000561&DISPLAY=DESC

Wong, J. G. (1996). Efficiency and effectiveness in the urgent care clinic. *Postgraduate Medicine*, *99*(4), 161–166.

Workman, P. (2001). New drug targets for genomic cancer: therapy successes, limitations, opportunities, and future challenges. *Current Cancer Drug Targets*, *1*(1), 33–47.

World Economic Forum, Eurasia Economic Summit 2002: Health and the Future of Business, the Global Health Initiative of the World Economic Forum. (2002, August 8th).

World Federation on Medical Education. (1998). International standards in medical education: assessment and accreditation of medical schools'--educational programmes. A WFME position paper. The Executive Council, The World Federation for Medical Education. *Medical Education*, *32*(5), 549–558.

World Federation on Medical Education. (2000). WFME task force on defining international standards in basic medical education. Report of the working party, Copenhagen, 14-16 October 1999. *Medical Education*, *34*(8), 665–675.

World Health Organization Report. (2004). *Changing History*, (pp. 1-167). Geneva: Author.

WS-Addressing. (n.d.). Retrieved from http://www.w3.org/TR/2006/REC-ws-addr-core-20060509/.

WS-Security. (n.d.). Retrieved from http://www.oasis-open.org/committees/tc_home.php?wg_abbrev=wss

Wyle, M. D., Lind, W. S., & Trainor, B. E. (1981). Maneuver/Fluid Warfare. *The Marine Corps Gazette*, *65*(April), 49–54.

Yasnoff, W. A. (2003). Privacy, confidentiality and security of public health information. In *Public Health Informatics and Information Systems*. New York: Springer. doi:10.1007/0-387-22745-8_10

Yates, J., & Campbell, K. (2005). Audiovestibular education and services via telemedicine technologies. *Seminars in Hearing*, *26*, 35–42. doi:10.1055/s-2005-863793

Yujie, Y. Shu, Wang (2005). The key research on integration wireless sensor network with Grid. In *Proc. Wireless communication networking and mobile computing*, (pp. 1477-1480).

Yunhong, G., & Robert, G. (2003). SABUL: A transport protocol for grid computing. *Journal of Grid Computing*, *1*(4), 377–386. doi:10.1023/B:GRID.0000037553.18581.3b

Zara, C., Torralba, M., Sotoca, J. M., Prat, A., Faixedas, M. T., & Gilalbert, A. (2004). The impact of new drug introduction on drug expenditure in primary health care in Catalunya, Spain. *The Annals of Pharmacotherapy*, *39*(1), 177–182.

Zou, L., Miller, S. N., & Schmidtmann, E. T. (2007). A GIS tool to estimate West Nile Virus Risk based on a degree-day model. *Environmental Monitoring and Assessment*, *129*(1-3), 413–420. doi:10.1007/s10661-006-9373-8

Zupan, J. (2003). Perinatal mortality and morbidity in developing countries: a global view. *Med Trop*, *63*(Mars), 366–368.

About the Contributors

Ekaterina Kldiashvili, PhD holds a MSc in Biology (1995) and PhD in Histology, Cytology and Embryology (2003) from the Tbilisi State University. Ekaterina works as Executive Director in Georgian Telemedicine Union (Association), Head of Lab and Telemedicine Group in Medical Center "Neoclinic", managing NATO Networking Infrastructure Project (2005-2006, 2007-2009), BSEC tender (2005-2006), telemedicine pilot actions, whole activity of GTU and also creation of eHealth network in Georgia. Prior to joining GTU Ekaterina worked at department of Pathology of Central Clinic of Tbilisi State Medical University, establishing and leading the electron microscopy laboratory. She was trained in cytological diagnosis of malignant tumors at department of Oncology of the Tbilisi State Medical Academy. Ekaterina also acted as Clinical Cytologist at department of pathology of Central Clinic of Tbilisi State Medical University and Virologist at Republic Center of AIDS and Clinical Immunology. She participated as researcher in Neuroscience project funded by Soros foundation. Ekaterina Kldiashvili represented GTU's activity and pilot actions at Med-e-Tel (2004, 2005, 2006, 2008).

* * *

I.H. Monrad Aas, is a Norwegian with doctoral degree from the University of Oslo (1983) and full professor competence (1994). He has done health services research on a broad number of issues, has authored close to 120 publications (including papers in international journals, books, chapters in books, papers in Norwegian, research reports), been a referee for international journals (e.g. British Medical Journal, Bulletin of the World Health Organization, Journal of Telemedicine and Telecare), opponent at doctoral dissertations, mentor and given feedback on more than 250 research works, invited speaker to international conferences in Europe, Australia, USA and the Middle East. At the Nordic School of Public Health in Gothenburg, he was leading courses at high level in health care management for health care personnel from all five Nordic countries and international courses for researchers. Has worked with the University of Oslo (1976-1984), The Norwegian Institute for Hospital Research (1985-1990), The Nordic School of Public Health (1990-1995), The Work Research Institute in Oslo (1995- 2006), and is presently with the Department of Research of Vestfold Mental Health Care Trust (2006-).

Thomas Clark, Initial Training and experience was acquired on with the US Military and Defense Departments and ranging from National Air Defense Computer Control Systems to Aircraft and Missile Control Systems. Additional Projects included (1)development of a 13.5 BEV Protron Synchrotron at Argonne National Laboratory, (2)design and development of a Multiprocessor Time Sharing Computer Systems and Networks, (3)parallel data processing systems, (4)advanced Office Automation Systems,

(5)Fault Tolerant and Highly Available Computer Systems and Networks, (5)Electronic Prescription Systems, (6)Telemedicine, (7)eHealth, (8)TeleCardiology, (9)TeleDiagnostics and (10)Patient Monitoring. This migration started at 'Control Systems Engineering', progressed through 'Enterprise Computer Systems and Networks', 'Advanced Computer Systems Applications' and 'System Theory and Design' arriving at 'Medical and Health Care Informatics'. A BSEE degree was acquired at the University of New Mexico followed by an MSEE degree at Wichita State University, both with emphasis upon Control Systems. These were followed by MSCS and ENGINEER degrees at the University of Southern California with focus upon Fault Tolerant and Highly Available Computer Systems. A cooperative diversion added BSL and JD degrees from Peninsula University thereby adding an understanding of California Common Law and Computer Systems and Networks. Current activities are focused upon all aspects of Local and International Telemedicine, eHealth, Medical Devices, Health Psychology, Patient Monitoring, Patient-Centric Health Care and Personalised Medicine. Home Territory is the Portland, Oregon, US region and the Northwest Territories, Canada and the US.

Michal Dzierzak was born in Warsaw, Poland on April 26, 1975. He received a Master of Science in Mechanics from Warsaw University of Technology in 2000. At that time he worked as IT specialist for Medical University of Warsaw. At present he is additionally teaching students Medical Informatics. After graduating from Warsaw University of Technology, he received Associate's Certificate in Project Management from George Washington University School of Business and Public Management. This certificate and work as a Project Manager in one of the International IT companies led him to become Project Management Professional (PMP). Work as an IT specialist and Project Manager helped him to understand almost all security aspects and business processes in healthcare area and especially: Public Key Infrastructure, Identity and Access Management, Security of Data in Distributed Systems.

Professor **Dag von Lubitz**, PhD, MD(Sc.): generalist and conceptualist recently retired from the posts of Chairman of the Board and Chief Scientist at MedSMART, Inc. Prior to his nearly decade-long affiliation with business industry, DvL had a distinguished academic career at the leading universities and research institutions of Europe and the US resulting in over 220 papers, book chapters, and books spanning medicine, molecular neuropharmacology, IT, leadership, and homeland defense and security. Laureate of the Smithsonian Institution Award, winner of Laval Prize, and holder of several other national and international scientific awards, DvL works currently as a consultant in the US and EU concentrating on global healthcare, decision-making and leadership in crises and disasters, and homeland defence and security. An avid mondialist, DvL specializes in developing effective collaboration and cooperation based on the combined people-technology approaches (including network-centricity and social networks) in worldwide business, politics, and education and training.

Gloria Bueno received her MsC from Universidad Complutense de Madrid in 1993, and her PhD from Coventry University in 1998. From 1998 to 2000 Gloria worked as a postdoctoral researcher at Université Louis Pasteur, Strasbourg. In 2000-2001 she worked at CNRS, Inst. de Physique Biologique-Hôpital Civil and from 2001 to 2003 she was a senior researcher at CEIT (Centro de Estudios e Investigaciones Técnicas de Gipuzkoa), San Sebastián, Spain. She is currently an Associate Professor at Universidad de Castilla-La Mancha (UCLM), Spain and she conducts the Machine Vision and Artificial Intelligence Group at UCLM. Her main research interests include image processing –particularly for biomedical engineering applications- computer vision, artificial intelligence, modeling and simulation.

Marcial García Rojo received his MsC from Universidad de Cádiz in 1987, and his PhD from Universidad Autónoma de Madrid in 1995. From 1988 to 1991 Marcial worked at Hospital La Paz in Madrid, and since 1992 he is at Hospital General de Ciudad Real (HGCR) in the Anatomical Pathology Department. He has also carried on activities in academic areas as Academic Coordinator in INTI, S.L. and he is currently conducting the Information Technology Department at HGCR. He is a research fellow of the Spanish Society for Anatomical Pathology (SEAP) and Spanish Society for Health Informatics (SEIS).

Roberto González received his MsC from Universidad de Castilla-La Mancha in 2004. He was an Assistant Professor at the Department of Control and System Engineering and a research member of the Machine Vision and Artificial Intelligence Group from 2004 to 2008. He is currently a research Engineering at REPSOL, S.A. His main research interests are computer vision and parallel programming.v

Oscar Deniz received his MsC and PhD from Universidad de Las Palmas de Gran Canaria, Spain, in 1999 and 2006, respectively. He has been associate professor at Universidad de Las Palmas de Gran Canaria from 2003 to 2007 and currently at Universidad de Castilla-La Mancha, Spain. His main research interests are computer vision and artificial intelligence. He is a research fellow of the Institute of Intelligent Systems and Numerical Applications in Engineering and member of IEEE, AEPIA and AERFAI.

Jesús García González received his MsC from Universidad de Granada in 1984. From 1986 to 1989 Jesús worked at Hospital Virgen de las Nieves in Granada, and since 1990 he is at Hospital General de Ciudad Real in the Anatomical Pathology Department.

Mita Lovalekar is an Assistant Professor in the Department of Sports Medicine and Nutrition within the School of Health and Rehabilitation Sciences, and an Assistant Professor of Epidemiology at the University of Pittsburgh. She is a physician trained in India, and completed both her Master's and Doctoral degrees in Epidemiology at the University of Pittsburgh. Her research interests include injury epidemiology and prevention, application of the Internet to dissemination of health information, and chronic disease epidemiology.

Olga Ferrer Roca working as pathologist in the Clinic Hospital of Barcelona since 1972 got the Assistance Professorship in Pathology in 1974 and the Chair of Pathology of the University of La Laguna in 1982. Commercialized a pathology image analysis system TEXCAN ® ™ specialized in visual textural analysis of the cell chromatin and DNA and immunohistochemical quantification. Founded the CATAI association in 1993, being the president since then. Got the UNESCO Chair of Telemedicine in 1999 for the University of La Laguna. Since 1996 train on Telemedicine the students of medicine and Computer Science, creating the European Master of Telemedicine and Bioengineering applied to Telemedicine in 2004, at distance. Editor of 8 books and 202 Publications is the author of the first textbook of Telemedicine Handbook of Telemedicine. Amsterdam: IOS-Press, 1998, containing the Ontology of Telemedicine

Francisco J. Marcano Serrano, Master in Telemedicine and Biotechnology applied to Telemedicina, University of La Laguna (ULL), Tenerife, Spain. Researcher in Telemedicine, Ontologies and biomedical image processing. Instructor at Computation and Information Technology Department – USB (1990-92) Senior Imaging Consultant - XEROX of Venezuela (1996-2004). Nowadays he is doing his PhD degree in biomedical research in the ULL. Fellow of UNESCO Chair in Telemedicine – ULL and CATAI (2005-).

Maria Esther Vidal, Master on Computer Science in 1991, and PhD on Computer Science in 2000 from the University Simón Bolívar, Caracas Venezuela. She is a Full Professor of the Computer Science department at the Simón Bolívar University and has been Assistant Researcher at the Institute of Advanced Computer Studies in the University of Maryland (UMIACS) (1995-1999), and Visitor Professor at UMIACS (2000-2007) and in University Politecnica of Catalunya (2003). She has reported her research on AAAI, IJCAI, SIGMOD, CoopIs, WIDM, WebDB, ICDE, DILS, DEXA, ALPWS, ACM SAC, CAISE, OTM, SIGMOD RECORD, JBCB and TPLP Journal. Current research interests are query rewriting and optimization in emerging infrastructures, and sampling techniques to efficiently evaluate queries on the Semantic Web. Prof. Vidal is member of SIGMOD.

Edna Ruckhaus, Master on Computer Science and Information Science, Syracuse University, 1986. Doctoral Candidate in Computer Science, Simón Bolívar University, under the supervision of Dr. María Esther Vidal in the area of Query Evaluation and Optimization Techniques in the Semantic Web. Member of the Database Group of the University Simón Bolívar. Visiting scholar at the MIND Lab, University of Maryland, 2004 2005. Consultant for the Venezuela Council of Science and Technology and the United Nations Development Programme. Over fifteen publications in international conferences and journals, in the areas of Ontologies and the Semantic Web and Metadata for Educational Environments in the Web.

Xiomara Santos Palacios, Researcher in Telemedicine, Ontologies and biomedical image processing. Senior Administrador Consultant – Globovisión Corporation (1997 – 2006). System analyst in Televen Corporation (1990-1997). Fellow of UNESCO Chair in Telemedicine – ULL and CATAI (2008-).

Enrique Iglesias, Master in Physics 1985 and Ph. D inPhysics 1987 from the University of Maryland, USA. He is Full Professor of the Physics Department at Simón Bolívar University and has been Assistant Research Scientist at IREAP (Institute for Research In Electronics and Applied Physics) 1995-1999 at the University of Maryland in College Park, and Visiting Scholar at NIST (National Institute of Science and Technology) 2005-2006. He has reported his research on Physical Review A, E, Nuclear Fusion, Physics of Plasmas, JQSRT, Applied Optics and Magazine Mexicana de Physical and Brazilian Journal of Physics. Current research is in the area of transient plasma diagnostics, and Spectroscopy from the Ultraviolet to the Infrared.Prof. Iglesias is member of the APS.

David Manset, born in 1978, holds a Mph from the University of Savoie in France, in Computer Sciences specialized in model driven engineering for distributed computing system architectures. David Manset is CEO of MAAT France and Director of Biomedical Applications for MAAT Gknowledge industrial group. During the last 7 years, he has contributed to European and international projects focusing on e-health and biomedical research, with a special emphasis on the application of grid technologies. In particular, he has architected grid-based platforms for projects such as the EU FP5 MammoGrid, the EU FP6 Health-e-Child, the EU FP7 neuGRID and the EU FP7 outGRID. His work and team have been awarded several times in major events (such as the International Inventions Symposium of Geneva in 2007, The international EGEE 2007 Conference, the international EGEE 2008 User Forum Conference, Europe's largest conference on Information and Communication Technologies, ICT 2008 and more recently the international EGEE 2009 Conference).

Dr. **Ribhi Hazin** is a John F. Kennedy fellow at Harvard University, where he is focusing on health policy and ethics.

Dr. **Ibrahim Qaddoumi** earned his medical degree in 1992 at Damascus University, Syria. In 1995 he did a Combined Medicine-Pediatric Residency Program in Michigan at St. Joseph Mercy Hospital and Henry Ford Hospital. His fellowship in Pediatric Hematology-Oncology was completed at the Medical University of South Carolina 1999-2002. He also obtained his Master's in Science at the Medical University of South Carolina in 2003. Dr. Qaddoumi joined the faculty at St. Jude Children's Research Hospital in the Department of Oncology in October of 2007. His clinical practice is focused primarily on low grade gliomas and retinoblastoma. In addition, Dr. Qaddoumi has practical interest in improving cancer in developing countries via utilization of twinning and telemedicine.

Dr. **Francisco Pedrosa** - Medical graduated from the Medical College of Pernambuco, Brazil, 1963. Initial training and experience in Pediatric Oncology in the Sloan-Kettering Cancer Center-Memorial Hospital, NY 1979 and St. Jude Children's Research Hospital, Memphis, 1982. Development of the Pediatric Oncology Unit at Hospital Barao de Lucena, Recife-Brazil 1980-2003. Degree in Pediatric Oncology acquired at Brazilian Society of Oncology, 1994. Founder of a support group for children with cancer, to give socio-economic support for the child with cancer and their families. Development of a new Pediatric Oncology Unit at Instituto Integrado de Medicina Prof.Fernando Figueira (IMIP), Recife Brazil. Director of the Twining Program between St.Jude Hospital (Memphis) and IMIP Hospital, Recife Brazil. to improve the care for children with cancer. Development of Telemedicine program in Pediatric Oncology. Current activities are focused upon all aspects in the care of children with cancer in Recife, Brazil. Medical Director of the Pediatric Oncology Center, Recife Brazil, Director of the program for Early Diagnosis in pediatric oncology. Director of the International Telemedicine Program at IMIP Hospital, Recife Brazil

Engr. **N.P Chowdhry** is an Assistant Professor, in the Dept. of Biomedical Engineering at Mehran University of Engineering & Technology, Jamshoro-Pakistan. He is Masters in Telemedicine & e-Health Systems from brunel university, west london, UK. He has participated in advanced learning workshop in the field of IT at AS-ICTP, Trieste, Italy in the capacity of junior Guest Scientist in (2001-2002). Mr. Chowdhry was awarded an honor of co-chair of the international conference on eHealth, Telemedicine & Health ICT of Med-e-Tel-2006 session on 'e-Health in developing countries' at Luxembourg. He has also contributed his research papers in the series of Med-e-Tel conference proceedings (2006-2009). He is an author of more than a dozen research papers at national & international level. Recently, he has been selected by Ministry of Science & Technology, PR.,C & participated in an international workshop on "Telemedicine Network Design, Development & Applications" in Kunming, China in the year 2009. He is member of an international society for telemedicine & ehealth (ISfTeH), IAENG (UK), IACSIT (Sing). His areas of research interests are medical engineering: includes: telemedicine/e-health, medical imaging, biosensors, vital sign monitoring and grid computing.

Engr. **Adnan Ashraf Arain** at his 29th year is the foundation member of CREST research group and Faculty Member at Mehran University of Engineering and Technology, Pakistan. The university awarded him all major academic credentials, including, B.Engg, M.Engg, & Ph.D in the area of network & communication security. His field of specialization is Security in Wireless & adhoc sensor networks.

Mr. Arain also possesses credit for publishing many research articles, book chapters, and delivering keynote speeches around the globe.

Professor **Bhawani Shankar Chowdhry** is Director Institute of Information & Communication Technologies, Mehran University of Engineering & Technology, JAMSHORO PAKISTAN. He did his Phd in 1990 from School of ECS, University of Southampton; UK. He has published more than 50 research papers in national and international journals. He is main author/coauthor of more than dozen books in the area of ICT. Recently, he has completed one year postdoctoral fellowship from one of the world's best Institution school of Electronics and Computer Science, University of Southampton, UK. He is co-editor of book "Wireless Networks, Information Processing and Systems", CCIS 20, recently published by Springer, Germany.

Professor Dr. **A. K. Baloch** is the Dean, Faculty of Electrical, Electronic & Computer Engineering at Mehran University of Engineering & Technology, Jamshoro, Pakistan. He received his M.Phil from University of Southampton (UK) and Ph.D form University of Bradford (UK). He is a recipient of Central Overseas Training Scholarship by Government of Pakistan for higher studies abroad. During his Ph.D Studies at Bradford University, UK. He was a fellow Ministry of Defence, UK. He was Fulbright Scholar at the University of Central Florida, Orlando USA during 2001-2002. He is a senior member IEEE USA, life member IEP and PEC. Dr. Baloch has published more than 30 research papers in journals and conferences of international repute. He has also visited more than 15 countries of the world.

Dr. **Stefane M. Kabene**, MPs, PhD, is a faculty member in the Aubrey Dan Program in Management and Organizational Studies with a cross appointment in the Faculty of Health Science at the University of Western Ontario, London, Ontario, Canada. His primary interests are in healthcare, information and communication technology and human resources for health. His focus is in Interprofessional collaborative practice, knowledge transfer, quality of care and patient involvement in clinical decision making. The future of health care lies in health professionals' capacity and willingness to develop new ways of working together for the benefit of the patient. Knowledge and power sharing, role valuing, use of information and communication technology and patients' participation in decision making are only a few of the variables we need to better understand. Dr. Kabene is involved in research projects with the Schulich School of Medicine and Dentistry, the School of Nursing, and the Faculty of Social Sciences.

Raymond W. Leduc, MBA, CGA, is a faculty member in the Aubrey Dan Program in Management and Organizational Studies at the University of Western Ontario, London, Ontario, Canada. His primary teaching areas are in strategic management and globalization. He is also a doctoral candidate interested in knowledge management, and in particular knowledge transfer and sharing, within interdisciplinary healthcare teams.

Dr. **Candace J. Gibson**, PhD, CHIM, is an associate professor in the Department of Pathology at the Schulich School of Medicine and Dentistry, the University of Western Ontario, in London, ON. She has been involved in medical research, teaching to undergraduate baccalaureate, medical, nursing and dental students, and administration in the department's graduate and undergraduate degree programs. Over the past decade she has been actively engaged in the introduction of teaching in health informatics as a medical school elective and in the health information management program in the Faculty of

Health Sciences. In the latter program she teaches courses in pathology, health informatics and health information management. Her current interests include the development of effective e-learning tools, HI and HIM curriculum development, and the introduction and use of the electronic health record.

Prof. **Robert Rudowski,** PhD Head of the Dept. of Medical Informatics and Telemedicine at the Medical University of Warsaw. Researcher at Karolinska Institute in Stockholm and Linkoping University, Sweden, Visiting Professor to Brown University, Providence, Rhode Island, Senior Position Fulbright Grant at the University of Utah (USA), Coordinator and Contractor of the Tempus Joint European Network (JEN-04272) Project "Computer Assisted Learning for Undergraduate Medical Students", Coordinator of Medical Education and Didactics Network II (MEDNET II) at the Medical University of Warsaw, Visiting Professor to University of Goettingen, Participant in the EU Project A -Cute -Tox. Member of : Board of Directors of the International Society for Telemedicine and e-Health (ISfTeH) (2003-2007), European Respiratory Society (ERS). His research interests include: medical data bases and their analysis (eg. database of thyroid diseases in Polish population after Tchernobyl accident, specialized database of in vitro and in vivo results for predicting human acute toxicity), decision support systems (eg. Kusivar system for mechanical ventilation of the lungs), modeling and optimization (eg. modeling of respiratory system and mechanical ventilation optimization), telemedicine/e-health (eg. telecardiological system for Acute Coronary Syndromes patients in Mazovia District), e-learning (multimedia educational programs for medical students).

Bartosz Kaczynski is a teaching assistant of medical informatics at the Medical University of Warsaw (Poland). He received his MSc in 2004 at the Warsaw University of Technology (Multimedia Techniques speciality at Faculty of Mechatronics). His research is focused on the development of teleradiology, image quality and compression. He is also IT administrator and help-desk support for the radiology department at Public Clinical Hospital of Medical University of Warsaw.

John E. Ribera obtained his Master's Degree in Communicative Disorders from Brigham Young University and his doctorate in Speech and Hearing Sciences from the University of Washington. He is currently an associate professor at Utah State University where he serves as the Director of Audiology. He has 29 years in the field of audiology and has worked in a variety of civilian and military settings. Assignments have included: (1) instructor in academia, (2) service provider in hospitals and medical centers, (3) researcher at a US Army research laboratory, (4) coordinator of speech and hearing services in a school district, (5) owner and operator of a private audiology practice, and (6) instructor and supervisor of a large hearing conservation program. He has served as the Director of Audiology at the House Ear Clinic in Los Angeles, California. His areas of interest are, speech intelligibility in noise, telehealth, hearing conservation, multicultural issues, balance disorders, tinnitus and traumatic brain injury. He is also the owner of Forensic Audiology Consulting Services (http://forensicaudiology.com) where he assists law firms as an expert witness. He has authored and co-authored several articles and presented at local and national conferences on telehealth in audiology. He serves on the American Academy of Audiology Telehealth Task Force. John has also served on the American Speech Language and Hearing Association Multicultural Issues Board, as president of the Utah Speech and Hearing Association and as a member of the Utah Brain Injury Council. He lives in rural Utah with his wife, Ann. They have 5 children and 12 grandchildren. In his spare time he sings in and manages a 280-voice symphonic chorus and annually conducts two large community choirs that perform at Christmas. His travels have taken him and his wife to Austria, Belgium, Czechoslovakia, England, France, Germany, Italy, Japan, Korea, Luxembourg, the Netherlands, and Spain, In addition he has organized several humanitarian hearing healthcare missions to remote locations in Mexico.

Dr. **Ronald LaPorte** is a Professor of Epidemiology at the Unversity of Pittsburgh Graduate School of Public Health. His PhD was in cognitive psychology. Dr. LaPorte's primary interest is the application of Internet Technology to the prevention of disease. Dr. LaPorte and his group are harnessing the Internet to improve knowledge sharing and prevention. They have created the Supercourse which has over 65,000 faculty world wide and a library of 4100 lectures from 174 countries. Dr. LaPorte published over 462 papers in the area of diabetes registries, chronic disease epidemiology, and the use of Internet technologies for prevention. Dr. LaPorte is a Director for Disease Monitoring and Telecommunications at the University of Pittsburgh WHO Collaborating center.

Faina Linkov is a Research Assistant Professor Of Medicine at the University of Pittsburgh School of Medicine. Dr. Linkov holds PhD in Epidemiology, MPH in the Community and Behavioral Health Sciences from the University of Pittsburgh. Her current research activities concentrate on the use of biological tumor markers to detect malignancies at early stages. She served as a peer reviewer for the British Medical Journal (BMJ), Journal of Medical Internet Research, and others. In the past nice years, Dr. Linkov has been working with Professor Ronald LaPorte in the Global Health Network Supercourse Project. One of the main goals of the Supercourse developers is to close the digital divide and deliver public health education materials to faculty members in the developing world. Dr. Linkov's research interests include cancer, early detection of cancer, global health, digital divide, and peer review mechanisms.

Dr. **A.W Ansari** is a professor at the Isra University, Hyderabad Sindh Pakistan and PhD from Bruel University London and Msc from Durham University north England UK. His is also MSc. Electronic from Sindh University jamshoro. PK. He remained as an advisor S&T Sindh Govt. and Director, IIT at University of Sindh, Jamshoro, PK. He has published more than a dozen papers in national & international journals & conference proceedings. His areas of research interests are: Artificial Intelligence, telemedicine, computer graphics, eHealth Grid and linguists.

Hermann de Meer is a full professor at the University of Passau and head of the chair of CNCC. He has led several national and international projects in computer communications related research. Prof. de Meer has chaired the first Intern. Workshop on Self-Organizing Systems in Passau. He is co-editor of the respective proceedings that appeared in the LNCS Springer-Verlag series. His research interests include performance modeling and simulation of computer and communication systems, Quality of Service, Internet protocols, self-organization, peer-to-peer networks, home networking, security and mobile computing.

Index

A

advancing clinico-genomic clinical trials on cancer (ACGT) 158, 162
agent-based modeling (ABM) 71
Alaska Federal Healthcare Access Network (AFHCAN) 206
Alzheimer's disease 130, 137
American Academy of Audiology (AAA) 206, 207, 212
American Association for Advancement in Science (AAAS) 220
American Cancer Society 220
American Speech Language and Hearing Association (ASHA) 206
asynchronous telehealth 214
Atlas On-Line 218
audiology 205, 206, 207, 208, 209, 210, 211, 212, 213, 214

B

biomedical 68, 69, 71, 94, 100, 101, 102, 153, 156, 161
Biomedical Informatics Research Network (BIRN) 106, 115
biomedicine 106
biometrics 192
BIOPATTERN 157, 158, 159
brain extraction tool (BET) 137, 138, 150
business process execution language (BPEL) 135, 136, 137, 151

C

Cancer Biomedical Informatics Grid (caBIG) 156, 157
cardiovascular diseases (CVD) 66, 215
collaborative grids 153
common object request broker architecture (CORBA) 111
communication satellites 4
computational grids 152, 153, 154, 156, 157, 158, 159, 160
computer-aided detection (CAD) 154, 155, 161, 162
computer retrieval of information on scientific projects (CRISP) 219, 222
computer virus 7
computing technology 17
Conditional Acceptance 43, 44, 48
content addressable storage (CAS) 195, 199, 200, 203
continuous medical education (CME) 11, 12, 13, 17

D

data fusion 165, 166, 168, 169, 170, 176, 180
data grids 153
data mining 153, 160
data security 182, 183, 185, 186, 189, 192
dermatology 21
diagnostic imaging 12
digital library 44, 45
digital pathology (D-AP) 117, 119
digital signatures 195, 196, 201, 202
direct attached storage (DAS) 198, 199
disaster recovery plans 42
distance learning 11, 12

E

e-Communication 181

e-era 14
eHealth 1-19, 31-36, 39, 41, 43, 46, 48, 50, 53-59, 65, 96, 164-168, 171-181, 184
eHealth Grid 164, 165, 166, 178, 180
e-infrastructures 129, 130
eLearning 10, 12, 13, 17, 19, 21, 30
electronic health records (EHR) 38, 49, 182, 183, 184, 185, 186, 187, 188, 189, 190, 191, 192, 193, 194
electronic mail (e-mail) 3, 208, 210
electronic medical record (EMR) 183
electronic paper records (EPR) 183
electronic pathology (e-AP) 117, 119
electronic patient record (EPR) 22
electronic programmable subsystems (PESS) 119, 126
embedded medical systems and networks 37, 44, 46, 47
enabling the grid for e-science (EGEE) project 130
enterprise level computing 39
European Institute for Telesurgery 47

F

fast fourier transform (FFT) 172

G

global area networks (GAN) 166, 181
global healthcare 65, 67, 76, 86, 90, 93
Global Health Network Supercourse 215, 219
Globus Alliance 116
Globus toolkit 111
graphical user interface (GUI) 111, 112
Grid 1-4, 9, 10, 16, 19, 32, 36-43, 46-50, 53-64, 105-115, 164-180, 195, 199, 201, 209, 212
Grid Computing , 68, 69, 70, 71, 73, 76, 79, 88, 91, 93, 165, 167, 168, 169, 170, 172, 174, 175, 179, 180
grid-enabled medical simulation services (GEMSS) 157
grid medical archive solution (GMAS) 42, 59

H

hardware 8, 15, 17
healthcare management 65
healthcare operations 65, 67, 72, 73, 74, 80, 81, 85, 87, 91, 93, 102, 103
healthcare technology
HealthGrid 41, 42
HealthGrid conference 41
Health Insurance Portability and Accountability Act (HIPAA) 188, 191, 193
hierarchical storage manager (HSM) 199
histology 114, 115, 116
histopathological 116
hospital information system (HIS) 121, 128
human papilloma virus (HPV) 216
human resources management (HRM) 185, 190, 192, 193

I

InfiniBand 116
information and communication technologies (ICT) 1, 2, 3, 4, 7, 10, 11, 17, 19, 129, 130
Information and Privacy Commissioner (IPC) 184, 187, 194
information, computer, and communication technologies (IC2T) 67, 93
information management (IM) 65, 71, 73, 79, 80, 81, 82, 83, 86, 87, 88, 89, 91, 96
information technology (IT) 39, 40, 56, 58, 63, 65, 82, 83, 85, 86, 87, 89, 91, 169, 174, 176
integrated advanced information management systems (IAIMS) 44
Integrated Services Digital Network (ISDN) 7
International Agency for Research on Cancer (IARC) 218, 222
International Business Machines (IBM) 42, 59, 60
International Cancer Research Portfolio 219, 223
International Covenant on Civil and Political Rights 185
internet 1, 2, 3, 9, 10, 11, 15, 17, 36, 37, 44, 45, 46, 49, 55, 56, 57, 67, 71, 95, 102, 165, 166, 167, 169, 173, 175
internet protocol (IP) 10, 17
intruder detection system (IDS) 174, 175, 196, 202

K

knowledge management (KM) 65, 71, 73, 74, 75, 79, 80, 81, 82, 83, 86, 87, 88, 89, 91, 92, 102

L

laboratory information system (LIS) 128
learning organizations 18, 19, 20, 23, 24, 29, 30
literature based discovery (LBD) 117, 122, 124
local area networks (LAN) 166, 168, 169, 181, 209

M

malicious scripts 7
medical device data system (MDDS) 120
medical imaging resource center (MIRC) 125, 128
Medici Effect 67, 98
message passing interface (MPI) 111, 116
metropolitan area networks (MAN) 181
minimum basic data set (MBDS) 22
Montreal Neurological Institute (MNI) 138, 139, 140, 146, 147

N

National Aeronautics and Space Administration (NASA) 4
National Cancer Institute (NCI) 216, 219, 220, 222
network attached storage (NAS) 198, 199
network-centric healthcare 72, 102
network-centric operations (NCO) , 72, 76, 79, 91, 106, 107, 108, 109
network organization 18, 19, 20, 23, 24, 29, 30
network storage 195, 197, 199
neuGRID 129, 130, 132, 135, 139, 141, 144, 147, 148, 149
Neurobase project 155, 156, 157
neuroimaging 137
neurologists 156
neuro-oncology 152, 156, 158, 159, 160

O

object oriented programming (OOP) 181
observation, orientation, decision, and action (OODA) loop 77, 79, 87, 88, 89, 102
ocular oncology 156
operating room of the future (ORF) 121
otolaryngology 21

P

Pakistan Educational and Research Network (PERN) 172, 176
parallel virtual machine (PVM) 111
patho-informatics 117, 119, 124
pathology information management system (PIMS) 117, 119, 120, 121
pathology information system (PIS) 121, 128
PC-based audiometers 208
personal health information 182, 184, 185, 186, 188, 189, 190, 192
Personal Information Protection and Electronic Documents Act (PIPEDA) 191, 193
Personal Medical Devices 38
petrol oil and logistic (POL) 173
pharmaco-pathology 118, 119
physiopathology 119
picture archiving and communication systems (PACS) 42, 107, 121, 124, 125, 128, 196, 197, 199, 200, 204
plain old telephone systems (POTS) 208
post operative care 164, 165, 169, 178, 180
privacy-enhancing technologies (PET) 187
public key infrastructure (PKI) 196, 201

Q

quality control 117, 121

R

radio frequency identification (RFID) 168, 179
radiology 20, 25, 26, 27, 30, 31, 32
redundant array of inexpensive disks (RAID) 196, 197, 198
remote computing 208, 213
remote controls 12
resource-sharing computing (RSC) 38
risk management 44
robotics 12

S

satellite technology 3
secure data transmission system (SDTS) 196
serial advanced technology attachment (SATA) 198
service oriented architecture 129, 130, 131, 132, 133, 135, 136, 141, 142, 144, 145, 147, 148, 149, 150
service oriented modelling and architecture (SOMA) 130
small computer system interface (SCSI) 198
software 2, 3, 4, 6, 8, 9, 10, 15, 17
solo-pathology 117, 118, 124
storage area network (SAN) 198, 199
structural image evaluation using normalisation of atrophy (SIENA) 137, 151
surveillance, epidemiology, and end results (SEER) 216, 217, 219, 221, 222, 223
synchronous telehealth 214
Systems for Health agency (SSH) 184

T

teams of leaders (ToL) 65, 80, 81, 83, 84, 85, 86, 87, 88, 89, 91, 92, 93, 96, 99, 102
tele-audiology 206, 208, 209, 210, 211, 212
telecommunications 3, 17, 19, 21, 24, 27, 29
teleconferencing 208
teleconsultations 20, 21, 25
teledermatology 21, 22, 25
telehealth 205, 206, 207, 208, 209, 210, 211, 212, 213, 214
telehealthcare 19, 21, 32
Tele-HealthCare system 167
telehomecare 21
telemedicine 1-4, 16-36, 39-43, 46-50, 53-59, 164, 166, 167, 172, 179, 180
tele-oncology 158
tele-pathology (TP) 119
telepreventive medicine 221
telepsychiatry 20, 21, 22, 25, 31, 33, 35
teleradiology 20, 22, 25, 26, 27, 29, 30, 31, 33, 195, 196, 200, 201, 202, 203
telesurgery 47, 50
tissue-based diagnosis 105, 106, 107, 108, 112, 114, 115
trust management systems (TMS) 187

U

UN Declaration of Human Rights 185
unified medical language system (UMLS) 44

V

videoconferences 3, 20, 21, 28
virtual autopsy 117, 119
virtual classrooms 21
virtual clinic 210, 211, 212
virtual groups 21, 35
virtual microscopes 112
virtual microscopy 108, 111, 115
virtual organizations (VO) 1, 3, 4, 5, 6, 7, 8, 9, 10, 11, 12, 13, 14, 15, 16, 17, 22
virtual private network (VPN) 195, 196, 202, 204, 209
virtual reality (VR) 68, 71, 95
virtual slide 116
virtual teams 22
voice-activating machines 12

W

web portals 174, 175, 178
web service description language (WSDL) 132, 136, 147, 151
web service resource framework (WSRF) 111
wide area networks (WAN) 209
wireless sensor networks (WSN) 164, 165, 166, 167, 168, 176, 178, 179
World Wide Web 3, 17, 44, 45, 67
worms 7

Breinigsville, PA USA
01 September 2010

244315BV00002BK/1/P